# Love's Home Run
## An African American Romance

### by Thomas Green

COPYRIGHT © 1995 BY THOMAS GREEN
ALL RIGHTS RESERVED
INCLUDING THE RIGHT OF REPRODUCTION
IN WHOLE OR IN PART IN ANY FORM


PUBLISHED BY Turtle Cove Books




BOOK DESIGN BY SOHEL AHMED



MANUFACTURED IN THE UNITED STATES OF AMERICA


ISBN: 0-9654742-1-6



This novel is a work of fiction. Any reference to real people, events, establishments, organizations, or locales are intended only to give the fiction a sense of reality and authenticity. Other names, characters and incidents are the product of the author's imagination.

*F*or Thomas Maxwell,
> Friends...
>> How many of us have them?

## Acknowledgments

*First and foremost I thank God for giving the strength to bounce back from mistakes, mistreatment and misunderstandings in the writing business. I am here to stay.*

*To Isaac and his staff at Playing To Win for teaching a dinosaur how to write in modern times. (Microsoft Word ain't so bad)*

*To my agent-slash-sister Valarie Benning. You knew...*

*To Renecia and Janice for welcoming me into the 2Friends family with open arms...and enough cheese to keep the pockets tight*

*To the staff at The City Sun...the best, most dedicated newspaper staff in the world. Things should have been better.*

*To Paul Ghiorzi and all the bouncers, bartenders and staffers at the West End and Audubon...two cool bars.*

*To my parents, Diane and Chip. And, all my family and friends in New York. It would take another novel to name y'all.*

*To my in-laws: Jason and Mable, Dexter and Shilla, Jahmal and Maiya, Teneka. Real family.*

*Last, but not least, my wife, Kenya, for loving me like no other.*

# 1

Djuana Pioneer stood on the stoop of 657 Tudor Street. The brick, six story building where Djuana grew up was the only structure standing on the south side of Tudor between 23rd and 24th Avenue. The opposite side of the street had a perfect string of tenement buildings.

Djuana was awaiting her man. As a treat, she was wearing his favorite dress; a blue lycra-knit, that hugged the curves of her plump thighs and shapely hips. A ballerina neckline highlighted her well-rounded, small breasts. She had a beautiful body. In that dress, she was radiant.

Djuana glanced at her watch; the gold timepiece was a gift from her man this past Christmas. It was now April, and that watch still had the sparkle of new in Djuana's eyes. True, she had only worn the watch a few times in the four months, but it was a special gift. The seven diamonds that encircled the face represented her seven year relationship with Dexter Forns. Her man.

Seven years. Djuana and Dexter met in the Galleria Mall when she was 18 years-old and he was a mature, well-liked 20 year-old. He was gorgeous and just about every girl in Djuana's high school wanted him; the boys at Hamilton paled in comparison. Dexter was tall, light and slender. He wore clothes well; expensive clothes. His voice was always a faint whisper and the correct words flowed off his tongue.

Dexter became Djuana's first lover two months after meeting her, and technically, her only. Djuana met other men during the seven years, but none could steal her heart from Dexter. She knew of his variety in women, yet hung on to the hope that he loved her as much as she loved him, and that she would be the one he married.

Dexter treated Djuana gallantly. Poured money and gifts her way. He was always patient and showed respect. He wasn't a good listener, but liked to share his dreams. Djuana believed that once he committed, he was going to make a good husband.

Dexter loved Djuana's body. Well, no man could resist looking. He could not find her eagerness to please him in other women he slept with. She was also a devoted, loving intelligent woman.

Yet, Dexter Forns did not choose Djuana to settle down with. He thought he had no choice but to pick someone else.

*1*

Djuana glanced at her watch. A second later she looked again. In another few seconds she didn't know what time it was. She was nervous; she had to tell him tonight. For three weeks she had instigated arguments by declaring he spend more time with her. She went as far as to tell Dexter to be a man and pick her or let her go. She never said what she really should have. That night was her deadline.

It seemed right to tell him that night. It was exactly a week since she found out for sure; a month since he had been out of reach. For some reason, suddenly, he did not answer his phone or return her calls.

A brisk, Oregon spring breeze ran a chill up the skin of Djuana's arms. She had on the navy colored collarless cardigan style jacket she had bought earlier, yet the wind still gave her goose bumps. She folded her arms and checked the watch again.

Dexter's burgundy Mazda pulled into the empty space in front of Djuana's building. She came down off the stoop and approached the sports car. Dexter opened the door from the inside. The sound of the Whispers singing one of their new tunes on his cassette tape deck guided Djuana into the car. She sat quietly after a weak hello kiss. Dexter was not much of a kisser, and that bothered Djuana.

At a traffic light, Dexter took a full view of Djuana's soft, round face. He smiled. Djuana had the most inviting eyes; they weren't cheerful, but warm. While still driving, he moved her dress up her leg with his right hand and gripped the inside of her thigh. Djuana didn't mind his hand, she wanted her body to be his. Also, she knew he would be turned on by the dress. She moved closer as to shorten his reach. The more pleased he was, the easier it would be to talk to him.

Before dinner arrived Djuana had sipped down two mixed drinks. Her courage would come from the Pina Coladas, she bargained. She found herself looking beyond Dexter into the wall-to-wall mirror at the back of the quiet soul food restaurant. She gazed at the other diners, her eyes fixed on a pretty light-skinned young lady holding a rose, cuddled across the table with her date. The guy, not handsome enough, Djuana thought, held both of the attractive, light-skinned woman's hands. He was kissing them finger by finger. The pretty lady's nice smile warmed Djuana.

Djuana sipped her drink. She felt a buzz after the fourth colada, yet couldn't resist when the waiter asked if she would like another. She looked in Dexter's eyes. Was he ready for this? Was she?

Dexter enjoyed seeing Djuana drink. He would try to get her to drink whiskey, rum or gin without the additives. Something strong. Two drinks would bring a glossy glow to her olive-brown eyes. Her smile would seem dreamy; a large blush, as he laid any bullshit he thought up on her. Sex that night would be great because all her silly inhibitions would dull.

But, when Djuana ordered her fifth colada through dinner Dexter became suspicious. He inquired, and Djuana flatly answered she needed to drink.

After a pause, she noticed the suspicion in his deep stare had not died down. She complained that it had been a long week at work and that she needed to unwind. It had been.

Dexter nodded, looking forward to some good sex. Djuana's dreamy look aroused him.

"You know something," he began, taking her soft hand and rubbing her knuckles. "I want to take you to the Bahamas this summer."

He went on to say more, about how nice he heard it was down there, but his words floated by Djuana. Now she was ready to talk. She gulped the remains of number six. The mixture shivered the nondrinker. The bartender had been making them stronger with every request, she believed. She squeezed her eyes shut and shook her head to regain her composure. She bit the piece of pineapple from the edge of the glass and waited for the perfect time to cut in. She only waited less than a minute before speaking softly, almost in a faint whisper.

"I have something to tell you," she forced her eyes to meet his. "I'm two months pregnant. We're going to have a baby."

She did it. She felt both relieved and scared. Her eyes watched her fingers part another slice of pineapple, then she bit it. Her eyes refused to look at Dexter until he replied to the bomb shell she had dropped.

Dexter's upper body tilted back in his chair. He stared through Djuana. His sniffed his upper lip to his nose. Djuana had pictured many different responses, but silence was not one of them.

Finally Dexter tossed his napkin over his near empty plate of food. With his elbows perched on the table, hands clasped and fingers crossed, he leaned toward Djuana.

"What do you mean you're pregnant?" He forced his voice into a whisper, his face distorted. "I thought you were on the pill?"

"I guess it didn't work," Djuana could have kicked herself. She reminded herself of the seemingly thousands of times she rehearsed her come back lines to muff them in the heat of the first questions.

"I can't believe you. How could you pull some shit like this?" Dexter's voice remained contained in a low vibe, and his fiery temper controlled. Djuana watched him stand. He continued, now raising his voice slightly. "What you're tryin' ain't gonna work. Get rid of it."

"It?" Djuana shouted. She rose and met him eye-to-eye from across the table. "I'm having our baby!" Her voice carried throughout the eatery.

"No you're not!"

Forks dropped, diners looked in their direction. Dexter stood, sifted through his wallet and tossed money on the table. Without another word, he turned to leave and Djuana sprinted after him.

She grabbed his arm, "We need to talk."

In a rage, Dexter spun Djuana from behind him and grabbed her face with his right hand and slammed her head into the wall near the restaurant's entrance. The sound of the back of her head hitting the plastic wood wall covering brought astonished cries from diners. Nobody moved toward the arguing couple, though.

Dexter held Djuana by her arms in a tight grip. She did not try to move. "Listen. 'Cause I am only gonna tell you this once. I ain't having no fuckin' baby. And I ain't getting married to you right now. Got it?"

With a shove, Dexter let Djuana hit the ground. He smoothly walked out.

Djuana was stunned. For a moment she thought she was in bed at home. Some men helped her up. Tears gathered in her eyes and drained slowly. She felt a thousand eyes upon her.

"Are you okay? Can I call you a taxi?"

It was the waiter that had served her all those drinks. Djuana struggled to get on her feet. Once standing she made her own way out. The Maitre d held open the door for her. She began the long walk home, staggering a bit on the wet pavement, immune to the soft drizzle for two blocks. Her legs guided the way and her mind followed. Tears? Only a few. Djuana Pioneer had done no wrong, she told herself.

# 2

Jack Newhouse slowly removed his dirty Portland Crowns uniform. The Crowns had just defeated New York in its first home game of the season. Most of Newhouse's Crowns teammates, and a few from the New York ballclub, had dressed and were leaving Adkins Stadium on their way to party. But the Crowns right fielder was moping at his locker.

This was to be the year the Crowns finally won a baseball championship. They had lost to the Las Vegas Gamblers in the title round of the playoffs two straight years. Vincent Slight had bought the Crowns five years ago with two intentions, making money and winning. Making money has been easy. He and his general manager/right-hand man, J.A. Honeywell, have put together a good team with plenty of character - and characters. Adkins is constantly sold out during the regular season where the Crowns win often. Beating Las Vegas has been Slight's only shortcoming.

For Jack Newhouse, this was supposed to be the year he finally settled down and got married. He was all set to propose to Vivian Woodward, whom he had been dating for two years. But, the night before the Crowns opened their home season, Vivian closed the door on their relationship.

Jack sat at his locker staring at Vivian's picture. The 6-foot-2, 215-pound right fielder stood and took the picture into his hand. He looked over Vivian's wide smile. A smirk cornered his lips. He thought back to the night before. The evening had been planned perfectly. Dinner and dancing at LeClair's, then back to his place. But at dinner Vivian admitted what Jack knew...or should have known. She still wanted her ex-fiancee.

"I like you a lot, Jack," Vivian said between forks full of salmon. "And I need you and you are good for me. But I am still in love with Bob."

Jack slid the picture of Vivian out of the frame and turned it around. He read the back aloud in the now empty clubhouse. "I'll always love you," were the words that stung his heart. He squeezed the picture and took a deep breath. A sleepless night and a long baseball game was wearing on him. But now he was going to get drunk with his teammates. He needed it, he thought. He left the empty, dark stadium and joined his teammates at the Tunnell nightclub.

The small building that housed the Tunnell was as loud and vibrant as ever. Jack entered the brick shack to find his teammates settled as if they had been there for hours. The players were dancing and drinking as if they had won more than just a game. But, that was such in the world of Crowns baseball. Of all the teams in major sports, the Portland Crowns were the most fluent in the art of partying. It stemmed from the family atmosphere that Vincent Slight began when he bought the team. You couldn't say the players on the team loved one another, but, when out, on the field or on the club scene, there was no tighter unit in sports.

The Tunnell's dance floor was jammed. The start of a new baseball season brought the crowd back to the club that was pretty much a Crowns hangout. It was located off Route 8, a small two-lane highway that ran from the city of Portland into its southern suburbs. The small, cabin looking building during the daylight hours seemed tranquil. Like a perfect spot to stop and have a meal with you family during a drive in the woods.

The thick aroma of marijuana, his stiff rum and Coke, and the bass in the house music combined to smother Jack. He had been there less than an hour, and already he was high. Mike Colbert, the Crowns' catcher, snatched Jack into a headlock from behind, shouting into his ear, "We win it this year or what?"

He kissed Jack on the neck.

Jack choked in agreement.

"I love you baby," Mike squeezed Jack's neck, pulling down the taller Jack.

Jack twisted out of the hold, and made his way out the front door. He slithered out to the parking lot in desperate need of fresh air and leaned on his car. He wanted to leave, but his desire to be among his teammates was stronger. He just needed more alcohol to dense his senses. He greeted people as they went in, nursing his drink. At times he looked up into the star-filled sky; but negative thoughts about Vivian forced him to stare elsewhere. He wanted her back badly.

Soon, his best friend and outfield mate, Oscar Taylor joined his mourning. Easy O, as Oscar likes to be called, and Jack were signed by the Crowns out of high school the same week nine years ago. They moved through the organization at the same pace, both being outfielders of different breed. O was a fleet-footed center fielder, whose speed was his weapon. Jack was a power hitter, but don't let him hear it said of him. His fans marveled at his long home runs and hard-stroked line drives, while Jack more appreciated his ability to get hits and play defense. He called himself a 'well-rounded ballplayer'.

O called Jack the best right fielder in the game. But that night, O called his friend foolish.

"What the fuck are you doing?" O spewed.

"What does it look like?" Jack's voice barely carried in the damp, pine smelling air.

O shook his head and hissed. He looked at Jack's drink. Two swallows were left in the glass. "Man, that heartbreak shit ain't gonna make it."

Jack gulped the remains. He parched his lips and finally acknowledged O's presence with eye contact. "Don't worry about it. I didn't ask you."

"Come on, New, you don't need the sweat. You got bitches on your dick all across the fuckin' country and you worrying about that silly hoe. I tried to tell you she wasn't the one."

Jack's eyes sliced through his inconsiderate friend. "Why reply?" he wondered.

O continued. "Look, Sondra said she has this new chick she has been wanting to hook you up with for the longest. Peep her out. Besides, you can't be acting like this when we get to Phoenix next week."

Jack became angry. He wondered how two guys with such difference in philosophies could be such good friends. Jack wanted so badly to be married, start a family and live the life of a father and husband.

"Listen, asshole, I want what you don't even know you have. I want to get married. Have the kinda wife you have in Sondra. Shit, man, I don't want to be sleeping with groupies all my life."

"Stop!" O put his open hand to Jack's face. "Stop dreaming about being married. It ain't all that you think it to be. I'm here to tell you. You got it going on. You can come and go as you please. Do who and what you want. Come on? Stop!"

Jack shook his head, watching his friend's dramatically spin his body. "Shit, Sometimes I wonder why do I try to talk to you?"

"'Cause you love me. Besides, if you get married then we have to pay for hotels when we have orgies. That would be terrible!" Jack finally loosened up and laughed with his friend. But the sight of Vivian's red sports car swinging into the Tunnell's parking lot suddenly sobered him. O watched Jack's face change in seconds. When the engine ceased and the headlights blinked, Jack's heart accelerated. He wanted to see her. Rising out of the driver's seat was Bob Haynes. Vivian had let her ex drive.

"I don't believe this shit," Jack whispered. The sight of her legs crushed his heart. He started toward her.

O sensed trouble, knowing his friends temper all to well. He lightly touched Jack's arm. "Let it go, man. Let's take a ride."

Jack nodded. "Yeah, I'll be right back."

Vivian hoped Jack would be there. Her plan was a dangerous one, but she wanted a confrontation to help her feel as if she had made the right choice. She wanted to see the two men together. But once she saw Jack approaching the car she knew she forgot one vital point. Jack was not a person to test.

Bob walked across the car, waiting on the passenger side while Vivian put on her jacket. Jack stopped at the hood of the car and asked to speak to her. She looked at Bob, who was looking at Jack suspiciously. She moved out to meet Jack.

"I thought you didn't like this place?" Jack asked.

"Jack, look, I don't want any trouble. We'll leave. I know this is a Crowns' hangout."

"Naw," Jack threw up his arms. "You and him ain't got to leave on my account. I just needed to say something to you..."

Vivian cut Jack off. "Listen, we'll always be friends. That is how I want it."

Jack looked into her eyes and was surprised to find he didn't mind agreeing. In the background, O winced and covered his eyes. He was afraid Jack was about to spill his guts. In the foreground, Bob could not wait any longer. He couldn't bear seeing Jack to cry for love.

"You ready baby," Bob said with his eyebrows raised.

"Yes." Vivian noticed Jack's smirk. "Good-bye, Jack."

She began toward the club. But, Bob was not pleased with the look on Jack's face.

"Problem?" Bob asked as he past Jack. He stopped as if to wait an answer.

Vivian stopped also. She recognized Bob's tone. It was his masculine, I'm gonna do something voice. She hoped Jack was calm, then slid her body between them.

Jack never replied to the question. But his eyes never left Bob and his smirk widened.

"What the fuck is he doing?" O mumbled as he approached the scene.

"Take a walk before you get hurt," Jack finally said.

Intimidated, Bob hit Jack quickly. The punch to Jack's left cheek stunned him more than it hurt. Bob moved in quickly. Jack grabbed him by his shoulders and forced him to the ground. Rolling around was all that really occurred before O and others separated the two non-fighters.

Vivian scolded Jack, "I knew your ass was immature. That's why I left you. Fight. That's all you want to do, is to hit somebody."

"Shut the fuck up!" Jack replied before he could control his anger.

"Yo, don't speak to my woman like that. I'll kill you," Bob threatened.

The three filled the damp night air with profanity.

Vivian fired the parting shot: "That's exactly why I left your ass! Your temper is going to get you hurt!"

O shoved his teammate from the club and toward his Pathfinder. "Walk. Just walk, New."

They walked back to Jack's ride. Jack ripped open the door of his Pathfinder and slammed himself inside as Vivian and Bob drove off in a cloud of dust and gravel. O leaned on the next car.

"I'm going to get us a beer," Oscar said, speaking through the truck's closed windows. "Do you think you can chill here for a minute?"

O took Jack's silence as agreement and disappeared into the club. Jack planted his head into his steering wheel and closed his eyes.

# 3

Jack left the Tunnell before his best friend returned. His desperate need for solitude hung over him like the odor of Mike Colbert's stale, sweaty baseball uniform after a doubleheader. He sped his Pathfinder across the wet streets of downtown Portland. The downpour had stopped as suddenly as it had began.

A stiff wind made the damp night air cool; yet Jack was riding with his window down. The steady breeze helped ease his anger. He felt that his chance to pound out his frustration was blown. The frustration of another lost relationship.

The Pathfinder hydroplaned across Main Street toward the Hawthorne Bridge. The highway would have been quicker to Jack's suburban home, but he felt a long ride would be helpful. He had anticipated the wet streets being empty. He was cruising at 70-miles-per-hour, rap music blaring, and he did not stop for many red lights. He thought about what he would say to the police if they pulled him over, he would say, in his best angry Negro voice: "Yeah, I was speeding. Whatcha going to do about it?"

More than likely, he'd take the ticket and pay it in the morning.

Approaching the intersection of Tenth Avenue and Main, Jack gained speed to make the changing street light. Gliding across the intersection his headlights picked up on a figure of a human frozen in the far crosswalk. In a sobering panic, Jack swerved the four-by to the right behind the person and then back to the left, avoiding parked cars. The black automobile skidded a circle across the double yellow lines and stopped.

After a deep breath, and thanking God there was no other traffic, Jack looked into the rearview mirror. He could see the pedestrian still standing in the crosswalk. Jack got out slowly, surveying the scene. Who had seen him run a light and almost kill someone? No one was in sight, still. He jogged over to find a woman with her hands covering her face. She was drenched from head to toe.

"Are you all right?" Jack asked.

The woman's lip stick was smeared across the corners of mouth, as if it had melted in the rain. Her hair was soak, dripping and hanging above her puffed eyes. She had been crying, and a heck of a lot, too, Jack deducted. Beads of rain drops, or tears, covered her round, milky brown colored cheeks. Jack caught himself staring, not stopping though. He took in a full view of her body.

Jack was instantly infatuated.

Djuana Pioneer did not answer the man who almost hit her with his speeding car. She was too tired and disoriented from the combination of her long walk, sleepless nights and the alcohol. Djuana hadn't slept much in the past three weeks due to a combination of nerves and sickness. This pregnancy was not going to be easy. Her upper body was heavy and legs weak from the steady walk. She wanted to say something and resume her journey home, but the sudden shivers caused by Jack's warm presence trembled her body.

She collapsed into Jack's shoulder and arms as he came closer, shaking her head side-to-side crying softly that she did nothing wrong.

Guilt stabbed at Jack the more he looked her over. He allowed her into his chest. Fighting the urge to squeeze her, he removed his jacket and placed it over Djuana's wet shoulders. She wrapped her arms around his waist and held on, her head embedded in his chest. Jack led her to the Pathfinder, asking if she would like a ride home. She did not respond. Jack awkwardly put her inside the front passenger's seat.

After getting the car started and moving it back on track, Jack checked on his passenger to find her asleep. "Now what do I do?" he wondered out loud.

He first lowered her seat to ensure her comfort, then looked through her purse. He watched her eyes, and the road, while sifting through the small pocketbook. He saw a small knife, seven single dollar bills, some change, tissue and a compact. Some other womanly junk, but no identification.

Jack sat under the traffic light at Second and Main through two changes before he decided to take the pretty lady to his home. The ride was quiet and quick... even though Jack's heart was pounding with anxiety.

Once in his garage, Jack shook Djuana lightly. With a stretch and a yawn, she rolled over to the door – her back to Jack.

Jack cursed.

He ended up carrying Djuana's plump body up the stairs to the townhouse. He angled her down the slim hallway and into his bedroom. Because he rarely had guests, the guest bedroom was filled with junk and trophies and the bed was sheetless. So, putting her in there was out of question. He laid her in his bed and Djuana spread herself out. He stood there wondering what he had gotten himself into.

Jack thought for a second about leaving her in her wet clothes, but he realized that idea was wrong. So, with care, Jack removed her dress. He undressed her down to her set of white lace panties and matching bra. The sight of her curved body choked Jack, freezing him in place. He stood tall.

Djuana's wet skin glowed in the dimly lit room. He hand dried whichever parts of her body he had the courage to touch. He patted her with a thick cotton towel, all the while dreaming of making love to her passionately.

Jack looked through his closet several times before settling on his first professional baseball jersey – a prized possession – to cover that body. It was also an extra large button-up that was in the best condition of any other jersey in his closet. He put it on her, one arm at a time. His knees on the bed, and towering over her, he slowly buttoned the jersey up her body. Djuana moaned once under the warm sheets, blanket and comforter. Her gentle smile and light snoring attracted Jack all the more. He stood over Djuana for a few minutes watching as she settled in.

Jack went into the living room on edge. Half his mind wondered why he wasn't in bed with his guest. The other half of his decent brain wondered why he had brought her home in the first place. He and his split-conscience sat up most of the night.

Jack only slept a few torrid hours. The aches in his back from sleeping on the sofa woke him for good near seven. Rising off the sofa, his body wanted to know why he hadn't slept in the guest room. Or in his own bed. He smiled at the last question. He began to make coffee in the kitchen when the telephone's ring pounded his heart. "Shit." He hoped it hadn't awaken his guest.

A loud voice told him to check the morning newspaper and abruptly hung up. It was Crowns pitcher, Danny Gross. Danny enjoyed the gossip reporters would write and would call the player it affected. He probably saw a trade rumor or story involving Jack, Jack imagined.

The small Saturday morning paper was laying across his welcome mat as if the paper boy had gotten out of his dad's car and placed it there with care. On the cover of the sports pages was a picture of Bob and Jack sprawled on the ground. The headline read: CROWN GETS CROWNED.

"Wonderful," a smirk cornered Jack's mouth as he reentered the house. Trouble loomed.

Djuana lay still in the large, comfortable yet foreign bed. The comforter on top of the sheets was a smooth fluff. Djuana's eyes had been open before the phone's ring completely woke her. A look around the room startled her. Her dress was hanging on the back of the door. Her stockings and slip in a chair. She ran her hands over the buttoned up baseball jersey on her body. She tried, but couldn't remember.

She climbed out of the bed and the thick, plush burgundy rug cushioned her toes. She walked to the door, enjoying the feel of the rug under her feet, and opened it slowly. The hallway was filled with the smell of bacon and freshly brewed coffee. She held her nose as the smells churned her stomach. Was it the affect from a night full of drinking, or was it the baby? She hoped neither, vomiting now would not be good timing.

Djuana followed the corridor to the opening. In front of her was a living room with leather sofas, an huge wall-unit stereo and television and an easy chair. On her left were steps leading down to the front door. And on the right, in the lit opening was the kitchen, with a tall, caramel-colored man wearing shorts and a t-shirt cooking breakfast.

Djuana startled Jack. "Good morning," he said with a thin smile. He didn't know what else to say.

Djuana placed her hand atop of the baseball shirt. Her bust held the v-neck jersey up, yet nothing was revealed. Anger chilled her bones. What was this man smiling about? she wondered. What had he done? What had he enjoyed? Hatred engulfed Djuana. She stepped to Jack and slapped him with all her 5-foot-7, 147 pound frame could muster.

"Bastard, I hope you enjoyed it!"

Djuana darted back to the bedroom. She forced the chair under the door's knob. She sat back on the bed; the soft comforter almost distracted her. She covered her nose and lips with her right hand.

"What is happening to me?"

She cried.

Jack sat at the kitchen table nursing a cold mug of coffee. What a pretty lady he had bolted-up in his bedroom, he mused.

Quickly, Djuana reappeared dressed and dashed down the stairs and fought open the front door. Jack bolted up after her. He met her on the porch; making sure not to touch her.

"Don't put your hands on me!" Djuana screamed as she finished the steps and was out on the sidewalk of the cul-de-sac.

"Look, you are too far to catch a bus or walk," Jack began to reason. "Come in and call a cab. Or, I can take you where you want to go."

Djuana stopped. Her eyes surveyed the scenery. All the homes were identical. The street signs were of a different color than she was accustomed. She felt alone and lost. She returned, walking past Jack and into the house. Jack entered seconds after to find her by the phone in the kitchen with her mini switch-blade out.

"Call me a cab."

Jack wheeled into his parking space at Adkins Stadium. Most of his teammates had arrived and the lot was filled. A few kids, some with parents, crowded the players' entrance. A daily ritual. Jack signed balls, gloves and assorted sized pieces of paper. He only gave his autograph to children; and only the polite.

Kristen Eisen greeted Jack in the corridor that led to the Crowns clubhouse. Kristen covered the Crowns for the Portland Gazette, the city's only daily newspaper. She possessed a combination of anchor-woman beauty and encyclopedic sports knowledge. The players enjoyed talking with her until she refused advances. Some believed she might, if asked right.

Kristen, a brunette, was small, yet her wide hips curved the many fitting the jeans and slacks she wore. During the playoffs she would stop hearts with knock-dead skirt suits.

Today, she approached Jack with her all-familiar quick smile and serious tone. "You want to talk?" she asked.

"About last night? Nope." Jack was expecting as much.

"No. Something more serious. The national media will get you on that." She took Jack by his arm and led him away from the clubhouse and toward the empty box seats in the stadium. They selected two, among the thousands of empties, three rows from the field.

She had his attention. Jack stared into her eyes wondering if she knew he had almost killed a woman and then took her to his home, and then wanted to sleep with, but didn't, and then had a knife pulled on him.

She began," I hear Slight is shopping you around. What do you know about this?"

"What are you talking about? Where did you hear this?"

"Come on, Jack. I am doing the story for my Sunday column tomorrow. Haven't you heard anything? Don't try to tell me you know nothing of this."

"I don't. It's news to me," Jack looked out across the playing field, where his teammates, and members of the New York ballclub were already dressed and practicing. "You tell me who your source is and we'll talk."

Kristen bit her bottom lip. She was good at bluffing. Secretly she had desired to ride on the laps of at least six Crowns' players. However, she was respected because no one knew.

"Jack, you know me better than that. I've been covering this team three years, and I have never betrayed any trust."

Kris shifted in her seat to mover closer to Jack. "But I will tell you this much. I know that Slight wants to give Hector Aponte right field this season and trade you for pitching prospects. I heard this from a source in Buffalo. They want you and Lee Spencer."

"Really?" was Jack's only response. He again turned and looked out across the outfield at his teammates jogging and laughing with players from New York. He became bitter, not against the question or the questioner, but at the fact the question had to be asked.

Jack felt he had produced for Slight, helping make the Crowns one of the best teams in the league. He felt he should be enjoying his time by now, with no worries. Last season he signed a three-year contract and expected to extend it beyond that. The thought of dumping him should not have crossed Slight's mind.

But he also understood baseball to be a business, more than a sport.

The Crowns manager caught a glimpse of Jack sitting in the stands with Kristen. "Shit. What the hell that boy think he doing?" Juris asked anyone near him stupid enough to answer. He yelled out to Jack, "New, get your ass dressed! Ain't you in enough fucking trouble?"

Jack waved and stood. Kristen grabbed his arm and almost begged for a reply.

"As of now, I am the Crowns right fielder. Have been for the last five years. That's that."

In the clubhouse, it was business was as usual. The game was three hours away and Don Cruz, Juan Santos, Mike and Oscar were playing cards. Neither man was fully in uniform. Floyd Young was at his locker reading the Bible. And, pitcher Scott Wilson went from person to person talking shit about the opposition.

Jack grabbed a couple of sandwiches and fruit drinks off the lunch table. He brushed off Scott, then a television crew. One interview was enough, until after the game, he told the media.

When he got to his locker he found the picture from the front page of the Gazette blown up and one of his teammates had written 'Clubber Lane Newhouse' in huge red letters below it.

The beer-bellied Juris came bustling into the clubhouse and made his usual announcement, "Saddle up, ladies! We got another ass to ride!" Then he approached Jack and barked at him to join him in his office.

Jack hesitated. He removed Vivian's picture, putting it on the floor of his locker. He put on his pearly white uniform slowly.

"Don't rush, Newhouse!" Juris barked.

Jack tucked in his jersey and belted his pants. He tied his high-top cleats and jogged into the smoke-filled office.

Juris removed his cigar. "You're benched for this game and Slight's gonna fine you. You can appeal if you want, but I wouldn't if I had done something that stupid."

"Whatever," Jack replied before spinning on his cleats and leaving the office. He didn't mind the day off. The money went to charity and the game was only the fifth of what was looking to him to be a long season.

# 4

Tudor Street was its lively self on a bright and warm April Saturday afternoon. Children had come from blocks away to play in Tudor park. The variety of swings, and the sand lot were major attractions in the mini playground centered between two tenements. Their parents and other elders would sit on the wide stoop of building 657 in folding chairs, or on the deep steps, and share gossip.

Djuana was in her own little world sitting on the fire escape of apartment 3B. Djuana sat, holding her knees and admiring the cloudless skies. Despite all the commotion below, she saw and heard different than the sounds of the neighborhood and the television blaring a baseball game inside the apartment. The fire escape had become Djuana's place of solitude.

It was where she could sit, and look beyond 656 and see her dreams played out in the ever present clouds. On that occasionally windy afternoon her thoughts were on the night before. *What happened?* she asked the darkening, churning clouds. They were ready to burst.

"How did I fuck it up?" she said aloud, in a high whisper. "I screwed up the most important conversation of my life with a man I knew I could never have, but wanted to marry."

She thought of how badly she wanted to get married. So badly that she proposed to Dexter; only to have him laugh at the idea. She thought of how she always wanted a baby to hold, love and raise. She thought of having a baby for Dexter; his light skin would combine with her creamy mocha-chocolate complexion to produce a pretty brown complexioned girl.

She wanted those things. Mostly in the old fashion order: marriage first, then babies. But it wasn't working out that way.

Djuana wiped her cheeks. The tears came easily, almost unnoticed until they reached her lips. "The bastard hit me," she said, almost as if to remind herself.

She looked up and wished for rain. In Portland, that's not so farfetched. She enjoyed feeling the drops hit her face and arms. She squeezed her arms together to ward off yet another strong breeze. Her mind zipped past those hurtful thoughts, as her arms and face goose-bumped, hoping for the phone to ring. She needed to talk this out with the only person that would understand.

Her mind tensed her body with the memory of the sudden fear she experienced when those high, beaming headlights appeared from nowhere. She remembered being frozen in place. Death was imminent. The vehicle swerved. A man with strong arms and a warm embrace gently melted her fears away. Then awakening in the firmest, warmest bed she had ever slept in.

"Djuana! Can't you hear Ma!" The roar of her brother belting out her name from inside the apartment snapped Djuana back to reality. It was time to make dinner. She ducked into the apartment to find Devon upset.

"What's up with you?" she asked him.

"These dag-on Crowns! I'm getting tired of 'em. That's why the Gamblers keep mashing 'em!"

The Crowns were not looking good, and were losing to New York.

The Crowns were Devon's favorite team, unless they were playing the World Champion Las Vegas Gamblers. His friends, who lived right there in Portland with him, all hated the 'Chokin' Crowns'. They would taunt him:

"You don't bet against the Gamblers!" and he would lie, "I don't like the Crowns anyway!"

She shrugged off his little crisis. To hell with sports, she thought. It's a man's thing. She began taking out the ingredients from the refrigerator and cupboards to prepare a fried chicken and rice dinner. Cooking was a joy to Djuana, and right then, it would be a nice distraction. While she prepared the simple meal, Tia finally called. Djuana was never more pleased to hear her best friend's voice.

Tia Williams was disappointed in Djuana for becoming pregnant. She had discussed having children with Djuana hundreds of times; it would be after marrying Mr. Right, then a baby boy first then a girl. Tia wanted five kids. Djuana would laugh at the thought of her slim friend baring five children.

It was Tia who had answered Djuana's questions about sex and love - not that she was an expert - but she was sensible and together they learned the difference in the two feelings. It was Tia who talked Djuana into birth control. Tia was the first person to interrogate prospective boyfriends.

Tia accepted her role as big sister, although two months younger than Djuana, because she saw Djuana as the woman she wanted to be in many ways.

At 5 foot 9, four inches taller than Djuana, and busty, Tia was noticeable. She had plain features, thin lips and dark skin. Her eyes were dark and seemed to lack fire, yet she was quick to smile and a master of telling jokes. Tia always felt underdeveloped, despite her large breasts, especially when out with her best friend. Compared to Djuana's arch shape and plump-where-it-should-be-plump body, Tia felt like a stilt with melons.

It was Tia who hated Dexter Forns from that first day in the old Galleria when the three met. Dexter was not Mr. Right, nor was he a good man to date; Tia told Djuana that. She told Dexter that she didn't trust him, and often threatened him not to hurt Djuana.

"Tee," Djuana whispered into the telephone. "Dex hit me so hard in that restaurant that I didn't know where I was for a minute."

Tia fell silent on the other end of the phone.

"Then, like I said, I just started walking."

"You walked all the way from the restaurant?"

Djuana paused. She stirred the brown rice. "I didn't make it home. The next thing I knew a jeep nearly hit me and I was standing in the middle of the street. This guy, who was driving the jeep, comes to me and comforts me like he..." Djuana raised the spoon. Her mouth moved yet no words came out. Then her hand dropped. She wanted to say the man held her with such tenderness. But it didn't seem appropriate.

Tia cut off her bedroom radio, this was more than she had expected. "Wait. What are you telling me? Dexter hit you, left you, then you ran into some strange man?"

"Do I sound stupid?" Djuana asked her best friend.

"No. I mean, I don't understand. What happened? He took you home? Shit, Dee, did he rape you?" Tia was fearful that some man had taken advantage of her friend.

"No. I don't think he did. You see, I remember he held me in the street, and took me to his car. I felt like a child in his arms. So secure. So comfortable. So at ease. I remember just crying myself to sleep while he drove."

"I did have too many drinks. And you know I can't drink."

Tia's mouth gaped open. Did she realized what she's saying?

"All I remember is waking in his bed," Djuana continued. "In his baseball shirt. In his house."

"Did he touch you, Djuana?" Tia's uneasiness became evident.

"No. I mean he undressed me, and when I awoke I did assume he had. But, to tell you the God's honest truth, I've been thinking about it, and I know that if he had, I would have known. I think he didn't do anything. And he well sure could have."

"Shit, Dee. Shit."

Djuana took a deep breath. "Well, when I got up I got out my cutter and made him call me a cab."

"What did he say? Do you think he slept with you?"

"He didn't say much. He tried to assure me that nothing happened. And I believed him in a way."

"I don't know what to say."

"Say I'm not stupid. Say I ain't crazy, nor has my life gone crazy."

"You're not crazy. But this is wild. Kinda unbelievable. It could've ended up worst. Thank God it didn't."

*17*

Jack sat in the dugout and watched his hungover teammates get whipped by New York most of the game. In between innings, Jack continued telling Oscar about his night with a visitor he found in the rain. O would shake his head in disbelief at each new detail.

"You didn't hammer the bitch?" O said in amazement.

"Nope." Jack said calmly, watching Mike strike out for the third time in the game, ending the seventh inning.

"You're a real ass," O said as he grabbed his glove and trotted out to center field.

Maybe he was an ass, Jack wasn't sure. He could have used some sex to ease his mind. He shook his head, "No, then I would have really been in trouble. But what the hell, she believes I did something anyway. Yeah, I shoulda boned her. Hold those big thighs, kiss those smooth lips, squeeze that ass..."

"Jack!" Bingo Wells snapped.

Jack had missed New York's at-bat. He looked up to find his teammates back in the dugout with him.

"Wake the fuck up! Shit, man, I'm trying to tell you somethin'!" Bingo waved off Jack in anger. "Fuck it!"

He stormed away leaving Jack disoriented. Bingo was the Crowns bread and butter. He was a 6-foot-6, 265 pound power hitting monster. He intimidated his teammates as well as opponents. He was a running partner of O and Jack's in the minor leagues. He made the big time a year before them, and had had an enormous season.

Bingo hit 57 home runs, the most ever by a Crown, until he topped himself with 63 the next year. He became a multimillionaire celebrity. The fun and frolicking he did with O and Jack became distant memories as he disassociated himself from them.

"You know something, Jack," Bingo said as he returned. "That's your fuckin' problem. You don't take shit seriously. That's why you can't keep a woman and got your ass busted last night!"

The players on the bench burst into a chorus of assorted laughs and giggles. Jack smiled. O raised his eyebrows and grinned at Jack.

The game entered the final inning with New York leading 7-5. Bingo had hit two long home runs, driving in all five Portland runs. In their last at bat, the Crowns players began playing with more spunk - their hangovers had eased. New York countered with its best relief pitcher, a big burly hard-thrower that the Crowns lost to twice the previous season, to preserve its lead and win the game. While he warmed up, the capacity crowd rocked Adkins Stadium in anticipation of a come-from-behind victory.

The Crowns' manager scratched his dry scalp. Hal Juris wanted this game. It being the fifth of the season, with 157 left, had no consequence. He looked down his bench at Jack, who was twirling a bat. Juris walked down the dugout to his talented outfielder. Juris knew Jack would go through a wall for him; if only he'd ask. Juris also understood that if he put Jack in this game — and lost — he would replace Jack in the owner's doghouse. But a hunch had the best of him.

Juris stopped in front of Jack; O was on Jack's left and Jim Finks on his right stuffing his mouth with tobacco.

"You own this guy, don't you?" the burly manager pleaded.

"Of course, Skip." Jack had gotten a few hits off that pitcher, but nothing great. But he knew the answer his boss wanted.

"Get ready," Juris said before returning to his favorite spot on the bench by the bat rack.

The Crowns put runners on first and second with one out, forcing the heralded pitcher to sweat profusely with each fastball he fired. The next batter roped a shot to the gap in right-center scoring a run, and pulling the Crowns within one score, 7-6. Runners then were on second and third. The roaring of the crowd shook the stadium.

While his teammates were at home plate congratulating Juan upon scoring and the crowd was jumping and shouting, Jack selected his bat from the rack. Juris grabbed his arm as he stepped from the rack onto the steps and pulled him back down. "You don't come through we both burn! Get a fuckin' hit!"

Jack smiled and entered the on-deck circle. Mike stopped on his way back to the dugout from cheerleading and grabbed Jack deep up between the cheeks of his buttocks; "Bust that ass, Boyieee!" he yelled. Jack tried not to laugh, but did.

The pots were simmering with the smells of appetizing food. The table was set. Djuana took a break. She wanted to watch television but sports and westerns had the stations tied up. Even with cable and more than 50 channels there was nothing on she took interest in. A minute of looking out of the window returned unpleasant thoughts.

She ended up standing in the entrance of the kitchen, which led to the living room, watching the baseball game over the body of her brother stretched out on the rug. The excitement in the announcer's voice had intrigued Djuana. He spouted on about a clutch situation. *Huh?* The man was raising his voice in order to be heard over the loud cheering.

Djuana marveled at how Jack Newhouse was so calm while the crowd and announcer were so ecstatic. *Is he aware?* The camera's close-up brought a spark of light to Djuana's memory. "Oh, shit. It's him." Her voice barely carried.

"Shhh! Be quiet!" Devon said. Then turned up the volume with the remote.

Djuana kicked her brother's foot. Her mind revealed vivid pictures from the night before: the name on the back of the jersey she slept in, Newhouse. Jack's dark eyes that seemed to glow with divine intentions, and those broad shoulders that held her and guided her to his car.

Djuana bolted into the living room from the kitchen when Jack went sprawling to the ground avoiding a wild pitch headed for his head.

"Is that legal? The guy threw the ball at him!" she asked her 11-year-old sports encyclopedia.

"He should've let it hit him!" The boy spoke without his eyes leaving the screen nor his head leaving his hands.

Jack rose slowly. He wasn't ready for the sudden dip to the dirt. He dusted off his once white uniform and spit out dirt. He regained his composure and hit the next pitch back at the pitcher, causing him to buckle and duck quickly as the ball passed over his head and into center field.

The cameras showed both runners racing home, with the crowd exploding in the background. The announcer yelled, "The Crowns win it! The Crowns win it!"

Djuana clapped and cheered. Devon looked behind him in amazement. She calmed, putting her hands over her ear-to-ear grin. She turned into the kitchen. She laughed at the look her brother gave her, "If he only knew."

Devon followed his sister into the kitchen. "Since when do you like baseball so much?"

"I don't. I just know Jack Newhouse, that's all," She became defensive as she worked around the sink and stove.

"Oh, really?"

"Yeah, so? Go wash up so you can eat."

Devon walked slowly through the kitchen and out toward the bathroom, a puzzled look across his face. He stopped, turned back to his sister, "So you know Jack Newhouse? So, then, get tickets, then."

"Shut up," Djuana frowned.

# 5

The next week was forgettable for Djuana. Four mornings in a row she was greeted with severe morning sickness. The fifth morning she awoke with an idea. She sipped ginger ale at room temperature and hoped for the best. She still vomited just before she had to leave to catch the 9:07 bus for work.

She disliked being sick and hated vomiting. She believed to die would have been better than suffering at the base of her commode while her head split open and her guts poured out.

Then, each day her brother would ask had she gotten tickets for a Crowns game, forcing her to relive that night. He would show her a schedule and pick the games he wanted to attend. His nagging not only made her sorry she had told him, but all the more upset at the reason she had met a baseball player.

Djuana did not want to go to a game, but she did want to see Jack Newhouse again. She wanted to ask him what he remembered from that night. What had he seen, what had he touched. She wanted to smack him again. And, she wanted him to hold her and make her whole life better.

One morning, the fear of spewing out her remaining insides was so strong Djuana couldn't get out of bed. She knew she should be going in to work that day, the monthly register reports had to be sent in, but her bones were reluctant. And, conjuring up scenarios with Jack Newhouse was more heartwarming than the disaster she saw her life to be.

She glanced across her bedroom at the digital clock on the high chest to see that she had better get moving if she was going. She had put the clock across the room to force herself to get out of bed to switch off the alarm. Now, if she could only remember to reset the clock before going to sleep each night.

Emma Pioneer burst into the room and announced the time. Emma was half dressed, in a bra and slip. It was nearing the time for her to leave for work, which meant Djuana was already behind schedule.

"You going to work, or what, Lady Day?" the round woman said.

"Yeah, Mother. I'm just a little beat." Djuana looked around her room. It was neat, but it always seemed untidy when her mother was in it.

Djuana found it incredible that her mother had not caught on to her predicament. Maybe she had. Maybe Emma was finally treating her 25-year-old daughter as a woman and letting her handle her own business. Djuana smiled at the thought. Naw, she had no clue.

Djuana sat up in the bed expecting the third-degree. Instead her mother moved across the room as if she was looking for something. She stopped at the vanity table, with her back to Djuana. Emma suddenly spun and approached Djuana.

"Why don't you take the day off and rest this weekend, you look like something the cat dragged in." Emma felt Djuana's forehead with her right hand. In her left was Djuana's bottle of Fantasy. That was the one perfume she did not like to share. But she was to weak to fight.

The feel of her mother's hand made Djuana feel 10 years old again. "You ain't warm. What's got you sick? Are you pregnant?"

Djuana's face froze. She fumbled an answer. "No, Ma. It's just probably something I ate."

"Yeah, see. I told you about all that grease. Have some salad for lunch sometime," with that she was gone, with the bottle of Fantasy.

Djuana tried to sleep but instead stared at the ceiling until her mother left for work. She called in sick. Mr. Thompson, her boss, said he understood. Had he noticed?

The Crowns left Los Angeles without a win in two games. They flew to Arizona, in the midst of a 10-game, 13-day road trip.

Jack loved traveling to other cities to play ball. In each city he had found restaurants, clubs and with O's help, women to sleep with. But, this trip came too soon. He would have rather been searching Portland for that 'woman'.

On the plane O sat with Jack in the aisle seat reading the Gazette. Jack could not remove himself from the thoughts of Djuana. He should have slept with her; should have made love to her. Gotten his hands on that soft body and — well, he should have at least gotten her phone number. His head shook side to side unconsciously.

O hissed and slammed the paper into his lap. "Shit! That fucking white hoe is nuts!"

Everyone heard him, but none of his teammates turned to acknowledge O. They were used to his outbursts.

"A little louder, please," Jack said. "The pilots didn't get the end of that."

"She is still writing about you being traded like she fucking slept with all the parties involved."

"Maybe she did. So? Who cares what she's writing? Why you sweatin' it?"

O mumbled a few words then got up. "I'll be right back."

Jack watched his best friend trot to first class. He knew O was about to blast the Crowns higher hierarchy, which on the road consisted of general manager J.A. Honeywell. Jack gave it little thought. What's her name in Portland was more enthralling.

Djuana enjoyed a day off in the middle of the week; her first in months. She spent the day home alone. She caught up on the soaps and got to see two movies on cable that she had missed in theaters. Pigging out on every and anything in the refrigerator and laying on the couch underneath her comforter was heaven.

The phone's ring late that afternoon startled her. Then, Dexter's voice scared her. They had not spoken since that night, and she didn't think they ever would again. She had called him three times, each leaving a message with his mother. And each time, Mrs. Forns - Djuana had heard the woman's first name once, and never used it - seemed more exasperated with Djuana. The woman was not rude, but she sure seemed unhappy to hear Djuana call. In the past, Mrs. Forns would tell Djuana things about her son. Nothing to telling, just hints that maybe she should leave Dexter alone and find someone else.

"Listen, Djuana. I'm coming by. We need to talk," Dexter said.

"Oh, so now you got time? No, Dexter. You can't come by."

"Uh huh. I'll be there in an hour."

Djuana didn't *really* mind he was coming. They did need to talk, she reasoned after he hung up. But, she was sure she didn't want to see him alone. She hoped Devon would come straight home, or even, that her mother would come home early. For the first time since junior high, she was afraid to be alone with a man.

Accepting his apology would not be the problem, she thought. Dexter had never hit Djuana before that night. But it was time to cut him loose and let the others have him. Lilly, with her high-yellow, loud self. And Jenny, with that big ass and big lips. Let them, and the others, have him. Djuana wanted to settle the pregnancy, then be out of his way. She wasn't sure she wanted to have an abortion, but it seemed the easiest route. And, an easy way out was what she was looking for.

Dexter's knock came nearly an hour after it was due; and the house was still empty. Devon was probably out playing and Emma didn't get off for at least two hours. Dexter eased into the apartment, surveying the scene. He took Djuana into his arms and kissed her cheek.

Djuana rolled her eyes. She didn't want to hear the bullshit. Only answers. Only the truth. Dexter watched Djuana enter the living room. His eyes could not get enough of her lips filling a pair of old jeans. Djuana moved the comforter to one side of the couch and sat. Dexter followed, sitting on most of the blanket. He understood the silence, he was to take charge, he thought.

"What do you want to do," he said as he removed his jacket while seated.

Djuana hissed and shook her head. She knew he wouldn't apologize. "It's all on me, huh?"

"Naw, Babe. We gotta handle this together. I ain't ready for no baby." Dexter reached into his jacket, which he had placed on the arm of the couch. He removed an envelope from an inner pocket and slipped it under her hand, on her thigh.

Dexter moved closer to Djuana and his voice lowered. The sound of tires hydroplaning on the wet street below came from the open window behind the couch to split Djuana's attention. She knew what she was about to hear, though.

"Look, Babe. You don't need nothing to tie you down right now. You got a good job, you want to get your own place and you always talkin' about traveling. We can have babies later, you know, like when we get married like we always talked about."

Dexter's guilt eased. He had made a winning presentation.

Djuana covered her face with both hands and leaned forward. The envelope slipped between her legs. She did not want to cry.

"Shit," she whispered. "Like *we* always talked about? Come on, Dexter. I was the only one interested in us being married."

"What the fuck that's got to do with this?"

Djuana stood up and crossed her arms in front of her chest. Her stomach churned, it was nerves she believed. Dexter stood behind her and planted a kiss her cheek. The feel of his penis rub against her ass infuriated Djuana. She pushed him.

"You hit me, Dex. You hit me and left me and accused me of trying to entrap you. Why? Haven't I loved you all these years? Haven't I cooked and cleaned for your ass after you've fucked those other whores, and they didn't do shit for you?"

"I understand all that. But, I ain't ready for no baby. It's as simple as that."

"Why don't you apologize? I ain't them other bitches that like to be smacked around."

"Whatever," he rolled his eyes and sighed. "I'm more than sorry. I ain't never raised my hand to you ever before. Let's just get this settled."

He sat.

A key in the door startled Djuana more than Dexter. She was pleased to see Devon walk in whistling. The kid stopped abruptly when he noticed his sister's tears and the visitor.

"What happen?" Devon said. He looked at Dexter.

Djuana slipped behind her brother and reopened the door. "Nothing. Dex is about to leave," she said. Her voice was dry. She felt the stares from both Dexter and Devon.

Dexter looked at the kid, then the kid's beautiful, yet mad, sister. He spoke, forcing his voice to a whisper.

"No. We need to get this out now."

"Good-bye, Dexter," Djuana said.

Dexter cursed, snatched up his jacket and bolted out the door. He abruptly stopped, chest to chest with Djuana. "I'll call you when I get to work."

He bent to kiss her and she bristled.

"No. I'll call you." She slammed the door and locked it.

"What's going on?" Devon asked. "What did he do? I'ma hurt him."

Djuana stopped her brother from questioning her and zipped back to the couch and under the comforter.

Devon fumed, "I'm gonna kick his ass one day. I promise."

"Watch your mouth!"

Devon went in his room and slammed the door behind him. He wished he were 18 or bigger. He wanted to defend his sister for a change. He remembered the times last summer she saved him from certain death at the hands of older boys in Tudor Park. Some day, he vowed, he will take care of his sister the way his mother wants him to.

# 6

Jack knew that if, and when, he died he would be prepared. Arizona could not be much less hotter than Hell.

The late April humidity had baked the artificial turf covering Aztec Stadium. The early evening sun was still potent as the Crowns took batting and infield practice before the game. Jack had hoped to wear shorts until game time, but Juris hit the roof and demanded he fully dress. The Crowns gray cotton button-up uniform did not repel heat too well.

After batting practice, which left Jack sweating profusely, he sat in the dugout shade watching the sun descend behind the hills out in the desert. Oscar came sweating over to where Jack sat.

"It's hot as Hell out there," O declared.

"Who you tellin'?" The thought of playing the outfield on a heated rug was not inviting to either outfielder.

"I don't know how-in-the-fuck they play down here all summer."

Jack grimaced, "Shit, I guess they handle it."

Jack's eyes locked onto his bat as he tapped his cleats with the barrel. He heard O laughing, and, without looking up, he knew it was because Mike was wetting Aztecs players with a water hose. The sight of Djuana wearing his minor league jersey was a vivid picture on the ground of the dugout. Damn, she was beautiful.

Better looking than Vivian. Much better looking. Probably more classy, too. He recalled how she gracefully held the top of his baseball jersey, that really wasn't revealing anything anyway, although she was highly upset. Then how she sat on his porch awaiting the cab, her legs crossed and ankle swinging. She refused money for the cab ride, that he knew would be in the $15 range. That's class.

Vivian's bones, he thought, paled in comparison to a body like Djuana's. Djuana's shapely thighs and hips was what he should have always wanted. Even though, he once loved the skinny physique of his ex. Or did he?

A female voice dragged Jack back to reality. She was standing directly in front of the setting sun. It was Kristen Eisen, reporter. She had confirmed her tip that Jack was trade bait, now she wanted him to comment.

She maneuvered her pumps step-by-step down the steep dugout steps. O leaped up to help her, but she brushed him away. He kissed her hand and told her how sexy her legs were without stockings. She thanked him without a smile and returned her attention to Jack.

She started right in. "Isn't it true you and Slight are having an dispute over your night life?"

Jack shrugged. He hadn't taken the situation seriously. "Slight and I are fine. He just wants the best from his players, on and off the field. Off the field I have been having problems meeting his idea of perfection. But on the field I have always been what he expects."

Kristen remained emotionless, jotting notes. "Slight said he is seriously shopping you and that he believes Hector Aponte is ready for your right field job. He mentioned Buffalo. I called them, and they want you."

Jack chuckled. "A lot of teams want me. So? Listen, Kristen. As of now I am the Crowns right fielder. Have been for the past five years. Five productive years."

He became bitter. "I don't have to defend myself. I should be relaxed, enjoying myself. I help Slight take first place three times. Played hurt. The thought of dumping me shouldn't cross that idiot's mind."

Kristen smirked a bit. She was imagining Slight calling her into his office after the story ran the next day. He would be furious that she wrote he was an idiot, even though one of his players had said it.

"So, you want to stay? What am I saying, of course you do. But, even if as Slight says, you are disgracing his team's name by fighting in public and getting arrested."

"I got arrested, what two years ago? Please. Forget that. It was a barroom brawl. Half of the Crowns were in it!"

"If he trades me, I'll go. And haunt him for the rest of my playing days."

Djuana stopped at the supermarket on Northwest Avenue after work. She bought a four-pack of wine coolers, she didn't expect to have the baby, so she felt like drinking, and three different bags of chips. She couldn't resist buying two pints of ice cream; chocolate and rum raisin. This was to be her first night of baseball on television and she wanted to be sure she had the snacks to last it through.

Turning the corner of 23rd Avenue onto Tudor, Djuana's eyes lit on Dexter's Mazda parked in front of her building.

"Shit." Djuana wanted to dash into the building and run up the stairs, but her legs slowed, almost wobbled.

Her eyes riveted on the car. Dexter rose out of the driver's seat. Anger rose from her toes and her fist balled around her groceries. She picked up speed and angled for the building's steps.

Dexter moved slowly. He looked over her body. Damn, he thought. Does all her dresses fit so well? Yeah. They do, he smiled. He loved how her hips looked firm, but he knew better. They would melt between his fingers like butter. The lavender dress she had on that day reached her knees and flared with her hips. He remembered that when she wore that dress he could stand in front of her and see one of her many lace bras struggling to support breasts that seemed to have been poured in. He hoped it was a front opening bra today.

Dexter jogged over to the stoop, a quick hop vaulted him up over the steps. Djuana wanted to kick him.

"We should talk," he said, standing as close to Djuana as possible, and not controlling his eyes.

Djuana wanted to be hard on Dexter. Let him feel some hurt, she thought. But, shit, he now was giving me attention. Have the baby and he'll always be there. Maybe he would even marry... STOP!

She finally spoke, "Just leave me alone, please, Dexter."

Dexter hated when she called him by his full name. It lacked her loving tone.

Djuana bolted into the building's front door with her elbow leading the way, and pain punctured her anger. The heavy door barely moved. She stepped back and kicked the door open and moved on toward the elevator.

Dexter laughed lightly and followed.

"Now what did that prove?"

"Fuck you. You're an ass, Dexter."

He let loose a devilish laugh. He had thought Djuana would act this way, but he wanted to remain the civil one. He was not going to let her have this baby. He stepped between the elevator and Djuana.

"Listen to me," he began.

Djuana erupted, "What!? Whatcha got to say, Dexter?! Huh?!"

"Dammit, just shut the fuck up and hear me out, shit!" He barked, then his voice abruptly lowered, "Use the money I left. I am not ready for no baby. I'm sorry. But I am just not ready. I do love you, but I ain't ready for this."

Djuana let him speak. All the while looking through him. It was as if she knew each and every word before it flowed off his tongue. She almost agreed. Before she realized it, Dexter held her chin and slid his tongue over hers. The sound of the elevator landing startled Djuana. Dexter held the door open and told her he'd call later.

Djuana pinned herself in the noiseless lift as the door closed. Her head titled back as her body leaned fully. She took in air through her nose, trying to prevent the sobs.

Once inside the apartment, Djuana had to relax her nerves in silence before cooking fried hamburgers and home fries for Devon and herself.

She caused her little brother to gag when she piled pickles, ketchup, mustard, lettuce, tomatoes, onions, and a dab of peanut butter – she had heard someone mention peanut butter on burgers on the bus – on the oversized hamburgers.

"You're crazy!" Devon declared.

"I just have a taste for this, that's all." When she spilled most of it on her t-shirt, Devon laughed so hard his Kool-Aid came out of his nose. They laughed at each other.

Djuana expected Devon would join her for the Crowns game and was thrilled when his favorite hang-out partner came and got him to play Nintendo at his apartment across the hall. She poured the onion and garlic chips into one Tupperware bowl, the pretzels in another and the corn chips in yet another bowl. The wine coolers were more than cold from their hour in the freezer. She was set.

The game began slowly. The Aztecs, what a name Djuana thought, led Jack's team 1-0, but the Crowns did make a nice double play. They threw the ball around the field and got two Aztecs out. Djuana applauded.

Jack hit a double, slid head first twice, as the Crowns rallied in the fourth inning to pull ahead 4-1. Djuana watched Jack's body while he ran the bases. His uniform was not tight enough, but his muscles were evident. His thighs flexed as he stretched his legs running. His forearms seem strong-his gentle hug came to mind. Djuana could have used a hug then. She was on the couch under her comforter, now into her ice cream.

Emma came into the house with a gush of cool air. She noticed the refreshments and tried to remember what movie she was missing. She crossed between Djuana and the floor model television, her coat half off, in time to see the score flash across the screen.

"Baseball?" she was puzzled.

Fright stabbed Djuana. She fumbled an answer. "There ain't nothing else on."

Emma sucked her teeth and threw her coat down in the chair near the door. She went through the house and returned with the TV Guide.

"Did you cook?" Emma asked, looking through the guide. "Oh, there is a Steven Segal movie on cable."

She reached for the remote.

"No, don't turn! I'm watching this."

"Well, you go ahead. I'll go in my room. Baseball is too boring for me."

Great, Djuana exhaled. The game wasn't boring at all. Jack hit the ball every time he batted. He ran the bases and made some nice catches. The announcers liked Jack as much as she did. Whenever he came to bat, they told another story about him that added to the collection of tidbits that made him seem all the more masterful. Despite having one of the best home run hitters to ever play in the league on his team, Jack Newhouse, one of the announcers said, once lead the league in homers.

Very impressive, Djuana glowed.

The Crowns put on a show for Djuana, winning 11-3. She felt privileged. She ate like a child, mixing the chips into a bag, shaking it, then digging her hand in every few seconds for a taste delight. She even licked her fingers.

But, Djuana could not get herself to drink the wine coolers.

During the Crowns victory, Vincent Slight and his team's general manager J.A. Honeywell were on a conference call with Ron Capton, owner of the Buffalo Soldiers. The three men talked for two hours on speaker phones about completing a trade that would help both teams.

Buffalo was the worst team in the Eastern conference for five years. Capton had bought them with little capital, but in the past year his fortunes had blossomed. Now he was prepared to compete with the big money teams for quality ballplayers. The only problem he faced was that no free agents wanted to play in Buffalo for him.

Capton decided to rebuild his team with young talent. He had collected an abundance of good young pitching, yet still lacked hitting to contend. He called Honeywell, knowing the Crowns could use pitching. Capton wanted Mike, the Crowns' crafty catcher, but Honeywell flatly said no. Slight intervened and offered Jack instead.

"Listen, Ron," Slight demanded as he tired of Capton's stubbornness. "You need us more than we need you! Shit, you have been watching my boys in the playoffs for the past five years. You take Jack Newhouse. He'll help you. He has got at least five years left in him. The change of scenery will help him. He's battle-tested and fearless."

"I am not an novice. Don't patronize me. Why are you so eager to dump him if he's made of gold?"

Honeywell almost laughed on the receiver - neither Slight or Capton knew what they were doing.

Slight paused, glaring at Honeywell. Honeywell caught his look, and killed the grinning. Those two, Slight and Honeywell, are the hardest working tandem in the business. Honeywell had the knowledge; he could tell if a player was both talented and could help the Crowns within ten minutes of seeing the person. While Slight had a wallet the size of Canada.

Capton continued. "Listen. I've got some good young arms. I could give you a Cy Young award winner for the next 10 years. All I want is Colbert and a farmhand."

"We can't do that. We are shopping Newhouse, you want him or not?"

A moment of silence. Then Capton's end of the line sounded muffled. He returned to say he needed time to confer with his aides.

"Thank God," Honeywell whispered too loud. Slight again glared over at him. The three men parted with pleasantries.

Slight hung up the phone staring at Honeywell. "What's with you?"

"We can't, I should say, we shouldn't be trading this early in the season."

"Who asked you? Jack has got to go. And I'd love to see him crying and losing in Buffalo. Besides, you should be helping me rob that asshole Capton."

"I thought my job was to worry about our team. We are fine right now."

"Fine!? Please! You're an ass if you really believe that."

Honeywell was thinking about all Jack had done for the team without ever complaining or demanding more money as did so many less talented Crowns.

He said, "I think you are letting personal feelings interfere with business. We could use some pitching from Capton, but not at the expense of an outfielder."

Slight fixed a stiff drink from the bar in the luxury visiting owners suite in Aztec Stadium. "I am going to say this to you once, and only once. Jack Newhouse is on the block. I don't won't him on my team anymore."

Honeywell looked out across the Aztecs' playing field. He thought of quitting, then starting his own business. Portland could use another Black book store. Or, maybe he'd buy a team.

He looked at Slight, who was fixing another drink.

Honeywell said, "You're right, Vinny. It's your team. Do what you think is best."

# 7

Sweat was packed. The small building was painted black, with a neon pink sign tall and wide across its roof. People were everywhere in the little downtown Phoenix club, a mile from the Crowns hotel. The small factory-type loft was painted all black; including the few windows facing the tiny side street it was on. The building looked about two stories high, but once you entered, the only stairs visible were the two you went down once you passed the three bouncers at the front door. The deejay was good, but the sound system was lacking the deep-bass that greeted you at the Tunnell in Portland.

Jack and Oscar were marathon drinking at the bar with teammate, Danny Gross. They weren't really discussing much, maybe a little baseball talk, before Brenda finally arrived. Jack noticed Brenda first. He rubbed his hands together, "Yeah buddy!" his loins tingled.

O knew what he meant. "Where? Where she at?" His head spun, circling the dance floor. Jack took O's head and moved it in the direction of Brenda dancing.

Brenda Smalls was Jack and Oscar's sex partner while in Arizona. She was short, 5 feet, little everywhere but big on energy. Her body was shapely and her legs curved; clothes did the body no justice. Her long hair, mostly a ponytail hairpiece, and thin lips highlighted perfect bronze skin. She was half Filipino, and half African-American. On that steamy, humid night, Brenda was wearing a olive green lycra dress which struggled to keep up with a swinging body.

O slid through the dancers with Jack in tow. He cut between Brenda and her partner. O picked her up by the waist, bending her over his shoulder. Jack told the guy to, "Just walk away quietly and nobody gets pummeled repeatedly."

The guy, head shaking, mumbled before walking in the other direction.

Talk was short. The three invaded the dance floor. O and Jack sandwiched Brenda while not spilling their drinks. Jack would break off on occasion to refill. O didn't let Brenda out of his sight.

On one of his trips to the bar, Jack stopped to roll his Tom Collins over his sweaty head. He laughed at his friend being out-danced yet not giving up. He scanned the dance floor for more teammates. Pitcher Lee Spencer was dancing slow to the high-powered rap music mix. He was grinding a light-skinned woman with long hair. Her dress caught Jack's attention. It was blue, and the same dress he had removed from Djuana Pioneer a week earlier.

How was she? he wondered. What guy could leave a woman of that beauty in a drunken state to walk home? Yeah, he chuckled, but I bet she's with the asshole right this minute, happy. He sipped his drink.

O cut Jack's vision and patted his shoulder. "Yo! We outta here!. You with us?"

Jack gulped his drink empty. "Definitely."

They grabbed a cab back to the hotel. In minutes the three were in bed together. Brenda enjoyed both men. Their unison while kissing, caressing and making love never ceased to amaze her. Neither man was selfish, yet both never seemed to get enough.

Jack sat up on his hotel bed. In the next bed lay Oscar and Brenda tangled in one. He wiped his face with his dry hands. The smell of sex filled the room. He got up slowly, two games in humid weather, two late nights of sex with Brenda, and about three hours of sleep had drained him. This was the type of behavior Slight was complaining about; Jack understood then.

He pulled up a shade and the bright orange sun burnt his eyes. He opened the window, took a deep breath, and closed it again. There was no breeze, or hint of fresh air to fumigate the room. Jack glanced over at Brenda's small, long breast and large, round nipples. Her nude body was near engulfed by O's long, muscular frame. An urge grabbed his thoughts - one more time. But, he thought better of it.

Jack took a quick shower and returned to find Brenda and Oscar in just about the same positions asleep. As he was dressing with his back to the sleepers, Jack could hear stirring. When he turned, Brenda was out of the bed. In the mirror, Jack watched O's reddened eyes scan the room, then he got up on one elbow.

Brenda zigzagged from spot to spot collecting her clothing. "Are we hanging tonight?"

"Naw," O said in a hoarse voice. "We outta here this morning." He fell back in the bed. "So, why don't you give me some jaw before you leave?"

Jack chuckled at his crude friend. Jack sat on his bed, tying his sneakers.

"O, please," Brenda said as she kicked open the bathroom door and went in. "You two fucked me like y'all ain't had none in awhile. Shit, O, you was hurting me!"

"Shut the fuck up and get back out here!" O said as he covered himself.

"Why don't you relax," Jack said, now fully dressed.

"No. I'm getting some before we leave. Where you headed?"

"Out," Jack said flatly. "I need a walk before the bus leaves for the airport."

O jumped up as the water started in the bathroom. He went in, grabbed Brenda and dragged her back into bed.

"No, Oscar, I've got to go," she was pleading.

"Yeah, in a minute." He maneuvered Brenda on top of him. She moaned and kissed him. Oscar's thin fingers guided Brenda's wide hips into motion; squeezing her ass. He had her ride him as Jack crept out the door.

The interview with Kristen had left Jack thinking, whenever he wasn't playing the Aztecs or screwing Brenda, about how, all of a sudden, his status with the Portland Crowns seemed to be shaken. He did understand the team's owner had vowed to never finish second again. The whole state of Oregon was tired of the Crowns losing to Las Vegas; twice was enough.

But, Jack didn't understand, what had he done wrong? He was the Crowns best hitter in both World Series. He had made the rainy town his home. Did more than his share of charity work; spent time and dollars on children in Oregon. He forced his fellow Black teammates to set up a college fund for minorities in Portland. In comparison, Jack hadn't been that involved in charity work in his hometown. In New York, all he really did was supplied his high school's athletic department with money and equipment.

Before Jack went out, he stopped two floors down at the general manager's suite. He didn't realize it was 7 a.m. until he had to knock more than once. J.A. Honeywell opened the door fully clothed. He had one a steel gray suit, except for the jacket. He was packing for the trip home.

"Sit down, Jack." Honeywell all but ordered as he returned to packing his traveling bags. "I know what you want. Eisen called me. And so did some idiot reporter from New York."

Jack slowly moved into the room, but didn't sit. He looked over Honeywell; Jack respected him not just because he was the only African American general manager in the majors, but because he was also the best in the business. Honeywell was tall and slender, with perfect shoulders for the Armani suits he loved to wear. He had dark, rich skin. He wore a full beard in the winter, but sported only a mustache during the season. He kept his graying hair short to the scalp. He was usually easy going for such a demanding job as the right hand man of Vincent Slight.

Honeywell went on, "Slight has been shopping you. He feels our payroll is too high not to have won a championship. Frankly, I agree."

"Fine," Jack said curtly. "But why me? I have produced for you."

"You know, that's probably why teams have been calling us more than we have been calling them. Teams want you. Not Danny, or Lee, or anybody else. When we call, it's 'How much for J-New.'"

"So, I'm gone?"

"No," Honeywell stood, out of breath from bending, packing and talking. "No. Actually, I'm trying to keep your ass. But, if I were you, and I wanted to stay in Portland, I'd clean up my act. Fucking hoes like that one you and O got upstairs now, is going to make it seem like the easy and right thing to do for Slight.

"Slight is trying to change the image; clean house. He will not trade Oscar Taylor."

Jack got that conversation off his mind almost as soon as he was out of the hotel. He strolled through downtown Phoenix in the early morning hours believing a long walk would remedy his blues. And, it helped. All he could think about was getting married and settling down. That would keep him in Portland.

That lead his mind to the woman back in Portland. She was beautiful enough to marry, he saw. She was soft and tough. He smiled at the thought of how her hand, the same smooth, satiny limb that he had held and touched along with other parts of her delicate body while changing her, was suddenly brandishing a knife.

The image of her naked body, glistening on his bed shook his heart. He wanted her more each day. He could picture, during his uneven paced saunter, dating this woman for no more than a month before making sweet love to her. He knew the sex would be good, because he desired that body so. Well, he imagined she had to know a thing or two. She could not have gotten that old, be that gorgeous, and not have had guys putting her through the whole book of positions.

Jack actually got jealous for the next minute or so.

He was going to get married in the next two years, he determined on his walk. His younger sister had done it. Married a guy after only four months of dating. O had even done it! And, in less time than his sister. Jack knew he could do it. He had turned down hundreds of wedding proposals. But, they were from golddiggers.

A few of the women he spent time with, tried to deal with and get to know them. But, it always came down to his money. And, he didn't fall in love with them.

Then he met Vivian. He didn't like her the night he met her, she seemed unapproachable. Vivian was sitting at the bar in the Tunnell alone, buying her own drinks. Jack asked her to dance because he liked the way her legs looked in the high-slit dress. She flatly said no. But she watched him for hours before introducing herself to him. They dance until the place closed.

She drove him home and invited herself in. "I don't usually do things like this, but..." They made passionate love until the next evening. Jack was late for an off-season work out and fined. Because Vivian didn't spend much time with Jack out of the bedroom, he had a difficult time seeing themselves as a couple. But, Vivian was persistent, loyal and loving through two years of dating, he believed.

Then, one night after Christmas, and before New Year's, Vivian popped the question.

"Jack, why don't we get married. I could live here with you and give up my apartment in town."

Jack was surprised. "Married? I thought you didn't want to be tied down after breaking off your engagement."

Jack now believed it was his hesitation that cost him Vivian. And, now he was back to sleeping with groupies with Oscar.

The walk only lasted twenty minutes before he was ready to return to the room. He thought about screwing Brenda a last time before leaving to release frustration. He turned a corner, three blocks south of the Hilton, and could see the entrance. There he saw a small gathering, and a burly man emerged dragging Brenda out of the lobby by her arm.

Oscar walked out behind them calmly. He stopped and stood to the side. He looked like he just got out of bed, wearing jeans and a t-shirt and his fade cluttered with lint. No shoes.

Jack walked to Oscar, "What's the deal?"

Oscar licked a cigar, surveyed it, then lit it. "That be her husband. And she be busted."

Brenda's husband grabbed her close to him as they neared the street. He hit her hard with a slap to her head. Jack moved, but Oscar grabbed him quickly.

"Leave it, New. That's her husband I said."

"Come on, you just gonna let him beat her?"

"New, that's his wife. Fuck that. She's been playin' wit' the fire too long. She's finally getting burnt.

"What is there to do?"

Jack snatched his arm free. He could see his father beating his mother in the same fierce fashion 15 years before. He should have done more to help his mother, he began thinking. He loved his mother. Why did she have to die first?

He could not bare watching any longer. He lunged forward as if shot out of a cannon.

"Shit." O whispered, then darted after his friend.

Jack stepped in between the man and his wife. "There's no need for that, chief," Jack said.

The man was ready to fight. "Who the fuck are you talkin' to? You a Crown too?"

He squared his shoulders to Jack's. "How 'bout I beat you up instead?"

Jack's eyes were riveted on Brenda. She was sitting in the passenger's side of the car crying uncontrollably and bleeding profusely. Jack's heart pounded in his chest. Where was the blood coming from? Common sense blended with the fear of getting his ass kicked, she had slept with two men in various positions. But it was his mother all over again.

*All Mom, and this hoe, wanted was to have fun.*

Jack allowed O to pull him away. And the man drove off with his wife.

The Crowns' chartered plane left Phoenix in a hush. Reporters and police had questioned each player, Jack and Oscar the most thorough, of course. Honeywell and the team's public relations person handled the details, Slight used the forum to vent his displeasure and plan to rid the Crowns of its "bad habits." Slight had read Kristen's exclusive interview with Jack in the Gazette. He told Honeywell on the plane that Jack was making trading him easy.

Slight's tirade on the plane was his usual captive audience speech.

"I was right, we don't need shit like this to hit the national papers. Do you hear about any Gamblers screwing married woman? No! He's got to go!"

Every passenger on the plane, a member of the Crowns or not, heard him. Honeywell sat quietly in the aisle seat next to Slight looking forward. Jack was near the rear, gazing out the window. He tried to drown out his boss with thoughts. His mind wondered from subject to subject. First of his mother. How she never fought back, like Brenda He wondered how bad his father would have whipped his ass had he intervened like he had hours before. Probably worse.

Then his mind shifted swiftly to the memory of the Portland woman's soft touch. Damn, he smiled, she was something else. It was fate, had to be. The woman he had carried, undressed, and let slap him was undoubtedly not a chance meeting.

"I'm going after her," he blurted almost to himself.

"Who?" Oscar asked puzzled. Then became agitated. "Not Brenda?"

"No, not that hoe. No." Jack turned to Oscar. "The one I took home that night, and she slapped me for screwing her; even though I didn't do nothing."

Oscar's forehead wrinkled. Then he remembered. "Ain't you in enough trouble?"

"So? I stay in trouble hanging' with you."

"Thanks."

"You have to see her. She's bad. So bad that I can't stop thinking about her."

"What's the big deal with her? First off, you don't know her name, nor where she lives and she thinks you fucked her while she was toasted"

"I can't stop thinking about her. She's, she's. O, she's all that."

"Please! Why? 'Cause you ain't hit it when you had the chance?"

"Naw. I know it's more than that. She's the first woman that I have felt intrigued by in years. Shit, man, it was refreshing to not have met her in a club or a stadium somewhere and have her know all about me."

Jack paused. Oscar was looking away, seemingly displeased. "She's all that, O. And a bag of onion and garlic chips."

Oscar's head shook side to side, and he laughed. "Are you mad? Are you? Tell me you are. Fuck that piece, er, I mean leave that shit alone. Ain't you got enough problems? Slight is up there trying to trade you to the worst team he can, and you want to add to it by going after a piece that thinks you raped her? Please! Just be happy she didn't recognize you or you'd be under the jail."

"I'm going for it."

"I'll visit you."

"Will you bring me a cake with a file?"

"Nope. God looks out for fools, not friends."

"Thanks."

# 8

The Galleria housed more than 50 specialty shops and restaurants. It was also the place where Djuana had met Dexter when it meant something to be seen in the Galleria. Now the more modern mega-mall, Pioneer Place with Sach's as its main store, has all the shoppers.

Djuana had worked at DeLux's for two years. She began as a part-time sales person. Through hard work and an unblemished attendance record, she became the linen section's manager three months before she found out about the change in her life.

Working directly under Djuana were two part-time stock clerks and two sales people. All four liked Djuana both as a person and their boss. The two stock clerks were high school boys that liked Djuana as a woman, more so. One of the two sales girls was in high school, also. The other, Charese Owens was a 22 year-old that loved men more than working. She was chronically late, and often called in sick on weekends. Still, Djuana kept her on.

Monday morning's bus ride to work was quicker than Djuana had ever remembered. That baseball player is making time fly, or is it the pregnancy, she wondered. Departing the bus she politely smiled at the bus driver, Omar, who stares at her every morning and asks her out every other.

Omar was an aged man, but very vibrant in his speaking manner. He had graying hair exposed from his bus company's cap, and his face was round and wide, with untrimmed whiskers. His uniforms were always too tight. His shirts and pants would bulge from aged, but well-formed muscles.

"That dress sure does bring life to that gorgeous body of yours," he said in his Southern accent.

Djuana shyly thanked him for the hard-handed compliment. He sprang out of his seat and jumped down the steps of the bus after her.

"Let me take you out this weekend?" he said.

"You know I'm seeing someone."

"Girl, please. You're not happy. Anybody can tell that. There was a time you'd smile to yourself the whole trip. Now, please, you barely grin. I'd make you happy. Real happy."

Djuana wanted to scream. "Listen, I respect my man, like you would want me to respect you if I were your woman."

Omar laughed. "Okay. Think that way. So, how about we exchange numbers and we talk and when you're tired of hanging on to nothing, we get together?"

"No, thanks." She felt his eyes staring.

"Damn, you have nice breasts," he muttered.

Djuana didn't bat an eye. "Good-bye."

He watched her natural walk force her ass to wiggle as if free from underwear beneath the rayon dress.

Djuana turned past the ice cream parlor on the ground floor of the mall as she did every morning. This morning, though, she felt an urge to rip down the gate and taste every flavor. Next door to the parlor was a record store, also yet to open. She stopped to look through the high glass windows. Toni Braxton's CD was on sale, again.

The record store's manager appeared suddenly and startled Djuana. They spoke lightly; greetings was all they had exchanged in the two years of seeing one another. She found herself staring at the short man's Portland Crowns baseball jacket. It was deep burgundy with gold trim. A large gold and white crown was on the front left side.

Nice she thought.

Djuana's mind clicked, she had better be moving if she didn't want to be late. She went to the newsstand to pick up the latest issue of *Essence*. On the rack next to the African American magazines were numerous sports magazines. She saw Jack's face on the cover of at least two, a couple of others had Crowns on their covers also. She picked up a few and looked them over. *Sports Illustrated* had more pictures of Jack inside and an in-depth story. She had to have it. But, her budget called for one magazine a week. And this week was suppose to be *Essence*. On the cover of *Essence* was Janet Jackson. No thanks Djuana groaned, and bought the sports periodical.

Phil, a lanky, young man, loved for women to browse through the magazines in his small shop. It gave him something else to look at. But, whenever Djuana came in it was an added delight. She would smile at him and offer conversation.

Phil sat behind the counter and smiled a hello to Djuana.

"So, no Ebony this week?" he said as he accepted her $10 bill.

"No. Not this week," Djuana politely replied. She had never bought *Ebony* in her life.

"What a loser," Phil groaned, holding up the magazine Djuana choose. He looked at Djuana. "I guess you didn't hear he and Oscar Taylor got busted in bed with some married woman."

"No. I didn't hear that. When did this happen?"
"Yesterday in Phoenix," Phil said proudly.
Djuana was hurt. "Really," was all she could say.
"Yes ma'am. A real loser. He and all his bum teammates."
"You don't like the Crowns?" she asked as he handed her change.
"Who likes losers?"

Jack sat in his Pathfinder in front of 656 Tudor waiting. Waiting for Djuana to show. He looked at the address he had written down. It had to be right; the cab company he called for her had given it to him. The driver, an avid Crowns fan, remember the trip well. Djuana sat speechless, and wiped her eyes often.

"657. This is it," he reassured himself. "So, where is she?"

He began watching the kids in Tudor Park, and he daydreamed back to when he was their age, seven or eight. He thought back to The Bronx and playing softball with his best buddies in a small parking lot between buildings.

He remembered how there were so many kids better than him. Where were they now? He refused to remember that some were on drugs, some were dead and others were struggling to make ends meet. He didn't recall at that moment that most of them resented his fame. He vowed to visit his old neighborhood as soon as the season was over.

Jack's plan was crumbling. He hoped to have seen her by now, after sitting in his car for four hours across from her building. He picked five O'clock in the afternoon to be sure to catch her coming home or leaving for work, whether she worked day or night.

But now he was wondering if she worked at all. Maybe her husband, or man worked. Maybe she took care of the kids during the day. Kids! Oh, boy. He needed to get out of there.

But the flowers? He looked at the dozen of roses in his passengers seat. He waited another hour.

After work Tia and Djuana sat outside of the ice cream parlor on the first floor of the Galleria talking. Djuana had accompanied Tia on a shoe-buying spree when she got off from work, and now she was forcing Tia to join her in an ice cream eating binge. All that day Djuana had craved butter pecan with whipped cream and fudge.

Tia watched intently as her friend scraped the bottom of her half-pint cup. "I need some more," Djuana said as she bolted up and reentered the parlor. Tia smirked and shook her head. The teenage girl in the shop giggled when Djuana returned so quickly.

Djuana came back to her seat with a different flavor. Mint chocolate chip deluxe.

"I thought you hated mint chocolate?"

"Not really," Djuana said blushing. "I just never tried it. You want some?" She held the spoon in her mouth and sucked it clean.

"No. You knock yourself out. So, have you heard from Dexter?" Tia asked. She was still laboring over her first half-pint.

"No," Djuana murmured. She wanted to talk about Jack Newhouse. She had read the article in Sports Illustrated and felt she knew him now. The article explained how Jack's mother had died in a car accident. She read his words, the way he described his feelings, three times. He loved his mother, and that was a good sign.

Tia pushed another question in the air, "I guess he still wants you to have the abortion?"

"Of course. Tee, I knew he would be ridiculous, but I really thought we would talk about it. Handle it together."

"Girlfriend, I don't know why you thought he would handle this maturely. Just forget that asshole, please. It's up to you, really. You do what is best for you."

"I haveta still keep him a part of it. If I keep the baby - asshole or not - I want him to be there. The baby will need him."

"Please," Tia sucked the roof of her mouth, releasing more flavor onto her tongue. She hated Dexter for hitting Djuana and wanted him out of her life more than ever.

Djuana's mind was set, yet she needed the closet person in her life to agree. She needed Tia to tell her she had the right plan.

"Tee, I can't kill my baby. I just can't do it." she said.

Tia heard her, but refused to say how she felt. She wanted Djuana to have an abortion just to have Dexter out of her life.

"I just couldn't," Djuana repeated, looking into her cup. More tears. "I cry too much."

Tia reached over and hugged Djuana and consoled her, whispering into her ear. The two ladies, still holding their ice cream and with the shopping bags at their feet, held one another; oblivious to the shoppers around.

Jack called Don Cruz on his car phone as he left Tudor. Don was the oldest player on the Crowns at 41. It was Don who had taught Jack how to play right field in Adkins Stadium; how to anticipate the caroms in the corner, and deal with bounces on that soft grass. He gladly took Jack under his wings, contrary to what was written in the newspapers about the rookie Jack Newhouse coming to Portland to take Don's job. Cruz was the Crowns right fielder for 14 years before Jack, and didn't resent losing his job to Jack, because Jack respected him.

Don answered the phone after nearly a dozen rings.

"What you up to?" Jack asked.

"Nada. Helping Damaris with her homework. Where you at? You coming over?"

"If you got time for me?"

"You kidding? Of course I got time for you, Poppy. Come on by."

When Jack arrived, Don was happy to get out of helping his 12-year-old daughter with her homework. "She's never gonna graduated sixth grade, that stuff is too difficult," he said to Jack.

They went into Don's den and Jack entered right into the conversation he needed to have with his mentor.

"You said you married Liela a month after you met her, right?"

"Yep. As you guys say, she was all that."

"How did you know you loved her?"

"I just knew. Every time I looked at her I wanted her." Don went to his personal refrigerator and got them beer.

"But," Jack eased up to the edge of the couch. Don was sitting in his easy chair on Jack's left. "You wanted her, right. I mean you didn't look at her and just want to bone her?"

"Kinda," Don got up and closed his door. All he needed was for one of his daughters to hear this. "You see, of course when I first saw her at that party, shit yeah, my shit was like, boing! She was beautiful. Gorgeous. The best looking woman I had ever seen in my life. Very feminine.

"Yo, bro', I just wanted to touch her hand, be next to her. I asked the guy's wife that threw the party to introduce us and we talked the rest of the night."

Don gulped his beer. "I was hooked."

Jack took a long swig. "When did you know you loved her?"

"I think I always knew. But love at first sight, nobody admits that exists. But, I spent that whole week after I met her with her, everyday. And I missed her when we were apart.

"When the baseball season was about to start, and we were about to go to Florida for camp, I was like, 'There's no way I want to be without you,' So I proposed and we got married and I've been one happy son of a bitch since."

Don drank his beer. Jack imagined Oscar doubting him if he told Oscar that he wanted to marry Djuana. Marry her. He thought about it a second and liked the idea.

Don got another beer and continued, "Yo, my teammates were all telling me that I was going to change. That my stats would go down. Bull. I hit like crazy that year. That was my best season!

"I love that woman."

Just then, as if on cue, Liela entered the den. She looked at Jack, and smiled. "Hi, New I didn't know you were here. I was in the basement doing laundry."

Jack stood and she gave him a kiss and hug.

She glared and pointed her finger at her husband. "That's not beer that you drinking, right Donnie?"

"Of course not, Momma," he put the can behind his feet. "No way."

"Uh huh. Well, anyway, Damaris has got to finish her homework before dinner. And, this time it has to be right."

"Of course, Momma," Don grabbed her and kissed her. "Of course."

Liela pushed him away. "You drunk that quick?"

Jack and Don laughed. "No I ain't!" Don said.

"Maybe I should break out?" Jack suggested.

"No," Liela protested. "Stay for dinner."

"Yeah, but you guys've got things to do."

Liela shook her head, "Please, I'll have to redo the homework anyway. He begs me to let him help the kids, then he has me send them to school looking like rare idiots from Bubblefuck or something."

"Oh, snap," Don said looking wide-eyed at Jack, then his wife. "Now was that nice, Momma?"

# 9

The rain tapped her window in a steady rhythm. The occasional lighting would illuminate the pitch-dark bedroom and the following thunder would slice through Djuana's body. She had been staring up at the ceiling for hours, picturing her future. To ease the pain of an uncertain future, she would turn her head and look at the many precious items in her room that female family members had given her.

The room was neat - most of the time. Her room was the master bedroom of the apartment, Emma allowed her to have it after Djuana's sweet-sixteen birthday party. The room was a wide square with a large double-window. She painted the room a yellowish-gold - the paint can read Sand - and the room was always bright. The Pioneer women took pride in handing down knickknacks to Djuana, the last girl born of the three very close sisters. Aunt Earline's hand-made lamp shades lay evenly atop Great grandma's hand-carved lamps. It was Aunt Cathy's canopy bed that was the talk of the room.

She was worried Dexter would kill her. He had been calling and threatening her at work; he had never called her at work before she got pregnant. She knew that when Dexter fought he was relentless. And evil. She remembered the little guy in McDonald's. He was staring at Djuana while she and Dexter sat eating in a booth. The guy finally came over and politely told Dexter he thought his wife was beautiful.

Dexter snapped, "Who the fuck asked you?" The guy cursed back and Dexter hit him, repeatedly. The guy bled so bad. Djuana never returned to that McDonald's.

Despite the worries, her mind was made. She was going to have the baby. But, who would keep Dexter from beating the baby out of her? Her mother would try, but she hoped not. The sudden crackle of thunder coupled with the thought of Emma getting hurt in the middle of this mess conjured more fear.

Her uncles would kill Dexter if they knew he had hit her. But, they had spent enough time in prison.

Djuana had spent that afternoon studying the pregnancy brochures Dr. Oppen's nurse had given her. The doctor was more thrilled than anyone else that knew. He was optimistic, even about Djuana some day getting married.

"You're a beautiful young lady," Dr. Oppen said that day. "You should be proud, and so should the father."

He was disturbed when she asked about an abortion. "Think heavily about this," he warned. "It is much bigger than you can imagine right now." Djuana had always known the doctor was against abortion, he spoke against it often during her visits.

"*Am I Parent Material?*" the small yellow pamphlet was called. Djuana read it carefully. It asked many questions to help in the decision of whether or not to have a baby. 'She wanted to call Dexter and have him go over this with her, but she didn't. Her door closed tight, she read the questions aloud from the yellow pamphlet. "Does having and raising a child fit the life-style I want?' " She thought for a second and said, "Why not?" She had always wanted to be a mother, have two boys and two girls.

"Could I handle a child and a job at the same time? Would I have time and energy for both?"

Djuana shrugged, "Please. People do it every day."

"Can I afford to support a child? Do I know how much it takes to raise a child?"

Again, she was confident. "I can do it."

"Am I patient enough to deal with the 24-hour-a-day responsibility?"

She paused to compare herself to Kenya, a pretty young woman with low self-esteem. She lived across the street in 340 Tudor, and had three children, from three different men. She leaves the two boys and girl with anyone just to go out clubbing. In the street, she barked at, or hit the children at the drop of a hat. Djuana, and Emma, considered the children to be no worse than Devon when he was a below double figures in age.

Djuana's hands massaged her stomach as she finally put the booklets down. Her mind was made up, again. She was not going to abort her baby. If Kenya could do it, she reasoned, she damn sure could become a mother. And, be a damn good one. Dexter would have to live with it in anyway he saw fit, she proclaimed.

Tears ran a steady, warm stream down the side of her face. Her reflexes wanted to wipe them but she forced her hands to remain over her tightened belly. "A boy, "she thought. "He's a boy. He's going to love me so much because his father ain't worth shit. He'll know the man that fathered him ain't shit without anyone telling him.

"I'll teach him everything, don't need no man."

Jack sat in his easy chair listening to Oprah and her guest psychologist tell how men don't understand the meaning of commitment. He wondered why Oprah didn't call him for that show, he knew plenty about the 'c' word. He had done it twice, he thought Vivian was committed to him, she wasn't. He thought the woman before her was ready for marriage, not quite.

He gulped two beers and popped open a third before the phone snapped his stupor. Drinking before noon wasn't his norm, but it was a full day off and he felt a need to relax his nerves with a couple of brews. His agent, Karl Berger yelled into his ear: "Why aren't you here in the Galleria?"

Jack had forgotten.

"C'mon, Jack. What the fuck are you doing to me? You wanted commercials, I got them. You gotta go to these personal appearances to get more ad execs interested. Shit, your image stinks right now, don't you understand that?"

"Yeah, okay. I'll be there in a minute."

"No. In a second. I've stalled enough."

"Berger, I pay you, remember? So chill."

They both hung up exasperated.

A barrage of hello's warmed Djuana as she entered DeLux's. The pleasant working atmosphere offset the low pay and long hours. Djuana was among the most personable and likable of the nearly one hundred employees.

Charese Owens watched Djuana lean against the counter stirring her hot tea while reading the same sports magazine as the day before. The part-timer looked up to Djuana like an older best friend, and respected how sensible her boss would make her frenzied life seem. Charese had a wide variety of men that she dated often. She would come to Djuana with such daily dilemmas as what to wear, what not to do and how to do it.

Charese couldn't wait for Djuana to put down the magazine. "Dee, I need to ask you something."

Djuana lowered the magazine. "Yeah?"

"Are you still dating Dexter?"

Djuana put the magazine down. "Why do you ask?"

"Well, he said you and him broke up. And he kinda gave me his number. You know I love you and I consider you my best friend, but the day you were off, he came here for you and he said you had broken up with him."

Djuana closed her eyes and took a deep breathe. she wanted to scream. "When was this?"

"Last Wednesday, the day you called in sick, you see, he..."

Djuana sprang up. "And what did you say when he 'sort-of' gave you his number?"

Charese became nervous. "Wait, you see, that's why I'm asking. If you and him are still together, then you should know what's up. I ain't trying to cut in. I swear. You my girl."

"Forget it. If you want to date him, I don't care. Go for it."

"No. I'm sorry I mentioned it. And I am sorry I took his number. Please, Dee, forgive me."

"Don't worry about it, Reese. No harm done. But, yeah, we're through."

Jack's Pathfinder glided into the mall's parking lot. For a second, he thought that he should have brought a jacket. He was dressed in black jeans and a white button-up shirt. He had contemplated wearing a jacket and tie, but shrugged it off.

He darted into the mall and found himself lost immediately. He forgot where he was suppose to met Berger. He knew it was a department store, not one of the smaller shops. He looked to his left and saw J.C. Penny - nope. On his right was DeLux's - that's it.

As soon as Berger saw his client, he ran to greet him with a phony smile and corny hug. He yanked Jack away from the hundreds of autograph seekers and executives. Berger forced his rant into a whisper, "Jesus fucking Christ, Jack. Why didn't you wear a damn jacket and tie??!!"

"Come on, Karl."

"Shit, Jack! I'm trying to save your ass and..."

"Look, before you bust a blood vessel, I'll go down to the men's department and buy a jacket and tie. Okay?"

"I don't know about you sometimes. Five minutes!" he said as Jack sprinted away. "You got five fucking minutes!"

Jack turned back, "You want anything?"

He laughed at Berger's reaction, Jack thought he saw steam rise out of Berger's collar.

Berger mumbled and went back to stalling for his client.

Djuana's mood for the day was set; she was bitchy after the conversation with Charese. Her mood dipped lower when she couldn't get Tia on the phone to complain. Nevertheless, Tia was to meet her after work anyway.

Because most of the shoppers were upstairs for the big toy sale and the celebrity hawking the merchandise, Djuana had too much time to herself. She jumped on the stock boys for not having their paper work done. She stayed on Charese to stop disappearing into the men's clothing department across the floor.

"You have enough men," Djuana said, before she could catch herself.

Djuana was rearranging the plaid linen display when she felt the presence of a customer. A man's voice said excuse me, right off she knew the sound, but couldn't place it. She turned to be startled, near frightened. Her eyes widened and her mouth parted open. She blinked. It was Jack Newhouse.

"It is you," Jack said quietly. "How are you?"

Djuana stood upright. Her frown was uninviting, but her voice was pleasantly soft. "What are you doing here?"

Jack laughed at the question. *If she only knew how I tried to hunt her down*, he thought. His smile remained as he recalled parking in front of her apartment building, scared to go inside. He thought of how easy it was to get the address from the cab company.

He said with the same smile, "I wasn't looking for you. I'm here for another reason. But, I am glad to see you."

Djuana's attention span drifted, listening to both the most attractive man she had ever been absorbed by, and one of her favorite songs playing over the store's speakers; the lyrics of Jodeci's *Come and Talk to Me* never seemed more appropriate. She watched his thick, not too thick, lips part and close with each word. He sounded so sincere as he told her how pleased he was to see her, how much he had thought about her.

"That's a very unusual name. How do you pronounce it?"

At first Djuana was puzzled, the question seemed sudden and well off the subject, then she remembered her name badge. "It's De-Juan-ah," she said flatly.

"That's nice. I like it. I'm Jack Newhouse. I think it's time we met."

Djuana stared at the open hand offered to her. What would it hurt, she wondered. Then she remembered the *night* and her thoughts soured. He may already know me too well, she groaned. She let his hand hang.

"I have work to do." She glided away from him.

Jack followed. He darted in front of her. This was his chance, the chance he had prayed for. He couldn't allow her to leave without giving it his all.

Avoiding contact, he blocked her path and she stopped. "Listen, I think about you so much. I worry about you and I really want to know you."

Djuana's arms folded across her breasts, a natural defense; even though this was the first man she could remember that looked her straight in the eyes when talking. Her head shook side to side as she fought the urge to let him in on how she really felt.

"I don't know what impression you got from our first meeting, but I ain't a groupie. I have a man and a job. I don't need anything from you."

"Cool. Great." Jack glided with Djuana as she moved defiantly, and continued to talk. "I am not looking to give you anything, yet. I'm just asking to spend some time with you."

"I said, I have a man. Besides, " her voice lowered, "didn't you get enough when you had me in your bed?"

"Spare me the dramatics," Jack turned serious. "I assure you, nothing happened at my place. You were drenched, and I changed your clothes. Nothing happen."

She almost believed him. And, almost liked him. She wanted to give in, and see him.

*The guy knows my name now, already knows my body, has seen me cry. Has held me. Shit. And, I know about him.*

Jack heard Berger yelling, but he didn't turn to acknowledge his agent. His eyes were riveted on Djuana's. She blinked often, seemingly trying to avoid his stare, knowing he was reading her eyes, looking for an invite. Jack was sure he had seen one. He took a step back to the counter top and found a pen near the register. He wrote out his phone numbers on the back of a credit card receipt. He offered the slip as he spoke to Djuana.

"These are my numbers. My pager, my car and my home number. I'd like to see you again, but I understand it is up to you. You call me, we go out. You don't, I won't bother you. I won't even shop here again."

She smiled, she relaxed. "Like you shopped here," she murmured under her breath.

"Thanks for the smile. I'll never forget it. It's the first one you gave me."

Slowly he turned to Berger and waved.

"Come on!" Berger whispered curses.

Jack returned his eyes to the now attentive lady.

"I hope to hear from you," Jack said, wanting to touch her. "Take care."

He nodded over at the sales people that had been staring at him and Djuana as he turned to leave.

Djuana didn't speak. She watched him leave, joining the shouting white man.

"He likes you," Charese appeared silently, startling Djuana. "After he bought that jacket and tie, he asked Jon about you; your name and if you were married."

Djuana finally looked at the numbers.

Charese continued. "You know who he is, right?"

"Yeah," she read the slip of paper, "Jack Newhouse, Portland Crowns."

"Damn, girlfriend, you got it made!"

Djuana's eyes circled across the second floor. He was gone.

"Yep. I got it made."

# 10

Dexter Forns lit his third cigarette in the last half hour. He hated down town Portland, most of all the mall. Use to be he could come to this same shopping center with his homeboys, Ice and G-Hard and pull at least four women's phone numbers. Those were the days. He met Djuana, and a couple other virgins, in that fashion. He sat on his car sporting a huge grin thinking about it all.

But, those days were gone. Now he received cold returns from women in expensive clothing to his witty greetings. The younger girls laughed at him; those immature bitches, would be his response. Still, he had his share of lovers. Today, though, none of that mattered. Dexter was waiting, parked at the bus stop, for Djuana to hear him out. She had hung up on him enough.

The glass building's revolving door constantly filled with bodies. Dexter's head struggled to keep pace with his eyes following women's legs and asses of all sizes and colors. Finally Djuana. Her walk was slow and deliberate. She was wearing slacks and the leather jacket he bought her two years ago. Why pants, he wondered.

Steps behind Djuana was Tia. Dexter wasn't thrilled at the sight of *that bony bitch*, as he called her. Dexter clogged their path and spoke as suddenly as he appeared.

"We need to get this straight. No more F-ing around..."

Djuana was not surprised to see Dexter; since his visit to her apartment all their phone conversations ended with him threatening to show up and beat her numerous times. Nor was she frightened, as he thought she would be. Standing a mere few steps away from the place they had first met, Djuana could see her past as his words flowed by her thoughts. A waste of seven years. Wasted on this man. A worthless man. A man who had given her hell for three weeks because of a pregnancy that he had something to do with.

"Are you listening?" Dexter was near losing the cool he drove to the Galleria with.

"No. So, does that mean you're going bust my ass like you said?"

"Cut the fucking around, this is serious. You see?" He glanced at Tia, who cut her eyes. "I have been trying to handle this and you fucking around. I'm the immature one?"

Tia tapped Djuana and whispered something. Dexter cut between them. "Why don't you mind your business?" He said pointing his finger at Tia.

Tia moved his hand and was about to lace into him before Djuana took control.

"What do you want, Dex? I'm having the baby. Period. So, what is there to talk about?"

Dexter scratched his head. This wasn't as easy as he pictured it. Time to take control, he decided.

"C'mon, let me take you home. Then we can talk in private."

He tugged Djuana's arm toward his car, not forcibly, yet, when she pulled away she lost her balance and stumbled.

Tia scolded him, "She ain't no doll! And, she ain't your slave!"

Dexter was furious. "You two are blowing this shit out of proportion. All I want to do is talk, so step, Tia, and find a man so you can have your own problems!"

Tia and Dexter exchanged heated words for a minute before Djuana had had enough of them fighting.

"Let's talk, Dexter," she said stepping to him. They walked a few more steps away from Tia.

Dexter began, "We have to do something about this, and soon."

"What is with you, Dex? I don't appreciate the way you have been treating me since I told you. I knew you wouldn't be all-that supportive, but damn! Shit, I can't believe you?

"Why are you pushing me to have an abortion?"

Dexter looked away. He scratched his head. Telling her the truth would be so much easier. But then, not only would she have an abortion, but there would be no more of that good sex. So, instead he said the speech he had prepared for the moment:

"Why would you want to do that? To have a baby and live with your moms? Come on, now. What happen to all those dreams you use to tell me? You want your own place, better clothes, a better job. And, what about college? You can't do all of that with a baby."

Djuana listened intently. She was stunned, he had paid attention to her dreams. Her voice lost its bite and she let him hold her hand.

"Dex, I have made up my mind. I want to have this baby. Please, Dex, just be supportive?"

Dexter squeezed her hand. "I don't want you to have this baby. I made up *my* mind. How I even know it's mine?"

"What?" She released his hand.

"You heard me."

"You bastard." In an instant Djuana landed an openhanded smack to the left side of Dexter's face.

Tia shook with fright. She clutched the bags, wanting to call her friend.

Dexter recovered and punched Djuana upside her head. She fell quickly. He stood over her, "Why you fucking with me?"

Tia ran to Djuana's aid, but before she could reach Djuana, Dexter pushed her back. He picked up Djuana, who was swinging wildly and screaming, and pinned her against his car.

Tia kept coming. She hit Dexter repeatedly about his back and head, but to no success. He would swat her away easily. Tia felt helpless, she cried for help. People slowed, some stopped, but nobody intervened. Her shopping bags had burst from use as weapons. Dexter hit Djuana a few more times while he had her pinned, but mostly he was telling her to get the abortion.

The sound of the police sirens froze Dexter. Djuana gained strength and pushed him off of her. Tia continued to hit him. He shoved her off her feet. He briskly walked around his car and got into the driver's seat. Before the police parked, he was gone.

One cop helped Tia, and assisted Djuana to her feet. Djuana was short with the two cops, Tia screamed Dexter's full name and the street he lived on. When the cops seemed to ignore her, she screamed it again and demanded they go after him.

The cops' attention was square on Djuana. The shorter officer stared at her bruised cheek and swelling. She felt his eyes, and her hand followed to find a sensation of pain.

"Do you want to go to the hospital?" the bigger cop asked.

"No," Djuana sniffed.

"So, tell us what happen," the short officer said, still staring at her face.

"Are you blind?" Tia blurted.

Djuana said, "He's just my boyfriend. We got out of hand arguing."

With that, the cops lost interest.

Emma Pioneer entered the apartment first; Devon was steps behind laboring with the family shopping cart full of groceries. Devon's bellyaching about the amount of muscle-work needed to push the cart was already distant when Emma saw her daughter and her daughter's best friend crying on the couch.

Devon stopped in the doorway. He walked around the cart for a better view.

"Take your narrow ass in the kitchen and put that food away before you get sweat and tears from that slavin' all over my food, boy!" Emma shouted. In rapid fire-fashion, she spewed several orders of what to do with the groceries at Devon. None of which included going near the living room.

Emma removed her jacket and handbag. She dumped them both into the recliner and slowly approached the young women. Djuana straightened. Tia picked up the used tissues, and felt an urge to disappear. Djuana was seated on the left side of the couch facing Tia. Her left leg was on top of her right leg, with her right foot exposed. Both hands were holding a tissue, her eyes studying the torn, used, sheet.

Emma slowly bent toward her daughter and gently lifted her jaw. She turned it slightly, and she saw the bruise.

"My Lord," she gasped.

"Dex and I had a fight," Djuana said in a hoarse voice. "It got out of hand."

"Where is the motherfucker? He's dead. I'ma kill his ass!"

Devon jumped over the empty bags he had scattered throughout the kitchen. He ran into the living room.

"What happened?"

Nobody answered him.

Emma examined her daughter, "Did you go to the hospital? Why didn't you call me? Damn, I'm in the market fooling around with that little asshole of a brother you have."

She went to the telephone and began dialing swiftly. She held the receiver with her shoulder, and asked again if Djuana had gone to the hospital.

"I said no, Ma. I'm okay, it's just a little swollen."

Emma seemed to not hear. "Hello, Cal, can you come over right now? I don't give a damn what you doing, just come over. That no good, high-yella whore done put his hands on Djuana. Yeah, that snake-ass motherfucker. Cut the Q&A and get over here."

Emma waved off her daughter's insistence not to bring Uncle Calvin into the conflict. When she hung up she addressed her daughter's concerns.

"Why not? What do you think you have an uncle for? When he gets here, you call that *man* of yours and tell him I want to speak with him. Then we'll see what kind of man he is."

"He hit you, Juanny?" Devon finally caught on.

"Shut your confused ass up, Devon!" Emma yelled. "You just worry your little ass about them groceries. They had better be put away!"

He took his cue to leave, kicking empty bags as he returned to the kitchen.

Djuana continued her disagreement about her uncle being involved. "Ma, this is between Dex and me."

"It was, before he took it there." She went into the kitchen and prepared a cold compress for her daughter. Devon was eating an orange and leaning out the window; in obvious defiance of what Emma had told him to do while in the kitchen. He got a beating meant for Dexter.

Emma returned to the living room, talking. "A man, if he is one, don't need to hit no woman. For no reason." She put the ice on the bruise. Wondering why the two younger women had not thought of it.

"I'm pregnant, Mom."

Through the silence Devon dropped a carton of eggs and blurted, "Oh, shit."

Emma took a long look at her beautiful daughter. Twenty-five-year-old daughter. Unmarried. Why? Because she had been in love with a no good man with her first lay.

Djuana couldn't look in her mother's eyes. She felt ashamed. "I'm sorry, Momma. I'm sorry," she sobbed. She stood and moved toward her mother. Emma met her and grabbed her firmly into her large bosom.

Tia put her head into her hands and between her legs and cried.

"Everything will work itself out," Emma whispered as her daughter cried loudly. "How could I have failed you so?"

"I love you, Mommy," Djuana sobbed. "I love you."

Emma Pioneer couldn't hold back the tears with the stubbornness people gave her credit for. In the kitchen, Devon held a box of cereal. He wondered if that was the last box he would pick alone.

# 11

Oscar wildly swerved his BMW into Jack's driveway. He leaped out of the car, slammed his door, and flung open the back door. He hauled two suit cases and a garment bag up the three steps to the front door. Jack was standing in the doorway frowning. "What? No frying pan?"

"You a funny guy. How about some help?"

"I am helping. I am holding the door open. Hurry up!"

Jack took Oscar to the second level of his townhouse, and into the den-turned-guess room. Oscar angrily put away his clothing. "That bitch had the nerve to put me out," he complained. "Me. Shit, she put me out of my own crib."

Jack smiled. "Like, you didn't put up a fuss?"

"Shit, she was standing at the door with the police talking shit; you know how she is. So, I just gathered some clothes and broke out."

Sondra loved Oscar. Loved him very much. And, she understood that as a professional baseball player, Oscar Taylor would be hard pressed to give her and their two-year-old son the attention she thought sufficient. But, then he began to cheat. Sondra had an idea, but Oscar was good at arguing her quiet. Then, her mother and three sisters had finally gotten to her conscience. For years they had been almost demanding she leave Oscar. Call the marriage a mistake and end it. Now that it was national news that he and Jack were sleeping with one woman in Arizona, she felt no choice.

"She called a few minutes ago," Jack said.

"What could she want? I ain't been gone an hour?"

"Basically, to do the same thing you're doing. Bad talk you and curse me out for helping you be the dog that you are."

Oscar sighed. "Fuck her. She'll probably call all damn night. Then she'll ask me to come home before we leave town. "

Oscar was right. Sondra was home in their large house, lonely. She called three times in two hours. Each time they argue over where Oscar had put something she needed right that minute.

"You need to take your behind home and settle this," Jack told Oscar.

"Nope. Ain't got the time."

"You stupid. Do you realize you cause most of this with her. She has been about as understanding as a woman can be, and then you stretch her some more."

"You don't know what she be doing to me. She's a pain in the ass."

"Come on, man. Who you talking to? When was the last time you took her out?"

"Yo, I try to take her places and she always got an excuse. Shit, I make four million dollars a year and she talking about we can't find a baby sitter.

"Fuck that."

Jack gave in. He knew better than what his friend was saying, but he didn't feel like going deeper into the subject.

At 12:30 a.m. while Jack and Oscar were watching X-rated movies and talking dirty - and after the seventh time Sondra called, this time to say some woman had called and hung up, someone rang Jack's door bell.

"That must be Janet," Oscar said as he rose and darted down the steps to the door.

"Why did you invite a hoe here?"

"Why not? Just chill and I will let you have some." He opened the door and the young lady gave him a long kiss.

Jack stood at the top of the stairs and when Oscar returned with the woman he pulled O to the side. "Listen, aren't you in enough trouble?"

"Fuck that!" Oscar pulled away. Then he turned back and whispered, "You got any condoms?"

"What if I said no?"

"Then you would feel guilty at my funeral."

"You know where. But, don't stay in my room. I'm sleeping in my *own* bed tonight."

An hour later O returned. He was grinning, and had on a pair of Jack's silk under pants; they were too big on him.

"You want some, G?"

Jack glared up from his easy chair. "Is she married?" he finally asked.

Oscar laughed and said, "No, but her daddy would kill us. She's 15."

Jack's heart leaped into his throat. "What are you doing to me?"

"Chill, New, chill! Does she look 15? Just come get your dick wet. I thought you said you needed some?"

"Yeah, but..."

"Stop looking at them flicks and cut the scared routine, we be doing this for years."

"I can't do that no more, O."

"Do what?"

"Bone groupies. I'm tired of that shit."

"You buggin'." Oscar stared at his teammate and felt the seriousness. "What's got into you? You worried about Slight? Fuck him! He ain't gonna trade you. He know we the team, shit. You here forever, like me."

Jack rolled his eyes. "Man, that's only the half. I just can't hang with the different bitches every night, in every city. Man, don't you know what you got at home? A wife, and a damn good one at that. That's what the fuck I am looking for. It's time to settle down."

The teenager called Oscar. He yelled, "I'll be there in a second." Oscar sat on the arm of the easy-chair Jack was in. He buckled his pants.

"You definitely buggin'," he began, pointing his whole hand at Jack with each sentence. "I here to tell you, the grass ain't greener. Fuck the married life! I should have never gotten married.

"Shit. Sondra is about to rob me blind. She's gonna take everything."

"Sondra ain't going nowhere. She loves the hell out of you. She ain't leaving you."

"I wish she would."

"No you don't."

Oscar sucked his teeth. He stood and shook his head at Jack.

"The grass ain't greener," he said as he returned to his teenager. He pounded the girl as hard as he could and ordered her to scream, being rough with her. He wanted Jack to hear them to make Jack jealous. He did, but Jack was serious about finding a steady lover.

Jack spent another sleepless night on his couch. When he did nod off around 2 a.m., he dreamt that instead of swerving to miss Djuana, he hit her. In his sleep, he squirmed at the sight of her body flying in air and landing on his hood, then the street. She moaned and groaned in his arms before dying when the cops arrived.

The nightmare woke him up just in time to see Oscar and Janet creeping down the steps to the front door. Jack noticed the headlights in his driveway, then the car left. Oscar came back in without a word and went to bed.

Djuana awoke hoping, praying, that the day before was a dream. It wasn't. The left side of her head was in pain. Next to her in the bed was Tia. Uncle Calvin was sleeping off a night of drinking on the couch. He and her mother had called Dexter's phone number most of the night.

And, she was both hungry and nauseous.

Djuana was the first up and about. She showered, cooked breakfast for all, then dressed for work. Tia and Emma tried to talk her into calling in sick; they wanted to begin plans for the abortion. Emma wanted her to call Dexter and invite him over. Djuana objected to all proposals.

"We need to talk," Emma declared. "That ain't gonna go away like a cold. We need to do something. And do it now."

"I know, I know," Djuana whined. She needed an escape. Going to work would be that outlet.

Djuana walked through the mall believing everybody knew of her bout the day before. She was greeted at her station by Anthony Thompson, the floor supervisor. He asked her about the bruise, which had darkened and began shrinking. She didn't want to have to explain to him, and she didn't. He seemed careless.

Mr. Thompson was all business that morning, very unusual. He was known throughout the mall as a flirt. He had taken Djuana out once, but when she refused to let the date end at his home, he backed off yet continue to make light passes. Two weeks prior to that morning he had invited her to a yacht party given by the store's vice presidents. Djuana said no.

Charese came in a few minutes late, her usual, and was burning to ask Djuana about the day before. "Are you all right?" she said before removing her jacket and punching in.

"I'm fine," Djuana said, a little annoyed that Charese would choose to be nosy instead of punching in.

"Shit, DJ, I saw from my man's car. I told his tired-ass to stop, but he said he shouldn't. Damn, I didn't know he was like that."

"Look, Reese, I rather not discuss yesterday. Okay. Let's just get to work." Charese disappeared.

Tia borrowed her father's car to use to pick up Djuana from work. She wanted to take her friend for a ride and talk.

When Tia told her parents the whole story about Djuana being pregnant, her father, Leonard Williams snapped, "Not by Dexter, I hope."

Tia's sister, Ansea, agreed: "Nobody likes him. He's a dog."

Tia's mother was distraught. "Poor child," Bernadette Williams proclaimed. "It's a shame. I know Emma is taking it hard."

"Ms. P wants Djuana to have an abortion."

"No way!" Bernadette said. "That would be a sin. I have got to talk with Emma."

"Mom, that's their decision. You can't step in."

Bernadette, ignoring her daughter, picked up the phone and called Emma at work. The two planned a meeting at Emma's apartment.

Tia parked in the first level of the mall's parking garage as a sudden cloudburst had unleashed buckets of raindrops. She browsed for a bit; she was a few minutes early. Once off the escalator, she spotted Djuana doing paperwork with her supervisor, Anthony Thompson. Tia unhooked the top two buttons on her loose cream-colored, long sleeve blouse, hoping Djuana's boss could catch a glimpse.

When Djuana saw her friend's bright smile it warmed her heart immediately. It signaled the end of another hectic day. Thoughts and worries were

# LOVE'S HOME RUN

constantly clouding her mind. And, Mr. Thompson's light passes were not helping. She glanced at her gold watch. Damn. *Why do I have this on?*

"You ready, Love?" Tia asked Djuana as she neared.

Djuana looked over at Thompson's wrist watch. "In a second. I just need to punch out and file these-"

"Hi. Tia, isn't it? Long time no see," Thompson cut in, smiling for the first time that day in Djuana's presence. His pupils darted up and down Tia's slim body.

Tia's smile widened, moving away from the counter so he could see all he cared to. "Yes. And how are you?"

"Oh, I'm fine." he turned to Djuana and told her he'd put away the paperwork. "I'm sorry you two have to rush off. Maybe I'll get to spend sometime with you one day, Tia."

Tia blushed. "Maybe."

"Okay, I'm ready. Let's go," Djuana said abruptly.

The two women made an ice cream stop before leaving the building.

"Miss, you are not going to gain weight alone," Tia said, steering with one hand, holding chocolate Fantasy ice cream in the other.

Djuana laughed. And thought about her belly widening and poking out from her small, yet plump, frame. No more size eight, she thought. Unconsciously, her free hand rubbed her stomach.

Actually, Djuana hadn't fit into a size eight in two years. She was a 10, 12 in many styles.

The low hush of soul music filled the car as traffic slowly moved in the steady rain. Tia abruptly turned right on Martin Luther King Jr. Boulevard, she has just about forgotten she had to turn, trying to figure out why her best friend, who hates no one, and there are many that she should, in Tia's eyes, doesn't seem to get along with her handsome boss.

"Why you hate Thompson?" Tia asked. surveying the traffic with a frown.

"I ain't never say I hated the man."

"You sure don't act like you like him."

"Well, he is my boss, you know. It's just all about business. That's all it should be. If you want him, go for him. Just don't ask me to help. I want no parts of him when I am off."

"Girl, don't tell me you still mad about that little date?" Tia looked at Djuana a full second. Djuana was looking away, at nothing in particular.

"He's a man," Tia said. "And, a handsome one at that, I might as well add. He just wanted some leg."

"Well, he ain't get none. And he won't."

"I'll give him some. Plenty!"

Djuana moved to end the conversation, "Let's stop at the grocery store. Maybe you can make me some of your brownies tonight."

"Okay," Tia sighed. She was in a talkative mood. She searched for a different topic. When she asked about Jack, Djuana brightened, to her surprise, and opened up.

"Did you say this guy plays for the Crowns? He's a baseball player?"

"Yep." Djuana stared out her window, catching the eye of a young man in a sports car across from them in traffic. He smiled. Djuana turned her head back to Tia, catching the end of her statement.

"And he was cool, I mean as far as you know?"

"Yes."

"You believe in fate?" Tia asked.

Djuana focused on the question. Was it fate? She thought it probably was sick fate, if any. She had met the man of her dreams while being pregnant by the man she always thought loved her.

Tia continued, "Things happen for reasons. Maybe he is a blessing in disguise."

"Maybe. I don't know. But, it's funny, when he came into the store I was bitter and at the same time glad to see him."

Tia shook her head and accelerated into open traffic. "He came to the store?"

"He was there for one of those promotionals we have," Djuana twisted her lips. "He didn't know I worked there, or so he claimed."

"I'm telling you, fate! Watch, you'll be telling your grand kids the story of how their grandfather almost ran you down, then fell in love with you."

"You a mess, Tia."

Superfood was crowded as usual on a early Friday evening. Tia pushed the cart while Djuana walked along side. A call home to Emma had extended their list of groceries; Emma had forgotten a few items the day before.

The two ladies shopped and gossiped. They looked over prices of baby products; Tia suggested they begin buying the stuff soon because the prices seemed high. Djuana was unsure. She was thinking Dexter would have to be a part of the money spending, heavily.

They put more snacks in their cart than food and joined the long checkout lines with a full cart. While on line, Djuana noticed the baseball cards mixed in with candies and gums underneath the *TV Guides*. She picked up a pack and opened it. A Portland Crown was the first she saw.

Tia elbowed Djuana, "You buying them? Or, are you looking for somebody?"

Djuana didn't reply, she just reached for another pack.

"Let me see," Tia took a pack and ripped open the shiny pack. She thumbed through the cards. "What's his name, again? Here's a Crown. Oh, he's white."

"Mr. Fate ain't white, is he?!"

"Tia! Quiet down. No he ain't white. Let me see those cards."

The women examined two more packs, with shoppers curiously watching, before Tia stumbled across Jack Newhouse. "Um. Nice. If you don't want him, I'll take him. Shit, he does have a job."

"What is of?" Tia winced.

"Not of, silly. O F. Outfield. He plays out there," Djuana pointed playfully. Tia looked and they both saw. Neither continued to smile.

Three aisles away, Dexter was pushing a shopping cart, turning down the canned food section, with a very pregnant woman on his arm. In the cart along with the groceries, was a young boy eating cookies. The sight of the happy-looking family caused a sharp slicing pain across Djuana's chest. She dropped the baseball cards into the cart. She began walking toward aisle six.

"Djuana?" Tia sternly called. "Don't ."

"Stay here on line," Djuana said, almost drifting. "I'll be right back."

Tia was enlivened, but she stayed with the cart. Kick his ass, she wished. *Please kick his ass. Fuck him up and the hoe with him*!

Djuana turned the corner, side stepping an elderly woman, and followed her man. She plotted out a plan. Hit him hard and walk away? No. Slap him and her? No, she's pregnant. Shit, she's pregnant, looked to be at least seven months pregnant. That no-good bastard has a nice little family. Shit. That was all I ever asked the motherfucker for, and what did he keep saying? 'I ain't ready', 'I ain't ready'.

Shit!

The family turned again and were going up the no-frills aisle. Djuana quickened her pace. Her heart lumped in her throat and thumped. She attempted to curb her anger before engaging the *happy-fucking-family*. A quick blink of her eyes, and Djuana realized she had been directly behind them a full second.

"Dex."

He didn't budge.

"Dexter," Djuana refused to yell and show anger. She wanted to be in control.

The woman looked up from the cart. She stared at Djuana, then turned to her man. "Dex, you know this woman?"

Dexter stared at the bags of dry peas on the shelf. It was next on the list. The hum of Djuana's light voice saying his name was deep in his memory. He had known it was her seconds before his woman spoke. He turned quickly, as if he hadn't heard the question; with his eyebrows raised.

"Huh?" was all he could say.

Djuana spoke in a controlled voice. "Dexter, you gotta explain this scene." Djuana looked at the *other* woman, waiting for her to protest. She was no competition, Djuana felt. Her mind went to fury: Why he want that no hair, no ass, no hips, no nails - the bitch's got a diamond ring!

Dexter stepped from the cart. "What do you want? You following me?" He pretended to be annoyed. He was fighting the shock, the fear.

Sahmara Forns continued to be disturbed. "Who is this, Dexter?"

"Just an ex," Dexter tried to hush his wife. A few shoppers had gathered. "I'll be a second," he said.

When Dexter stepped near Djuana she slapped him with every ounce of anger and body weight she could put behind her small, soft hand. Dexter, although not strongly built, barely moved.

"Just an ex? That's all I am? Huh, Dex?" She hit him again.

Dexter grabbed Djuana into a bear hug from behind. Djuana struggled to free herself, all the while cursing. Sahmara was pushing Djuana, trying to force her to fall into the canned goods. Dexter held on, and at the same time pushed his wife away.

"Come on, bitch! I'll fuck you up too!" Djuana yelled and struggled. She began calling to Tia as her friend neared.

"Get him off of me so I can kill both these motherfuckers!"

The supermarket became a one-aisle show; the crowd swelled deep from both entrances of aisle five. Tia slithered her way to Djuana's aid. Security came running; and Dexter released Djuana as the guards asked. His very pregnant wife pushed Tia to the ground. She sprang up, wildly swinging her arms, but a guard had stepped in between them.

Dexter was cool. He berated Djuana from behind the guards: "See? Now do you under-fucking-stand? I am through with you. Just let it go."

Djuana was unruly, "Yeah, you played me once, that's it! I'ma kill the fucking baby, you besta believe that shit. Your baby, this one, is dead. Believe that. I don't want shit from you! Ever!"

A gasp silenced the attentive crowd. Tia pushed and pulled her friend away. Djuana kept the verbal shots flying as they left. Dexter's very pregnant woman held their crying son and glared at Dexter. He shook his head, and almost begged, "That bitch is lying. Don't you see she's jealous? She's just trying to ruin what we have, Babe."

Dexter's wife walked away, leaving her husband with his arms spread.

"Two damn fools and one dog," said one older female in the crowd.

"Disgusting," another female said.

A man, shopping with his wife and infant shook his head while his wife frowned at him.

"You see?" she said to her husband. "That's the stupidness that men do that I'm was talking about."

Djuana didn't want to shed a tear, yet she cried the whole car trip to her apartment. Tia wept in anger and drove. They had left the cart full on groceries on the checkout line.

"How didn't I know? How?" Djuana broke the silence. She thought about how for the last year or so she could not get him on the phone unless he returned a call. He seemed to never be home. At his job at the Post Office, it was impossible to get him on the phone. His co-workers had become cold, but Djuana thought little of those men and women because he rarely spoke of them.

She caught Tia off-guard when she said she felt like a huge part of her life had been lost.

"When I was with him, I was lonely, but not alone. I know he wasn't there for me as much as he could or should have been, but I always knew he was there."

Tia felt like shouting, waking her friend up. Instead, she just calmly tried to reason with Djuana.

"Dexter was never faithful, Djuana. Never. Nor was his ass ever respectful towards you. He never treated you like a woman. Just like some fucking trophy, and shit." Tia steered the car through traffic, in a rush to get to Djuana's.

"You gave that man your all, and all he ever gave you in return was grief."

"You don't understand," Djuana said quietly. "It's not that I want to be with him, I just miss the feeling of having someone that was mine when he was with me."

Tia exhaled. "Please."

Djuana leaned her head on the window, wanting to kick herself. The man who caused the pregnancy doesn't want her to have the baby. Her best friend, whose opinion she cherishes, isn't ready to be a Godmother. So, Djuana wondered, why have the baby?

"Tomorrow. Tomorrow I am getting rid of this baby," Djuana fiddled with the tissue she had used up. "Am I some kind of ass? I can't have a baby by him and be connected to that ass my whole life. I can't."

Tia felt more hate for Dexter that moment than the night his hand held and squeezed Tia's ass while dancing at Djuana's last birthday party.

# 12

Bill Courtnall took his job as a private investigator very seriously. He had solid contacts in the small, but deadly underground world of Portland, Oregon, and had a working relationship with the Portland Police Department. He used the latest gadgets, no matter what the cost, and had quick access to three guns; a .357 magnum in a shoulder holster, a .22 pistol in an ankle holster and had a .38 under the driver's seat in his Ford Taurus. He wore a slick white fadora, a dark gray raincoat, and always sneakers.

When Courtnall first received a call from Vincent Slight, he thought it would be marital problems. What else would the imposing and grand owner of the Portland Crowns baseball team want from a private investigator? Slight gave him orders to follow seven of his players and give him the reports. Slight paid him double his usual fee for all seven in advance, with more money promised, as long as the operation was covert.

Courtnall sat alone in Slight's office studying the crowded trophy case. Division championships, conference championships. No league title. He grinned, "They'll never beat the Gamblers," he mumbled. Just then Slight startled him by bustling in. With him was the team's general manager.

Courtnall stood to greet the men. Slight introduced the two men and barked at them to sit.

"Let's get to it," Slight said as he sat.

Courtnall was mesmerized by Honeywell's dark, well-groomed features. "You're J.A. Honeywell?"

Slight looked at the two men. "Yeah. So? Let's get this on. We are not here to get acquainted."

Honeywell smirked at Slight. He knew what was about to be said.

"I never knew you were... I mean, I saw you on television, but you were always in the background. I didn't know you were Honeywell." Courtnall continued to stare. "I mean, I just didn't expect..."

Courtnall thought about his next sentence. "I have a great deal of admiration for you. You did a great job building the Crowns."

Honeywell nodded his head slowly, crossed his legs, unbuttoned one of his many dark, double-breasted suits. "So this is the private eye you hired. Quick guy."

Slight was fuming, "Courtnall, you got anything for me, or not?"

Courtnall pulled out three red folders with names taped to each. He handed the 'Spencer' folder to Slight first. He looked through his notes as Slight open it.

Honeywell squirmed in his seat. "This is ridiculous."

Slight put on his thick reading specs, "But, who asked you?"

Courtnall guided Slight through the folder, reading from his notes: "I had one of my best operatives follow this guy. He's something else! First, he is a big time coke user, as you can see from the photos. We have him buying, usually late night, from the same supplier."

Slight cut in, "Did you know about this, J.A.?"

"Yes. We all knew."

Courtnall continued, but Slight cut him off again. "There's only three folders, what about the others?"

"We only have something on three of them," Courtnall explained, looking to Honeywell for approval. "The others are basically clean. Oscar Taylor has been put out of his house by his wife. He's been staying with Jack Newhouse. Mike Colbert is physically abusing his wife, and it seems, has been for sometime."

Courtnall shifted papers in the file until he found his report on Lee.

"Your pitcher, Lee Spencer is a serious sniffin' machine. Good thing you guys pay him well, 'cause his is spending serious bread on the stuff."

Spencer was the league's best pitcher. He had won more than 20 games in three straight seasons. He was the league's MVP two of those seasons. His problems with cocaine were never substantiated into common knowledge. In the past season's playoffs, a friend of Honeywell's in the league office warned him that president of the league wanted Lee tested for drugs before he pitched. Honeywell cleaned him up.

That season, though, he was off to a 1-5 start. Personally, his worst beginning of a season since coming to Portland. His poor start, had plenty to do with the team's weak record through May.

Slight continued looking through the notes. "What about Newhouse?" he asked

"Nothing," Courtnall said.

"Impossible, keep after him."

Honeywell stood, "I've had enough. You are losing it, Vinny."

Slight grinned his sly smile. "On the contrary, I'm gaining control. Don't you see? It's time we made some changes before the ship sinks."

What could have Honeywell said? Not what he was thinking, for sure. He had seen the Portland Crowns' ship float with holes in her for years. He wasn't sure how the team would fair with repairs.

The Crowns flew out of Portland with a six-game losing streak. The team's first six-game skid in three years. Slight was in an outrage, to say the least. He lashed into his players on the plane, singling out Jack and Lee.

Lee glared out of his window and into the clouds while Slight yelled at him from across his seating partner, fellow pitcher Danny Gross. Lee couldn't have cared less; he was getting paid the second highest salary for a pitcher in the majors.

"I know what your problem is, Spencer!" barked Slight. "I know what all of you on this plane's problem is. You are all spoiled! That's right! Spoiled. I am sick of the sight of you. Sick to my stomach."

The owner finally sat.

Jack was suffering more than any of his teammates. He had no hits during the last 10 games in Portland. He was worried. The Crowns had decided to call up Hector Aponte, a minor league phenom. Slight loves the guy for two reasons: he's cheaper and, right now, hotter than Jack. Aponte was to meet the team in Milwaukee.

To make matters worst, he believed, his mind was steadily on Djuana Pioneer. Why hadn't she called? he sat and wondered on the plane. Will she? Will she be mine? Will she let me make hot, passionate love to her? If she does, will I be able to handle it? Shit yeah, I'd hold those soft thighs and pound away. Kiss those soft lips, lick and suck those inviting nipples and just taste her...

"You hear me, Newhouse!?" Unbeknownst to Jack, Slight had returned to lecture his players.

Slight leaned over Oscar seated in the aisle seat to get into Jack's face, and slipped. He fell into Jack's lap. Oscar cracked up in laughter. A few other players laughed.

Slight pushed himself upright, using Oscar's groin and Jack's thigh for support.

"Get your hand off my dick!" Oscar laughed and turned to Jack. "Your owner is a bologna smuggler!"

Slight mumbled a few curses and headed back to first class.

Three sleepless nights and two zombie-like days passed before Djuana's appointment with Dr. Oppen to abort Dexter's would be third child. He called and admitted that the little boy in the shopping cart was his, and the pregnant woman was his wife of seven months.

His wife. Those words hurt Djuana more than the sight of Dexter's son, and another one on the way. It hurt her that he had bought another woman a diamond – and married her. She and Tia tried to figure out how they hadn't picked up on it sooner. They couldn't, really. He had done a good job fooling them.

The night before the planned abortion saw the Pioneer household its saddest. Devon cried himself to sleep with Emma over him explaining why it had to be done. Emma herself couldn't sleep. She stayed in her room, praying most of the night. Tia slept on the couch because Djuana felt a need to be alone with it.

Toni Braxton's soulful voice and lyrics full of feminine hurt had kept Djuana's face and pillow wet with tears all evening. Guilt had Djuana believing that if she had allowed him to leave her when she choose a New Year's Eve party instead of being at home alone two years ago none of this would be happening. Dexter had called three times, from some pay phone, when he found out about the party.

"I don't think you should go alone," he tried to reason.

"Tia will be there," Djuana replied.

"That's not what I mean. You ain't going. I'll take you out tomorrow."

"What are you worried about, Dex? Have I ever disrespected you? Never. I just want to go out with some friends instead of being at home with mom and her bunch."

She never did ask him where he went. Nor did she push the issue when she heard a female voice call his name. He said the woman was talking to someone else.

She also thought about all the men, some very handsome, some wealthy, she turned away because she was dedicated to him. She wished he died a painful death.

In the early morning, before 8 a.m., Devon's light knock at her door broke Djuana's concentration. He came in and announced he had made breakfast for everyone. His sad tone of voice warmed his sister's heart. For a second she thought about changing her mind and having the baby.

She gave her brother a reassuring smile. "Since when do you cook?"

"I know how to cook. Y'all just never let a kid do the job. Come on and eat 'fore it gets cold."

Djuana was hungry, but she hated the violent illness that she suffered after eating in the morning. She couldn't remember if she could eat before the operation, and she didn't care. She entered the bright yellow kitchen to see Devon spooning scrambled eggs out of the skillet. At the set table was very dark and crispy bacon, lumpy grits, and toast as dark as the bacon. Seated at the table and frowning were Emma and Tia.

Devon looked at his sister. "What? Ain't nothing burnt. Just a little dark that's all."

He got the orange juice out of the refrigerator.

Djuana sat grimacing. Her stomach was turning. Tia covered her laugh.

Emma examined the bacon. "Damn, boy, could you have at least saved one piece?"

Devon sucked his teeth. "Please, Ma."

"I can't eat, Devo. I don't feel too well."

"Me neither," Tia chimed in.

"Yeah, I know," he said, his mouth full of his cooking. "But Ma said you have to eat no matter how hard you barfed chunks back up."

Tia gasped.

Djuana selected a lighter piece of toast and buttered it. The phone rang and all the women jumped for it. Devon sat munching away. Emma answered it laughing at how none of the women wanted to eat. But her smile disappeared. It was Dexter. Djuana spoke with him. The conversation lasted a second. He offered a ride to the hospital, she declined.

Southwest General Hospital had a small lobby with a comfortable waiting area. Five love seats were spaced out in a circle around a large glass table. Behind the half moon reception desk sat two polite women in street clothes with white medic coats and stethoscopes.

Djuana and Tia checked in at that desk and were told Dr. Oppen had not yet arrived. They sat in the empty waiting area. Tia watched Djuana become nervous instantly. She fidgeted, twitched and rubbed her hands together. She looked around and claimed to need a drink. Tia got her a soda pop.

Djuana sipped out of the can twice before putting it down for good. She then asked what was taking so long; fifteen minutes after they sat.

Tia inhaled then exhaled deeply. "Take it easy, Dee," she said.

"You hate me, don't you, Tia?" Djuana was serious.

"Come on, DJ," Tia became agitated. "No I don't hate you. I hate what we are doing. What if something goes wrong?"

"I shouldn't do this, right? We shouldn't be here? Right?" All those hours spent making this decision, and still Djuana wasn't sure.

Tia did not want Djuana to have the baby, yet she would never say so. She had felt strongly against her best friend having Dexter's child since she was told. She would wonder to herself how would Djuana, a beautiful woman, find a good man with a already made family. Most good men would not want to take care of another man's child, she felt.

Tia wiped her eyes and shook her head. She looked down into her own hands on her lap. "It's your choice, Dee. I don't know what to say."

"Help me decide?" Djuana pleaded. "I don't know what to do. I don't want to kill my baby, but. Damn."

"What does your heart say? Go with your heart."

After fifteen minutes of hard thinking, what-ifs and battling her nerves, Djuana blurted, "I want to go home."

Tia wanted to object. "You sure?"

"Yeah."

"Dee? I don't know. I mean, I'm worried that the baby would make everything you always wanted harder to obtain. What about going back to school? What about your own apartment? I want to be able to see you get married."

"It can happen. It can all happen. Women do it everyday. The baby won't kill my future. Just make me work harder, that's all. I can do this."

Djuana hugged Tia. "Don't worry, Tee. I can do it. But I will need your help. I know I will."

Tia kissed Djuana. "Me and you, kid. We can do this."

# 13

The Milwaukee baseball team swept three games from the Crowns in Wisconsin. Jack hardly remembered the two nights and three days. He and Oscar rarely spoke. Oscar had women in the room each night, over emphasizing his pleasures and making the women moan as loud as possible. Jack ignored them. The team took a bus to Detroit, and lost two games there. The sorry trip ended in Minnesota. The Crowns won the last game of three there before returning to Portland.

Jack's slump continued. He managed only four hits during the 10-game road trip. When the Crowns returned home he was determined to work his way out of the slump. He spent his first day home, a day off for the players, with the Crowns batting coach at the batting cage under Adkins Stadium. He hit a thousand balls under the watchful eye of his coach. He sprayed line drives all over the hollow basement. Still, afterwards his confidence did not rise.

Kristen was at the stadium to interview Honeywell for a off-day story when she saw Jack's Pathfinder sitting alone in the parking lot. She went down stairs and watched Jack hit balls hard. She approached him after the workout as a friend, not a reporter. Jack warmed to that advance.

Kristen said, "You seem very frustrated, what's up?"

Jack quietly nodded. "Yeah. I'm just out of it."

"You want to talk about it?"

"Off the record?" Jack's thick eyebrows rose.

"Maybe. Let's have lunch."

Kristen's smile eased him. He showered and changed.

They agreed to eat at Digger O'Dell's, an Cajun cuisine eatery. They drove in their own cars, with Jack following. Once inside, Kristen maintain the lead, she picked the table and ordered two orders of jambalaya. Then, she began the conversation: "So, Jack, what's bothering you? It's kinda obvious."

"Is it? And you think your readers want to know also?"

"Inquiring minds? Ease up! You know me better than that."

Jack smiled. She was right. Other writers have burned him before, but never Kristen. Yet, he still wanted to know if she had a story planned or real conversation.

"Jack, I've always liked you despite the way you and O dog-out women."

"Yeah, that's part of the problem. I can't deal with that anymore. I'm ready to settle down, but I don't have anyone to do it with."

Kristen fell back in her booth seat. "Please. Is that it? You want to settle down? Then why don't you? You have women all over the country that would do backhand springs to marry into your dough. And, you're not bad to look at."

"Exactly," Jack smiled.

Kris playfully kicked him under the table.

"But, seriously, I want real love. Somebody I can love and will love me. To hell with the money."

"Money *is* important. That is what makes, or breaks, a lot of marriages."

"I guess," Jack exhaled. "But, I just want a good woman I can be with."

"Well, what is your definition of a good woman?" Kris batted her eyes. She sat upright.

He sighed again. Blinking his eyes off of her milky-white, smooth cheeks. "One that will love me for me. And, take the time to find out who I am. One I could trust. One that would be there for me."

The food arrived. The waiter, a tall slender, light-skinned young man asked Jack for his autograph without a hint of excitement; just a wide grin. Jack quickly signed his name to the blank check the waiter offered.

"I don't know," Jack continued after the food was placed. "Sometimes I feel like I am never gonna find her. Or that I already have and don't know it."

"That happens. Just be patient, Jack. I would advise you, though, to leave those groupies alone. I fear for you and O. I know others screw around also, but you guys are really wild. I'm afraid that I am going to hear one or both of you have contracted AIDS."

Jack picked at his food. "Yeah. You're right."

The ball was hit hard. Very hard. So hard that the usually boisterous crowd at Adkins Stadium fell silent. Jack was playing the left-handed power hitter close to the right field line as to not allow an extra base hit - a usual move in the late innings of a tied game. San Francisco had rallied to tie the game at two the previous inning. When Jack saw the ball leave the bat he instinctively moved to his right, in the direction he knew the ball was heading.

Jack took three steps toward center field before he glanced away from the ball looking for Oscar. Oscar was jogging yelling to Jack, "It's you! It's you, New!!"

Oscar had already given up chasing the ball. He began circling yards away from the spot where it might land, preparing to back up Jack.

"Thanks, buddy," Jack grumbled. Jack shifted gears and emotions. His anger went from Oscar to the ball. He was going to catch it. After furious strides toward the middle of the outfield, he headed for the wall behind him. The ball was in his sight, lowering in the sky and still traveling quickly. When Jack reached up with his gloved hand he could feel dirt under his cleats, he was no longer on the soft grass. He had entered onto the warning track. His mind panicked, the warning track? Then the wall must be a few... CRASH.

Jack hit the wall with a loud thump, his head driven straight into the padded wall snapping back. The ball hit the wall a second later. It hit inches below the top and rolled rapidly to Oscar. He relayed the ball in. The batter was on second base, as if he had not run hard. The jolt with the wall had left Jack semiconscious. His head, right shoulder and right knee all swelled.

He didn't try to stand, but felt an urge to sit upright. He could not hear his best friend speaking, yet knew O was there.

"I'm all fucked up," Jack said before passing out.

O grabbed Jack by his jersey to prevent him from tumbling over. Jack was sitting on his buttocks, legs sprawled, arms limp and mouth open. Quickly, teammates, dropping their gloves as they ran, and the club's medical personnel sprinter to the scene. The Crowns' head doctor flicked on his radio and ordered a neck brace and ambulance while he ran to Jack. Tim Pugsley Garcia, the Crowns second-baseman was crying. It was Jack who nicknamed Tim because of his short, round physique. The accident look much more fierce than it was. The players and the fans, both at the game and watching on televisions, thought Jack had broke his neck.

After the game, Bingo Wells stormed into Slight's office. The secretary didn't budge, although there was an important meeting going on. She had witnessed that scene much too often in her three years there. Slight would handle it. Slight and Honeywell were sipping scotch when their superstar exploded in. "What the fuck are you going to do about Newhouse?!" Bingo demanded. "He done cost us with his slow ass! He should not be out there.

"Shit, he almost got Oscar killed!"

Slight peacefully sipped more scotch.

Honeywell rose from the leather chair. "What do you want done?" he asked, standing eye to eye with the Crowns number one superstar.

"Bring up Aponte," Bingo said staring down Honeywell. He turned to Slight, "What are you waiting for? Us to be in last place? Aponte can hit and play the field better than Jack could ever. O is always saving his ass, in more ways than one!"

Honeywell defended Jack. "The guy will come around."

"He ain't shit, never was," Bingo laced into Honeywell. "If you didn't want him and defended all the shit he has done, he would have been gone. You traded others for doing less."

Slight finally interrupted, "Gentlemen. Aponte is on his way. If he produces, he stays. Buffalo wants Jack. They can well have him. That's that. Good-bye, Bingo."

Bingo smiled. "Perfect." He left.

"Vinny, your making a mistake. New will still produce for us."

"Jack Newhouse is finished here. And, the sooner Buffalo ups the ante, the quicker he can pack." Slight poured more liquor into his glass.

Honeywell rubbed his pointer finger over his top lip. He was defeated, only because it was Slight who owned the team. He did not want to see Jack traded. He thought of an excuse to keep him that Slight would find legit. None came to mind.

Slight gulped his drink. Fixed another. "The guy drinks and screws in every city we visit. He fights with fans, and over those whores at that! I thought he was going to marry that chick he was seeing, what's her name? But he lost her.

Let him go."

Slight shuffled papers on his desk. "Look at these numbers," he held up Aponte's updated minor league stats. "This is gold. Solid gold with O in front of him and Bingo behind him.

"Shit, we'll run the Gamblers off the field."

"Vinny, fine, I understand Aponte is going play either way, especially since Jack's hurt, but I am against trading him. The man carried us in '90. He was the only one that didn't piss on himself against Las Vegas."

Slight became enraged. "Cut the sentimental bullshit! Did we win in '90? Have we won a championship with Jack Newhouse? No. When was the last time he stole a base? When was the last time he had an assist?"

"Christ! the slowing hump left lip marks on my outfield wall! He used to eat those balls up!"

Slight looked at Aponte's stats again. He already knew them by heart. "Call Buffalo. Aponte can do the job."

Jack spent that night in the hospital. He stayed in the intensive care unit with a concussion. The team's doctor ran tests on his vision, memory and reflexes, then had numerous x-rays performed. All through the day of exams, Jack rarely spoke.

The nurses were overly polite and attentive to the star patient, but he ignored them. Tons of flowers and get well wishes were sent to him from fans, yet he was not cheerful. He was worried that the injury had opened the door for Slight to replace him. The reality of the situation depressed him.

The Portland Crowns were a very close-knit ball club. Most of the players had matured as ballplayers together in the minor leagues, and had lost lots of games together before becoming a dominant force. Slight had allowed

Honeywell full administrative control in forming the team, but now he felt his presence was needed to push the team over its last hurdle before stardom. Beating the Gamblers, Slight believed, would call for changes.

Jack was watching the soaps when his private room's door flung opened and slammed against the wall. Mike had kicked it open because his hands were full with boxes of pizza.

"Is this the Jack Newhouse suite?" He barked.

In barged 18 of Jack's 24 teammates. The rest sent their solace, yet had other engagements. Except Bingo. He ripped Jack in the media, saying the Crowns would never win with him. Along with Mike's pizza, Danny and Pugsley had brought beer.

Don came straight to Jack and kissed his forehead. "I would have had that," he said.

Don, once the best right fielder in the game, was now the slowest outfielder on the Crowns.

O carried a brown package that contained six X-rated movies that the team chipped in to buy. O sent a rookie to get a VCR.

"What if I can't find one?" Luis Ratz asked puzzled.

"Then go out and buy one!" O yelled. "Don't stand there, hurry the-fuck-up! These are goodies!"

Jack had to grin. "You butts are going to get me put out." The room, large and gloomy before, became small, loud and crowded.

"Doubt it," Mike said. "O's slept with just about every nurse in the joint." The room roared with laughter.

"I must tell you Jack," said Cris Carpenter, the other Crowns starting outfielder, as the chuckling ceased. "We were going to get you a stripping nurse, but we only collected $8.95."

"You cheap-ass millionaires," Jack frowned.

Don said, "We asked Bingo to chip in and he said to tell you to kiss his ass."

"Kick his ass, he said? Why, sure I will," Jack laughed so hard it hurt.

# 14

Djuana opened her mind and heart to the fact that she was having a baby in the fall. She cashed her check as she usually did at the end of her shift on Thursday's and went out on a clothes shopping spree. She went to two different maternity stores, spending almost all of her two week's earnings. Most of the clothes she bought were for the upcoming months, she hadn't any noticeable physical changes at that time. She went back into DeLux's, and using her 20% discount, spent the rest of her money. She went to the ATM and took out money to cover her expenses to and from work. She planned to wait until the next pay day for her bills.

Djuana even began the process of telling people. She called her true friends and by the end of the day she had received numerous phone calls. The news spread through Djuana's small chain of friends, and soon word reached Tia. Everyone expected Tia to have known, she was the tightest of all of them to Djuana. But, Tia, afraid of breaking Djuana's trust in her, denied the story. She was caught off guard when the women said it was Djuana that told them.

Tia called Djuana disturbed. "Thanks for telling me you handed out fliers telling of your predicament."

Djuana laughed, "Don't worry about it. I let the cat out of the bag, and it feels good."

Djuana was surprised to have found so many nice styles in the maternity stores. She was also sadly surprised to find she had gone up a size from an eight in most styles to 10 in maternity clothes. It was then it dawn on her seriously that she was three months pregnant. She bought various colors of stirrups and pullover and button-up blouses to match. She bought underwear, including a few wire bras. Her breasts had become tender and heavy, and the nipples were tingling constantly.

Djuana's metamorphosis into being a proud pregnant woman helped ease her mind. She began to take serious notice to the changes her body had been going through while she moped. She told Dr. Oppen, who was glad she changed her mind and wanted to have the baby, and he described all her little discomforts and bodily changes.

The dull ache, a feeling of fullness, in her belly, the doctor explained, was the cause of fibrous and elastic tissue was forming in the external muscle layer of the uterus. The uterine muscle cells were stretching and the shape of the uterus was changing from pear to round as the fetus grew. Some of the processes were internal, he went on to explain, but others she would see.

Dr. Oppen gave Djuana a tight hug and kiss on the cheek, he was happy she stood him up at the hospital. They had enjoyed a fine relationship, he was a good listener and always offered Christian advice. Djuana had been using him as her gynecologist for six years and his bed side manner was what kept her loyal. Djuana took to the way her approached the many subjects they disgusted. He would come off as a concerned father sometimes, and other times as a knowing doctor. Emma, though, didn't like him. She wanted her daughter to go to a African-American female doctor instead.

Emma would complain, "She would understand you better. And she wouldn't be so happy to see you with your legs cocked open."

Djuana left the mall, jumped into a cab on the taxi-line and rode to her hair dresser on Burnside. Even though a bus would have been free, she didn't feel like being bothered with lugging those shopping bags off the bus and hauling them the four blocks to the shop. And, more importantly, she could relax in peace in the cab.

The city of Portland was dedicated to making its downtown area the least congested as possible. The Tri-Met public buses and the Metropolitan Area Express, Portland's above -ground light rail system, are free if a person travels within a 300-block radius of downtown, known as Fareless Square.

In the cab, the short driver was listening to Portland's news radio station. The sports report began with news of Jack Newhouse being in stable condition. Djuana sprang forward.

"What happen to him?" she blurted.

The driver looked into the mirror and brightly said, "He ran into the wall last night. It looked pretty bad, but they say he'll be back soon."

Djuana frowned. "What wall? Was he driving?"

The driver let loose a mocking chuckle. "No. No. The outfield wall. He was chasing a fly ball and ran out of room. They'll probably show it tonight on the news again."

Djuana's mind went to work. "Which hospital is he in?"

"University. But I think they said he'll be getting out today."

"Thanks."

"No problem."

Djuana sat back. She dug through her purse and found Jack's number. She couldn't wait to get home to use it.

Pamela Kirke was shocked to see Djuana come through the hair salon's door. She greeted her friend and customer with a long hug and light kiss - her hands away from Djuana though. In one hand she was holding a curling iron, the other a comb with globs of conditioner.

"Girl, where you been? Did Dex have you on lock down?"

"Not even. I was just a little busy," Djuana looked around. The small, six-booth, store front shop was crowded for a Thursday night. Each booth was being used. The other women all smiled or spoke to Djuana as she found a seat.

"I'm sorry I didn't make an appointment."

Pam shrugged. "Your in luck, after I set Fran I'm free. The crowd's not for me this time!"

Djuana put her bags in Pam's office and sat among the waiting women. Most she knew casually. For a second she wondered where everybody was going. She didn't want to ask, because she knew that most of the women there were either married or dating seriously. That would be all she needed to hear about: a couple's affair. The talk of the shop that night was of Denzel Washington's new movie and inattentive boyfriends. Djuana chose to not enter in either debate.

She instead looked around at the posters of men around the shop. There were movie stars, television actors and sports figures. But, no Jack Newhouse. She was looking at the basketball poster wishing it was Jack, changing each feature until the player was in a Crowns uniform and more handsome. She hoped he was feeling fine.

Then, Dexter arrived.

Dexter's Mazda double parked outside of the shop. He had checked all over town for Djuana, at many of the spots where he had picked her up from before. He had almost forgotten about Pam's.

Pam, standing over Fran, setting her hair, saw him first. "Um. He's early tonight."

Djuana followed Pam's eyes to see Dexter as he opened the door and came in. The sight reminded her of the life long connection she would have with him. It was then, for the first time in seven years, she looked at him and felt no passion; no urge to touch him. No love.

She walked directly to him. He stopped and greeted her. "What are you doing here, Dexter?" She coldly whispered. Every eye was on him.

"We ain't talked. I think we should, even though 'you' made the decision."

"Then, talk."

Dexter's head spanned the shop. "Not here. Come outside."

As soon as the door closed, the women began to whisper.

"Problems in paradise?" a round woman said.

Another, her hair being weaved, quipped "He ain't bad looking, but those be the one's."

Pam quieted the audience. "Y'all need to mind your own. That's why some of you ain't got a man."

Dexter tried to hold Djuana's hand. "Don't touch me," she said.

"Come on, Babe. Ease up a little. I never wanted any of this to happen."

"Any of what, Dexter? Me to get pregnant, or me to find out about your family. Or all of the above?"

"Juanny, you got it all wrong," he said, but Djuana had not stopped speaking.

"You jerked me, lied to me, for what? Seven years? I hate you with a passion."

The parlor fell silent, and motionless. It was hard to catch every word, but Djuana helped with her anger.

Dexter folded his arms. Djuana bit her bottom lip and looked away and into the leaving buses' lights. They both knew they were being watched.

"I'm sorry," Dexter near mumbled. "But you just don't know the half. You don't know why or how these situations occurred."

"You called me a bitch. A lying bitch," the tears began slowly. "You put your hands on me. Twice."

"I'm sorry. You know I always loved you, no matter what."

"Don't," Djuana's voice carried in the brisk night air. "Don't even go there."

Dexter moved closer. "I never hit you before in my life. I am sorry and I wished it was you I married."

Djuana pushed him before he touched her. "You sure are sorry. A sorry excuse for a man. You don't know how I wish at night that this was somebody else's baby."

Dexter looked away while Djuana took tissue out of her handbag. She wiped her eyes and nose. He was becoming agitated.

"Why you fucking with me?" he said. "All you want to do is argue. I'm here trying to talk with you."

"Stop. Save it for your wife. We don't have anything to discuss. You do as you please. You want to be a father to this baby, do it. Don't ask me shit. You know my address. Mail whatever you want, and you will be welcome wherever the baby is. Just don't be expecting me to listen to your shit."

Djuana wrenched open the door and stepped in. All eyes froze in any direction but hers. Dexter darted in ahead of her. He pleaded with her, "Babe, I know you are going to be a good mother. But, I still don't think this is the right time or situation for you. Think about it."

A few looked directly at them, but most of 12 or 13 women in the shop tried to be oblivious.

"Bye, Dexter." She bullied by him, hoping he would brush her so she would have a reason to fight him. He side-stepped her. She returned to her seat. The lady next to her forced her head into the magazine.

Dexter watched her soft, beautifully shaped legs cross angrily. She will be a gorgeous pregnant woman, he imagined. His wife was, and is again, unattractive while expecting.

He knew Djuana would be celibate until long after birth. He felt his bugle rise as he remembered how true she was to him, how snug her vagina was the times he disappeared for two weeks, or after her period.

"Fine. Be like that," he said as he stormed out with his head high.

"The Virgin Mother," Dexter grinned as he got into his ride. "Shit. That pussy's gonna be sweet."

He began plotting a way to be first again.

# 15

The telephone's ring startled Jack out of a dead sleep. Its second ring irritated him, causing him to rise off the pillow. The third ring caused a sharp pain in his still aching head. He and his headache had finally fell asleep minutes before. He was home now, and felt relaxed in his own bed, but the constant phone calls were more disturbing than the hospital.

Jack snatched up the cordless phone on the fifth ring. He had forgotten to cut on the answering machine. He grumbled a hello into the receiver. The voice on the line was soft and unsure. She asked for Jack by his full name. He was pissed, he didn't recognize the voice, and didn't want to be bothered.

"Jack, this is Djuana Pioneer. I hope it's not too late?"

Jack popped up, pain rushed to his forehead. "No, not really." He looked at the digital clock on the night table. 10:49 was not late at all.

Djuana listened intently. "You sound like you were sleep. Maybe I should call back tomorrow."

"No, no. I'm up. I was just laying down. I was watching the game."

Djuana perked. "Yeah, I just came in and caught the tail end of it. How did you like it?"

"It was all right." Jack hated the game. His replacement, Hector Aponte, broke into the big leagues with two doubles and a home run. Jack cringed when the crowd at Adkins gave the kid a standing ovation.

"Just all right? You say that because you are not playing. Are you feeling better? They showed a replay of the accident. It looked pretty bad, but they say you'll be back soon."

"I hope so. I feel a lot better, although I still have a slight headache," Jack leaned an elbow on his pillows. "So, you saw the play, huh? The wall kinda snuck up on me. I had it all the way."

"Sure," Djuana chuckled.

Jack smiled.

"You watch baseball often?"

Djuana was relaxed, but not comfortable enough to say what she felt. She wanted to tell Jack she hated baseball until she met him. But a better answer came to mind.

"My brother is a big fan."

"That's good. Does he go to games?"

"Sometimes. His uncles take him sometimes."

"Well, maybe you can bring him and the two of you can be my guest."

"Oh, he'd go crazy. He's been asking me about going since I told him..."

Jack could hear the disturbance in her silence. "Are you still upset about that? About how we met?"

"No. To tell the truth, I don't think you did anything. That's why I think about you."

"Think about *me*? That's good to hear, because you are all I wonder, dream and think about."

"What's with you, Jack Newhouse? Are you as nice and sincere as I think you are? Or are you the guy I've read about that sleeps with many women in other cities?"

"Do you want to take the time to find out for yourself?"

"Maybe," she tested him more.

She wanted to tell him how bored she'd been that night. How she wanted to speak with him ever since she heard about the injury. How she needed a different, unknowing ear.

She began: "Jack, when I heard about you being hurt I felt an urge to call you. You see, that night you made me feel so warm and secure. Then I see you in my store and you make me feel the same way. When you said you had been thinking about me and worried about me, you sounded sincere."

Jack found himself in unfamiliar territory: A woman was talking to him about her own feelings. Not baseball, not pay checks and not what sex act they would be glad to perform. He was full of questions. He spoke without thinking; the words had been there waiting for Djuana. They continued to discuss favorites, their jobs and families. Djuana surprised him by asking about an article that Kristen wrote in the Sunday paper about his need for a female companion.

"She wrote that? Damn." Jack worried about the hundreds of letters he will receive from single women in Oregon.

"Do you really want to get married?"

Jack was happy to reveal how single he was, "I thought I was going to. The last woman I dated dumped me for her ex. I was surprised, but I am kinda happy she did it. Now I can find someone to really love and really love me."

Djuana became silent. She thought about the stories she had heard from numerous people, including her mother, about Jack and his teammates. She wanted to ask, but felt he would be forced to lie.

*Would he lie?*

Probably. But, it should not matter, she reasoned with herself. When she became his woman, then she would need to know.

She laughed to herself. *When* she became his woman.

Djuana told of how Dexter hurt her, revealing how she loved him deeply for seven years. She twirled the phone's cord, laying on in bed, between the sheets and staring at the ceiling. She was thinking of how deeply she loved Dexter. She couldn't envision loving that strongly ever again.

"Is that the man from the night I met you?" Jack was curious, but hesitant. He didn't want their pleasant conversation to turn because he was being noisy

"Yes. He left me at a restaurant, and I was walking home when I walked in front of your car."

"He sounds like a real loser."

"He is, I'm sorry to say."

"Why?"

"Because I spent seven years trying to make him mine. What a waste."

"Do you want him back?"

"No. No way."

"Really?"

"Really. I do miss him sometimes, only because I'm lonely..." Oops. She patted her forehead with her soft, tight fist.

"But, I know I deserve better," she recovered.

Jack wanted to leap through the phone and make her feel loved.

Djuana did feel exhilarated, though. Both her heart and mind were ablaze. Jack was a wonderful talker with so much to say. He told her peculiar stories that opened an effusive part of Djuana's soul she had never showed a man. Dexter, the one man she spent most of her time with, was not fond of her sense of humor. He would tell her to shut up at times she was playful or talkative. Thus, she began to not share thoughts with him.

Jack and Djuana spent nine hours on the phone. Not more than a minute of silence passed between them. Djuana checked the clock when she heard Devon in the bathroom. "Do you realize how long we've been on the phone," she sat up and notice the light seeping in the window shades.

"Not really," Jack looked and was shocked.

"It's almost seven in the morning!"

"I'm sorry. You better go. Don't you have to leave for work soon?"

"I really get up about eight," Djuana didn't want to hang up. "What about you, how's your head?"

"Lady, your voice has soothed my brain cells."

"Oh, really," Djuana blushed.

"Yep," Jack's voice had cleared. Djuana liked it hoarse.

"I wish I could see you today. How about lunch?" He asked.

"That's possible. If you can."

"I don't know why not."

The two planned to meet at the Galleria for lunch during Djuana's lunch hour. She warned him, though, that they are meeting as friends. Jack agreed.

Both were exhausted and sore from holding the phone for nine hours, yet they were at the same time more alive than ever. Djuana waited less than five minutes before calling Tia and giving her a near word-for-word recount.

As Jack twirled his Pathfinder into a parking spot at the Galleria his car phone beeped. His heart raced, was she calling to cancel? He snatched up the phone. It was his agent.

"Where are you," Berger demanded to know.

"The Galleria mall."

"For what?"

"Lunch."

Berger blew air through his nose. "Geezus! How fast can you get across town to my office. You can have lunch with me."

"I could in twenty minutes. But I ain't. I am not breaking this date."

"Shit. Okay, okay. But we have to talk. It's very important."

"Shoot. You got seven seconds."

"Lee has been traded to Buffalo. They want you next. I made a few calls, and Buffalo called me. They want to know if you'll play first if they make the trade."

Jack's heart dropped. "I am not going to Buffalo."

"So, first base is out of the question?"

"Berger, you deaf? I ain't going to Buffalo."

"If you say no to playing first for them, then it won't matter."

Jack felt the hollow pit in his stomach deepen, a combination of hunger and nerves. He looked up at the Red Dragon's sign.

"I've got to go."

"Don't worry about it, but we need to meet with Slight and Honeywell real soon."

"Yeah, hook it up. I'll call you in two hours."

Djuana sat nervously at a booth in the Red Dragon Chinese restaurant. She had watched the clocks in DeLux's all morning. Now she sat and watched the Red Dragon's clock tick a second past two. She needed a watch since she threw away the diamond timepiece Dexter had bought her.

He'll be here any second, she warned herself. She wondered what more could they discuss after nine hours on the phone; besides her pregnancy. No, not that. She wasn't ready to discuss that. It might scare him away. She hoped he wouldn't notice her belly. But, her belly at that time was not protruding at all. It was well hidden by the oversized, black cotton long-sleeve blouse.

*When should I tell him? When would be the right time?* Tia told her to tell him that day, at lunch. She would try, she promised Tia. As she sat there awaiting Jack, she planned to control the conversation; letting him know she was not available, but would like his friendship. He would understand. He seemed so nice and refreshing on the phone. He didn't once direct their conversation toward sex.

Then, there he was. Dressed causal, as Djuana had directed, with a yellow rose in his right hand. He wore a two-buttoned, navy blue polo shirt, jeans, sneakers and a navy blue field jacket. He smiled at Djuana, she was already blushing, as the host escorted him over.

Quickly, he took Djuana's hand to his lips and kissed it. Then he handed her the rose.

"That's for allowing me to have lunch with you," Jack whispered.

Djuana blushed.

"Drinks, Juana?" The Matre'D asked.

She looked at Jack, "Would you like anything?"

"Sure, let me get a Bud, and plenty of water."

Djuana ordered a ginger ale with lemon and the valet disappeared.

"You must come here often," Jack said.

"Oh, because he called me by my name? We order food about twice a week to the store."

"So, people call you Juana?"

"Not many. I don't think he can pronounce it with the D. You can if you want to."

"No. I like Djuana."

She liked how he pronounced it, with the Juan very prominent. She looked into his face. He was handsome. More so than the pictures she had studied. She liked his dark eyes, full eye brows and inviting lips. They were rounded, not big, and soft. She recalled his light kiss on her knuckles minutes before and unconsciously licked her lips. A sprinkle of goose bumps covered her body.

"Since this is your hangout, what do you suggest?" Jack said. Looking down at the menu, Jack could feel Djuana giving him the once over.

*A long kiss*, she wished she had nerve to say. Instead she giggled.

"Something wrong?" Jack asked. "Do I have a hair out of place or something." He patted his low-cut fade.

"No. Not at all." She continued to giggle.

A different waiter brought water, Jack's beer and Djuana's soda. He also took their order. Jack let Djuana order for him. She was delighted and made a quick choice. How many times had she wanted to order for Dexter just to be different?

Jack glanced at Djuana. Why is this woman single? he wondered. He looked at her black blouse; nothing was revealed. Then he looked over her hairstyle.

Quietly, leaning over to her, he said, "I like your hair that way." he remembered the wide, soft, bright rust curls that were drenched and hanging down her face the night he first saw her. Now Djuana's hair was auburn brown with a mid-length bob, coaxed from her crown into a super smooth drop, covering her ears and reaching her neck.

Djuana thanked him. Omar, the bus driver, had said the same exact words hours before, yet not as calmly nor sincerely as Jack did.

"How's your head," she asked. She was trying to be in control. Keep him from noticing her nerves, or the baby.

"It's much better. I took the horse pills the Doc gave me, and took a nap this morning."

"That's good. I want to thank you for coming out here. I know you probably had things to do." She tried not to smile, but did.

"It's my pleasure. I am serious about wanting to get to know you. It starts with spending time with you."

"Yeah."

Damn, he's making it hard to keep to the script, her forehead wrinkled as she studied her glass. She twirled her straw. Tell him, her conscious nudged. But she feared he would upturn the table and dash out the door. Why would a major league baseball star, making millions, want to date a pregnant woman. Pregnant by an asshole. He would run out the door.

Suddenly a penny bounced on the table near Djuana. "If your thoughts are more expensive, I'll pay."

She had to smile. *He is something else.* "I was just thinking about something," she finally said as the food came.

Saved.

"I figured you were thinking. But what about so deeply. Am I boring you?"

"No. When we get to know each other better, I'll have plenty to tell you," Djuana said as she spread soy sauce over her chow mien.

Jack was apprehensive. "Are you married to this guy you told me about last night?"

"No," Djuana was startled. "I am not married. Where did that come from?"

"Your ring," Jack pointed to her left hand. He wanted to touch it, hold it. On the ring finger was a onyx in a thin gold setting.

"Your kidding me?" She laughed heartily. The ring, something she was sure Jack wouldn't buy for a child, was a Christmas gift from Dexter two years ago. That fall she had been nagging him about getting married.

The ring, Dexter explained, ''Friends Forever'' bond. She like it, but not for what it symbolized. Putting it on every morning had been become a devoted part of her daily routine.

"Well, it is on that finger."

"No, Jack. I am far from being married."

She noticed his gold chain, a simple herringbone, and decided to pick on him. "That's a nice chain," she commented.

"It's cute."

"Cute?" Jack laughed.

"Oh, I'm sorry," she deepened her voice. "That's manly, Dude." She laughed a hearty giggle. To Jack it seemed a bit much, but it was refreshing to Djuana.

"Oh, boy. It feels so good to laugh again."

Jack's grin dimmed. It had been more than a year since Vivian gave him the chain for his birthday. He touched it, and planned to get rid of it that night.

He watched Djuana for a few seconds, thinking of the correct way to ask her about the night they met. He had an idea it was a man that sent her into the mood she was in at the time. He left that thought alone; observing her eat was a warming sight.

Her hands and mouth never stopped moving, yet with respectful manners. She kept her napkin handy and wiped her lip quickly between fork visits. Djuana devoured her food, and most of their appetizer, within minutes.

"You were hungry," Jack finally said.

Djuana looked down at her spotless plate and small portion left on the serving platter. Then she saw he had barely touch his plate. She sipped the last of her soda.

"Yeah, I was. I didn't have breakfast because I didn't want to seem like one of those conceited women who only have salads."

Djuana had eaten hearty that morning, and she had two candy bars while working.

The sudden appearance of a pretty woman and a bright-eyed young boy startled Djuana.

The lady excused herself and the boy, then turned to Jack and said, "Mr. Newhouse, my son is a big fan and he wants to know if you would sign this for him?"

She handed Jack a small piece of paper.

Jack glanced at Djuana as he took the paper and pen. She seemed uptight.

"I'm sorry about this." He asked the boy his name and signed: Always strive to be the best.

Djuana was speechless. She was impressed, and at the same time in awe of her lunch mate. She enjoyed how careful he was with the youngster, and respectful to the parent. When they walked away, thanking her also, she finally spoke.

"You are really something else. I know you must have thousands of fans."

"I hope so," Jack grinned. "But, thanks for your patience, anyway. You know, I hate when that happens. I hope it didn't bother you too much. I have to tell you, its apart of what I am."

"No problem, no bother to me. Hey, it's you they want."

"Yeah, but it's you it will probably bother more. But, I promise, if we do get together like I hope we will, we will have plenty of privacy. I have learned how."

"Really." She wanted to question him about the getting together statement, but held off. She imagined sitting through a baseball game, yuck! "I have to admit something, though, I am not that crazy about baseball."

"That's all right," Jack replied knowingly.

His answer seemed dry. She quickly blurted, "I'll be glad to learn if you teach me."

Jack was pleased with the compromise, "Sure. I'd like that. And I'd like to see you at some games."

Djuana smiled.

Jack had to bring up marriage again. He was intrigue by the fact that such an attractive African-American woman hadn't been snatched up. He ate a fork full of Egg Foo Young, then sipped ice water.

"Tell me something, why isn't a beautiful young lady like yourself married?"

"Thank you. My mother asks me the same question every single day. I just can't answer that."

"Do you want to be?"

Djuana took a second to think. The answer was obvious to her, but should she tell him? He is a well-to-do baseball player, women have probably been trying to hook him into marriage for years. Would he understand the answer? She looked him in the eye, one of the few times that afternoon, and said, "I would like to someday. If I met the right person."

"Have you ever been engaged?"

"You mean with a ring and a date? No." Djuana began eating the orange slices and fortune cookies.

"What, you were verbally engaged or something."

"Kinda. I really wouldn't like to get into that."

"Sorry." Jack watched her again.

Djuana ran her finger up and down her glass, thinking how terrible Dexter is compared with Jack. When she looked up she noticed Jack watching her.

"You're staring at me."

"You're beautiful," instantly he responded.

"Thanks." Djuana decided to take control of the conversation. "What about you, have you ever been engaged?"

"Nope. I thought I was close to it, but that didn't quite work out."

"What happen?"

"Well, she went back to her ex. Something I thought might happen."

The bill came, and out of custom or habit, the waiter placed it at Jack's side. He removed the plates. Jack asked Djuana if she wanted anything else.

She said no thank you, and dragged the bill to her side of the table, "I'll handle this. My treat. Do *you* want anything else."

"No thanks. But, Djuana, let me pay the bill."

"Jack, I invited you. Next time can be all yours."

Jack figured she didn't make much money in the mall, but didn't push it. He watched her go through her handbag and remove her purse. She took money out and slid out of the booth. She dropped a $3 tip and took the tab to the counter. Jack followed, eyes on hips. Djuana's curved torso was hid in a knee-length, hunter green knit skirt with a modest slit in the back.

Her black, small heeled, leather sling-backs revealed smooth ankles and heels. Jack marveled at those legs. No stockings! Perfectly rounded calves with a hint of hair on the legs.

Djuana felt his eyes, and hoped he enjoyed the sight. She paid the bill and allowed him to escort her out the double doors. Before they could leave, a man cut them off, grabbing Jack's hand. He shook it heartily and asked for Jack's autograph.

"He's the best, lady, the damn best there is!" The fan said to Djuana.

"I know," Djuana said. She believed it.

Jack signed the man's piece of paper quickly.

Outside, she instantly recognized the black Pathfinder. Suddenly, a ride seemed alluring.

"Well," she exhaled. "Thanks again for joining me. You are a pleasure to be with."

"And, you too. Would you like me to walk you back to work?"

Djuana said no, but was glad he asked. Her doubts about his sincerity were diminishing. They approached his car, he pressed his alarm releasing the locks and Djuana opened the driver's door for him.

"Drive safely. Oh, I already know you can handle this thing." Djuana chuckled, but she felt stupid for saying that.

Jack slid behind the wheel with a sharp grin. "I want to see you again."

Djuana closed the door. The car's engine turned and the windows slid down.

"You will," she said. "I promise you that." Again she felt she was saying too much, but her words were flowing freely.

Jack took her hand off the door and kissed it. "Thanks again for a great lunch."

Djuana's hand numbed. *I want a kiss. I want a kiss. Kiss him!*

She leaned in, and Jack craned his head to meet her tender lips. Her tongue parted his lips and searched his mouth for his tongue. She held on to his jacket, grasping tightly, and raised to her tiptoes. Passion brought light moans from the pit of her heart to her vocal cords. The kiss was the best first kiss in either one of their memories. His tongue was patient, and hers was aggressive.

The kiss lasted seconds, but neither knew the true flow of time. They separated to a soft plop. Djuana licked her mouth dry. The sight enhanced Jack's arousement. He rubbed his chin with his hands. Djuana smiled and wiped his chin, "I'm sorry. I wet up your face."

Jack was flabbergasted, all he could do was shake his head. After a second or two he said, "Call me?"

"Yes, Jack. I will call you."

The Pathfinder glided slowly away, leaving Djuana on the verge of madness. Her body had never given her any trouble - in fact, she'd never felt that she just *had* to have a man make love to her during the lonely nights Dexter caused. But the thought of Jack Newhouse touching her... making love to her, made her ache with desire. She didn't know how many nights she'd awakened from a dream in which his body possessed hers, to find herself trembling, her breasts hurting for his touch.

"No. No," she babbled walking across the parking lot of the mall. "Shit! I just met him. Just kissed him and just really talked with him."

Jack and Djuana had walked out of the Red Dragon ten minutes to three o'clock. Ten minutes before Djuana was due back at DeLux's. When she punched back in she was fifteen minutes late. And in love.

# 16

Emma Pioneer took a deep drag of her sixth cigarette in the last half of an hour. She wasn't used to having company, and it was making her nervous. Emma had been a chain smoker for 23 years before quitting. The circumstances surrounding her only daughter, and first born, caused her to return to smoking, she told herself. That pack of Pall Malls she was emptying was the first she had bought in a year. She had to, she needed a smoke when her only daughter dropped the bomb shell of being pregnant.

Emma's only brother Calvin sat across from her at the small kitchen table quietly drinking his beer. Emma was drinking vodka mixed with orange juice; her favorite. Also at the table, but not drinking anything, was Tia's mother, Bernadette Williams. In the living room were Tia and Calvin's wife, Marla. Tia and Marla were discussing a baby shower for Djuana.

The quiet in the kitchen brought the shower plans to the attention of Emma. She sipped out of her mug.

"I don't believe this," she moaned. "My baby. I just don't believe this."

Calvin gulped his brew, turning his neck up. It was times like this, when his sisters were crying for simple reasons, that Cal disliked being the only man around the family.

"I'm getting sick of this shit. Emma, the girl is in her twenties! Late twenties at that! Shit. You actin' like she be 15 or 16. Come on. She'll be all right."

Emma cringed at Calvin. "Thank you, Cal. You fucking genius. Why don't you go in the other room before I crack your skull with this Absolut bottle?"

Calvin snatched up his beer and stormed into the living room. Bernadette watched him leave, picking her next words carefully.

Emma spoke first, fighting tears, "That man don't understand. My daughter is all fucked up, and I did it."

Bernadette switched seats, getting closer to Emma and taking her hand, "Come now, Emma. You worked hard in raising two fine children on your own. And everybody knows you did a damn fine job."

"Sure I did," Emma answered sarcastically. "I lost my baby to her first lay. He turned her from an energetic young woman with dreams into a lovesick zombie waiting for his call. She had dreams. She wanted to be something, but she instead waited for him."

She poured the remainder of her mug down her dry throat. She mixed another drink and continued.

"Then he knocks her up and wants to beat it out of her because he is already married. He's gonna get his."

Bernadette squeezed Emma's fat hand.

"It will be okay, you can't go thinking like that. It won't solve anything. God will give him his due." Bernadette moved closer, "Listen, me and Lenny will help in any way we can."

The booze began unleashing Emma's feelings. She began crying loudly, and the sobbing brought everyone into the kitchen.

"My baby could have been anything. She was so smart in school. She could've gone back to college, but no." She sobbed and looked up at everyone trying to console her. "But no. Now she's all fucked up 'cause of a first-dick she couldn't shake."

"Don't say that, Emma," Marla said. "She'll be all right."

"You know better than that. Djuana is still very bright and oh so beautiful," Bernadette said, patting Emma's back and handing her a fresh tissue.

Emma rose and became defensive. "Yeah, like I don't know what the fuck I'm saying?! What the fuck did I go through?! Ain't no man gonna want her with baggage!"

No one acknowledged the sound of a key in the front door. Djuana floated directly into the kitchen and brightly smiled at her family and closest friends. The sight could have been the climax to a wonderful day. She had been gleeful the remainder of the afternoon. But when she saw the tears on her mother's face and the near-empty liquor bottle, she stiffened.

"What's up?" Djuana frowned.

Emma bullied her way through Marla and Bernadette to Djuana, then gently held her daughter's face. The smell of alcohol on her mother's breath churned Djuana's delicate stomach.

"Why Baby, why?" Emma began. "Why have this man's baby? Don't do this to yourself. No, please, Juanny, baby, don't do this."

Calvin pulled his melodramatic sister by her arms, "Come on, Em', just sit down for a second." He lead her back to her seat at the table.

He then kissed Djuana's forehead, she had begun to cry. "Don't worry about it, Dee. You a grown woman."

"Oh, no you don't! That's my fuckin' daughter!" Emma exploded from her seat. "If you want to be Uncle Helper, then go out and bust that yella nigger's ass!"

Marla replaced Calvin trying to quiet Emma. It was no easy task. Tia tried to console Djuana, but the hurt had already seeped in. Calvin kissed his niece again.

"I love you, and you know your mom does too. Forget what you heard. Do what you think is best. You know we'll all be behind you. She just wanted things to be different and shit, you know. That whole marriage thing and all.

"But watch, she'd be the one spoiling the baby the most."

"What, she think I did this on purpose?" Djuana cried. "That I wanted it this way? I didn't. I didn't."

Emma tapped on her daughter's bedroom door, then entered without waiting for the okay. The visitors had gone home, and Devon was asleep.

"You feelin' all right, baby," she said to Djuana, who was sitting on the edge of her bed, in the darken room, looking out the window. Djuana didn't answer. Emma walked over and sat on the other end of the bed. She looked over her daughter.

Djuana was angry, more so hurt, by her mother's words. The rest of the family, including Tia's mother, wanted the words excused because Emma had been drinking, but Djuana felt the words were true to heart; believing a person under the influence of alcohol spoke truth.

She was also embarrassed. Her sudden and extreme mood swings were disturbing. She was worried that she no longer had control over her emotions. Emma spoke after a few minutes of silence and looking at the back of her daughter's body. "This ain't how I want this to happen," she began. "Why didn't you marry Alfred? He had a good job and loved the ground you walked on. I just want you to be happy. And to have it easier than I did. I want you to get married, and experience real love.

"You have a baby, and your chances of finding a good man lower."

Djuana stubbornly heard only what she wanted to. Her mother didn't know what she was saying. She felt that when she was without a baby there were no good men. The few men that seemed decent, disappeared, if they didn't get any pussy, or after they did.

Emma continued, placing a hand on Djuana's shoulder, "I love you, DJ. Do you know that? I know I don't say it enough, but you should know. I want you to go back to school, start at a career and not work at DeLux's the rest of your life.

"Get out of Portland. Do things."

Djuana finally faced her mother. "You did it, Mom. You stayed, took care of us. Did you hate it? I know you did, but you did it and raised us well. We always ate well, and were dressed right." She sucked the roof of her mouth and hit the window seal with a close fist.

"I wish I wasn't pregnant," she turned, back looking out the window, crying. "But I am. And I ain't gonna kill my baby. I don't know what's gonna happen, but I'ma do what I have to do. I'ma have the baby and go on."

She wiped her eyes, folded her arms across her chest, and faced her mother, "Mom, I know you didn't have that much help, but I am gonna need you. I know I am because I'm scared. And if you're not there like you've always been..." The tears flowed and she sobbed loudly. "Then, I don't know what I'm going to do."

Emma squeezed her daughter into her bosom with pride. Her mind hadn't changed, she still wanted Djuana to have an abortion, but it felt good that her daughter needed her. She kissed Jay on the top of her head, holding her and telling her to cry it out.

"Don't worry, You know I'll be there," Emma said. "Ain't I always?"

Jack had little time to savor the sweet moments with Djuana. As soon as he drove off the car's phone beeped, letting him know he had a backlog of phone messages. Most were from women. Oscar called twice, and Berger, not a patient man, left four messages of urgency during the hour-long lunch. Jack called him back as he drove to the Stadium.

"Jack, where are you?"

"On my way to Adkins, why?"

"Have you notice a shadow?"

"A what? What are you talkin' about?"

"Slight has someone tailing you, Lee and Mike. I just found out. Lee punched his tail in the face and the guy is pressing charges."

Jack looked in his rearview mirror. A long line of cars were behind him at a red light.

"Damn. What's this about?"

"Slight is trying to prove you guys are fuckin' up. And, he probably can by now. Lee's agent called me and said Lee knew the guy was following him for a least a week."

"Shit," Jack whispered. He tried to remember each of his moves the last week. "I haven't done shit in the past week."

"I hope not. I talked with Buffalo and I told them you refuse to play first, and they want you no matter what. I think you better start packing."

"You speak with Honeywell yet?"

"No. He hasn't returned my calls."

"Meet me at the stadium. We'll talk to him before the game."

Jack put down the phone and sped the car up. He screeched into the parking lot and bolted into the building. Reporters were waiting for him as he approached the clubhouse. The four men began slowly, asking about his health, then hit hard while Jack put on his uniform. Kristen stood to the side, waiting to catch Jack alone. Jack's short answers didn't please the journalists; he promised to say more after he talked with Honeywell.

Kris crept up behind Jack when the other reporters moved away. He was sitting on his stool, tying his cleats when he felt the light touch of Kris' hand on his shoulder. He looked up, knowing it had to be her, she was the only woman with a clubhouse pass.

"You think Slight is finally going to trade you?"

Jack bent back down to finish lacing. "I really don't know, Kristen."

"I heard you met a woman here, how's that going?"

Jack looked up into her eyes. "Excuse me?"

"No," she put her recorder and pad in her handbag. "This isn't for publication. I was just wondering if you had found Lady Right, like we had discussed."

"How did you hear about this?"

"Your teammates can't keep secrets."

"Well, I like her, but I am still getting to know her."

Oscar came into the clubhouse with a scowl. The reporters scurried to him, but he spewed venom, "Don't ask me shit! You bunch of asses!"

They quietly scattered, picking other players as soon the clubhouse became saturated with Crowns. Kris stepped back, as Oscar began stripping off his street clothes.

O glared at Jack. "Why didn't you call me back?"

"I had a date," Jack poured a lemon-lime Gatorade down his throat. He put on his maroon Crowns' warm-up jacket and put his batting gloves in his uniform pants pockets.

"With who?" Oscar began undressing.

"The one I told you about."

"Not that nonsexual one night stand?"

"Yeah. That one."

"Well, lover boy, did you hear about Lee?"

"Yeah."

"I would have done the same thing. Bust that Dick Tracy motherfucker in his private eye." Oscar pulled his under shirt over his head. "The youth movement has begun. I told you! If we had won last year, none of this shit would have been happening."

A reporter inched closer to them.

"Fuck off before I stab you with your own pen, asshole!" Oscar barked.

"Chill, O," Jack said.

Oscar hated reporters more than anything associated with baseball. He rarely spoke to one, unless another player recommended them. His attitude toward writers and other media types stems from an article written about him three season ago. He contends that the reporter misquoted him on purpose, the reporter denied it.

"Those mutherfuckas are like leeches! Look at 'em, trying to get something so they're editors will kiss them in the morning."

"Whatcha get on da niggers, Roscoe?" O mocked them. "Oh, we gots lots, Boss. They's makin' soooo much money!"

Oscar kicked his stool across the room, hitting Luis. He was aiming for Jim Nesbitt, from the Beaverton newspaper. Luis pushed the chair aside, saying something in Spanish.

"I ain't sorry!" O yelled. He then booted Jack's stool in the same direction, missing Luis and everybody else.

Jack shook his head, "Man, will you relax?"

"If they trade you to Buffalo, I'm quitting. Period!"

"Take it easy," Jack became agitated. "I ain't going nowhere. Just fucking relax, please?"

Berger sat in Honeywell's office quietly. He tried to discuss his client's position, how Jack loved Portland, how he wanted to end his career where he started it, how Jack had made his home here, how Jack had done everything asked of him. But, Honeywell didn't want to hear it.

Jack arrived and Honeywell began the meeting in a stern manner. "If Aponte produces, you're gone. End of discussion."

Berger had begun to reply, but Jack drowned him out, "Why you coming like that?"

"Jack, it's out of my hands. Slight wants to take the team in another direction."

"So, that's what the P.I.'s were all about?"

"For the most part, yes. Jack, I warned you in Phoenix. Your shit has stunk for too long and Slight hates the smell."

Berger finally cut in, "Not only was it unethical, but it violated my client's right to privacy."

Honeywell sat up behind his desk. "Do I care? Slight's office is down the hall. It's almost game time, gentlemen."

Berger stood slowly, then the other two men stood. Honeywell motioned to Jack, and he told Berger he'd meet him outside.

Honeywell bit one of his cigars. He lit it and the aroma engulfed the huge office quickly. He sat on his desk and grinned at Jack.

"I remember my first day on the job," he said, turning from Jack, and looking out across the field outside his window. "Slight told me, we don't win in five years, I lose my job. It's been seven years. And, we still haven't won.

"It's not just you Jack, Slight is putting everybody on alert. The message is straight up: defeat Las Vegas, or be out."

Honeywell blew smoke at his wall-to-wall window. "I don't plan on breaking out until I'm ready. If I were you, and you loved it here in Portland, I'd clean up my act.

"If you want to fuck, do it. But, learn some discretion, at least. Hanging with O is going to get you traded.

"Slight ain't gonna trade him."

# 17

Leonard Williams kept his eyes on the road yet his ears were focused on his cheerful passengers. He had expected to be chauffeuring weeping women. Instead Djuana and his daughter, Tia sat in the back of his Buick giggling as if they were teenagers again. Pregnancy is no joke, he fumed.

Tia was surprised at Djuana's joyous mood, also. But, she was happy to have her friend back to her old self. "So, details, details!" she forced her voice below that of the radio.

"He's something else, Tee. You know I can't pick 'em, but he makes me feel like I'm..." She almost said it. "I mean, he makes me feel so comfortable around him."

"Dee. You like him?"

Djuana blushed. "Yeah. He makes me forget and feel good about myself. Is that bad? No, right?"

"Naw, not at all. Did you tell him?"

"No. I can't. I mean, I wanted to."

"Djuana!"

Leonard looked back. Tia began whispering and he looked forward again.

He heard his daughter say, "Sooner or later he'll be able to tell for himself. Don't you think he should hear it from you?"

"I just want to enjoy the good feelings for a little while. Is that wrong?"

"Naw, girl, you deserve it. But be careful. Don't use him. It could get ugly. He's a pro athlete."

"Exactly. How do I know he's not trying to use me? He can get some anytime he wants. He might get some of this and dip."

"Don't prejudge."

Djuana was happy Tia said that. She blushed.

"I read in the newspaper that what he needs is to settle down, so I don't think he's trying to just get some. I believe him when he says he is looking to settle down."

"We're here," Leonard finally cut in. He wasn't fond of the conversation.

He parked in Dr. Oppen's gravel lot, at the side of his office-home. It was a short visit, as the doctor had explained they would be after the first. He weighed Djuana, took a urine sample and blood pressure. She complained of back and leg aches, and he told her it was normal and to lay down more often after work. He begged her to eat the right foods, and take in more carbohydrates and Vitamin D.

Leonard and Tia waited less than an hour before Djuana returned with two prescriptions for vitamins. Leonard watched through the rearview mirror every chance he got. He became angry as Tia rubbed Djuana's firm, expanded stomach. He mumbled to himself as the he drove. He thanked the Lord that it wasn't his baby with baby. He prayed Djuana would have the strength to make it, and in the same prayer, his daughter would get married soon.

Djuana relaxed with a large glass of Kool-Aid and a bag of potato chips. She sat in front of the television prepared to watch a movie on cable, but a news flash changed her agenda. She loved TBS, but hated June Franz. When the reporter, with the Valley Girl accent did sports, her voice would rise to an even more irritating tone.

Before Djuana could grab the remote, June Franz mentioned 'The latest on the Jack Newhouse trade-rumor saga that now said Jack could be going to Buffalo as soon as the weekend because he was asked to miss a road trip. She said he was left behind because of his injury, but some felt otherwise.

Djuana was so disturbed she jumped from the couch and searched her handbag for Jack's number. Seconds later she was dialing. She listen to the rings, anxiously hoping he would be there. Jack answered in the same hoarse, baritone voice she enjoyed fantasizing about.

"Hi Jack, this is Djuana. I hope I didn't wake you?"

Jack pushed his way out of the bed. Stacie asked if it was Vivian, Jack quickly put his finger to his lips to hush her.

"No. Djuana, I'm up. I was just laying down." He sat up, hoping she didn't hear Stacie.

"I just heard that you didn't travel with the team. Is everything okay?"

"I hope so. I mean, I feel like everything will be fine."

"Is it true you may get traded?"

"That's a good question, I sure hope not," Jack muffled a squeal into a groan. Stacie had pinched his buttocks.

Djuana wondered, but didn't ask. "Me neither," she said. "I still haven't seen you play in person."

Jack smiled. He felt Stacie's hand slide under his arm and between his legs. "Ah, Djuana, can I call you back? I was about to grab something to eat."

"Sure, but I was wondering if you were interested in tasting my cooking. I made some homemade chicken soup, and my mom says it can heal any ailment."

Stacie pulled herself to Jack and engulfed his penis into her mouth. Jack hesitated, then pushed her away, and stood up.

He answered Djuana, "That sounds good, do you want me to drive over there?"

"No. I'll come out there," Djuana scrambled for paper and a pen. "Give me the directions."

Of all the Crowns Stacie had sex with in her three years living in Portland, Jack and Don Cruz were the more brutish in bed, and she liked it like that. But she had to stop calling Don; his wife, Liela, boxed Stacie's face pretty bad after their last encounter.

Jack, on the other hand, would stop seeing Stacie if he was in a serious relationship - although they spent a few nights in bed together during his turbulent period with Vivian. Stacie respected this about Jack - that was the reason she would often tell him that she would marry him. Jack would laugh and reply, "That's nice, but I don't think so."

Stacie had grown tired of hearing no from the Crowns, Jack in particular. Lee Spencer would say yes anytime, but he was too much of a coke head. No other Crown would touch her. She did have success with visiting baseball players, and members of Portland's professional basketball team in the winter.

Jack looked over at Stacie sprawled out across his bed. She was all ass, no chest and not pretty, but she sure was talented in the bed. Jack closed his eyes, he felt weak. Why hadn't he stuck to his plan? He was supposed to wait for Djuana. He shook his head in disgust at the sight of Stacie fingering herself. He turned his head.

"Get up, it's time to go," he sternly told Stacie.

She was not ready to leave. "Who is this you dumping me for?" she asked.

"Not you worry, lady. Just beat it."

"Well, I don't have any cab fare, you driving me?"

Jack went to his wallet, tossed her a twenty, then called a cab.

"Damn. This must be somebody special, usually I get a five and shown the door!"

"Whatever. Just start stepping."

Djuana called Tia as soon as her phone cleared. Tia was doing a paper for school and was happy for the distraction. Djuana asked her to drive her to Southwest Portland.

"They think he's going to be traded real soon!"

Tia was careful not to sound as careless as she was. She thought her friend had enough to worry about. "Those are just rumors, like the news report said. Why don't you call him?"

"Yeah, I did. You gonna drive me or what? I don't want to go over there alone."

Tia needed a break. She also wanted to meet Jack Newhouse. "Okay, I'll ask Dad, he'll say yeah, then I'll be over there in about an hour. I've got to get dressed."

"No rush, I told him that I made some chicken soup from scratch. Well, it ain't exactly done yet."

Tia laughed. "No you didn't."

"Yeah. I did. I'ma start it right now. Call me when you are on your way."

Stacie was long gone, but Jack still felt uneasy. Women can tell, he worried. He popped the top off of the Lysol and sprayed again. He looked over his bedroom - he hoped the evening ended in there - and all seemed in tact. Jack gathered up his collection of X-rated videos and tossed them down the steps leading into the garage. He set up his compact disc player with six different artist - all smooth.

The bathroom! He had almost forgot. He dashed through the house and barged into the large cubicle. He snatched down Stacie's towel and wash cloth and dumped them in the laundry room out back.

"Anything else? Anything else?" He was near panic. Finally, the headlights of a car glared into his living room from the driveway.

Djuana almost lost her breathe from anxiety. Tia laughed, then became worried.

"You okay?"

Djuana patted her chest. "Yeah. I guess it's been a long time since I've done this. Let's wait a second."

Tia looked up the steps and saw him first. "I don't think we can. He's heeere!"

Djuana looked up wide-eyed. Jack walked to her door, the car was nose-first in the driveway and the passenger's side of the car faced his walkway.

Jack opened her door. "Hey. How was the trip?"

"It was shaky a bit, but once we got off the highway I sorta remembered."

Tia stood out of the car. Djuana looked to her, they both smiled. "Jack, this is my best friend, Tia Williams."

Jack met her at the trunk and shook her hand, "It's a pleasure," he said. Djuana went in the back of the car and got the chicken soup. "So, that's the good stuff, huh?" Jack said as he lead them up to the house.

Djuana grinned and muttered a yes. Tia, walking up the steps behind her, pinched her plump butt. Djuana jerked her head back to see her friend giving the sign of her approval. Once inside, Djuana let Jack know they wouldn't stay long.

He took the soup and put it in the refrigerator and offered them snacks. Tia accepted a glass of iced tea, and Djuana took the tea and some pretzels.

They sat in the spacious, high-ceiling living room, Tia looking around like a tourist. Djuana was uneasy that she remembered so much of the layout. The plush wall-to-wall rug was as she cushioned as she recalled. She had an urge to remove her shoes. The couch was dark green and leather. There was two leather recliners and an exotic glass coffee table. No of this Djuana remembered.

Then, the phone began to ring. First it was Jack's agent, a quick call. Vivian called within seconds to tell Jack she had a dream about him.

"Are you doing okay?" she asked.

"Fine. What do you want?" Jack asked, standing by the entrance of the living room with the cordless.

"I dreamt that you were stabbed."

"I'm fine. Listen. I have company..."

Vivian abruptly hung up.

"The phone hadn't rang in hours," he pleaded with his two guests. They both smiled, then looked at one another. Djuana was concerned when the phone rang again. It was Oscar's wife looking for him. After Jack said he wasn't there, she tried to begin a conversation.

"Sondra, can I call you back?" Jack asked.

"Oh, you've got company?" She said in a confrontational manner.

"Yes. I'll call you later," Jack was exasperated.

"Is Oscar there? Are you two fucking together again? Why you doing this to me, Jack? Why?"

Sweat formed on Jack's brow. "Listen, So', it ain't like that at all. He is not here. The team left Portland for the Midwest. I wasn't invited."

Sondra began to cry. "Shit. I'm sorry, Jack. That man has me all mixed up. I don't know whether I'm coming or going."

Tia again looked over at Djuana. Djuana was concerned, but hid it from her expressions. She sipped her iced tea and took in more of her dream home. She pictured hosting her friends from uptown her in the valley. Oh, they would fry green with envy, she gushed.

Less than an hour after they arrived, Djuana stood to announce they were leaving. Tia rose after her and told Jack it was nice meeting him. He said likewise.

At the door, Tia darted down the steps, saying goodnight.

Djuana stopped at the landing, "It was nice seeing you again. I hope you like the soup."

Jack stood close to her, "Maybe we can get together soon?"

"Maybe. I'll call you."

Jack touched her hand, lowering his voice he said, "Thanks for coming out here to bring me your remedy. I'm sure it will be delicious."

"Be honest with me," she leaned closer. Jack wanted to bite her cheek and suck it. But he forced himself to hear her so he could answer.

"Did you touch me that night?"

Jack felt at ease, not only because he hadn't done anything wrong, but because of Djuana's light smirk.

"You know I didn't. And you know I sure could have."

Djuana stared at Jack's somber expression. She sobered. "I don't know why I trust you."

Jack took her hand, rubbing his thumb over her soft knuckles. His touch was more gentle than any Djuana had ever felt.

"Maybe 'cause I earned it," he whispered.

Djuana reached to his height with her lips leading the way and Jack accepted her into his arms. He kissed her lightly, but her tongue pierced his mouth with such force that it startled him. He held her closer, his arms around her ribs and hands at her waist. He tried to get her to kiss in a slow rhythm.

Djuana slid her arms around his neck and held on. When his tongue slowed, she licked his lips and searched his mouth, kissing him with passion.

Tia's mouth dropped open. She unconsciously licked her lips and shook her head.

"Wow," she muttered. "Damn, girl."

Djuana returned to the car with a plop into the seat and a slam of the door.

Tia was still amazed. "Damn, DJ. What up with that?"

Djuana looked up at Jack on the steps waving. She waved. "Let's split."

The car zipped out of the driveway and back the way it came. Tia reframed from the questions burning her lips. She looked over at her best friend and admired the way Jack had returned to Djuana the pleasure of a smile.

When Djuana got home she called Jack to let him know they arrived safely. They began to talk, neither wanting to be alone. Jack had felt lonely as soon as the car pulled out. His teammates were on the rode without him for the first time in his career. Before Djuana called, a reporter called and nagged Jack with questions about his pending trade. Djuana's voice and the refreshing way she didn't speak about baseball were welcome.

Djuana wanted to avoid being lonely also. Tia asked to spend the night, and that would have been nice, but Djuana planned to talk with Jack for a while and knew that would be awkward with Tia around. Djuana came in, dropped her jacket on her bed, and dialed Jack's number in seconds. Jack had just finished heating up the soup.

"It tastes really good. I like the seasoning," he said between spoonfuls.

Djuana was proud. She gleamed a blushing smile from ear to ear. It was nearing 1 a.m. when the conversation began with Djuana doing the most talking. But, she worked to getting the discussion on him. And, she found, Jack's family was large, yet not as close-knit as hers.

When Jack talked of his mother, he was vibrant and lively. Djuana had thought the topic would be morbid. She told him how she read about her death in a magazine.

But, he explained, his mother wouldn't want him mourning her forever.

"My mother didn't want me to play baseball for a living," Jack told. "Sheez, she wanted me to get a city job, get married and that sort of thing right in New York. To never leave and have my family right there in front of her for her to enjoy! "

Djuana laughed. "That would have been nice, too," she began undressing and was to her underwear, shifting the phone from ear to ear.

"Yeah, for her. I hope she's up there proud anyway."

"But, I'm sure she's bragging to all the other Angels about you and your admirable accomplishments."

Jack smiled at the thought. "Yeah. Probably so."

"You have a sister in New York, right?"

"Yeah. She lives in Queens," Jack spooned through the large pieces of vegetables and chicken and sipped more broth. The taste pleased his grumbling belly.

"She's two years younger, right?" Djuana was remembering the article.

"Where was this story? In *Jet* ?"

Djuana sucked her teeth. "No! Women read sports magazines also, you know."

Jack laughed.

"Hold on for a second, please?" Djuana pulled the brand new Crowns t-shirt with Jack's number on the back carefully over her hair. She got the rollers out of her top draw then flopped on the bed. When she retained the phone, Jack asked her if she was getting ready for bed.

The question caught Djuana off guard. She wondered what he might be thinking. "Yeah. I've changed and am rolling my hair now."

"Hmm." Jack was wondering what she was wearing - he dared not ask.

"What was that for?"

"Nothing. Just enjoying your soup."

Djuana didn't believe him.

Jack quickly changed the subject; Djuana would never forget, though.

He asked her about her plans for the upcoming day. She had none, so they set up a movie date in the late afternoon. Jack said he'd call.

"Thanks again for the soup. It was great. I hope I can get you to cook for me again soon."

"Maybe. If you play your cards right," Djuana said, holding the phone on her shoulder and rolling her hair in the mirror. "The soup was nothing. I hope it went straight to your head so you can get back to playing."

"Oh, it did. I feel much better."

Neither went directly to sleep after hanging up. Both, more so Djuana, had an urge to call back just to say good night again.

# 18

Before Jack could get himself to sleep; dreaming Djuana was in the bed with him, Oscar phoned. He was in his hotel room in Milwaukee with a woman he and Jack had once enjoyed together. It was 4 a.m. in Portland, and 6 a.m. in Milwaukee.

"If you get traded, Blood, I'm dead," Oscar said, voice hoarse, and a limp body on top of him.

"Ain't gonna happen," Jack said, almost wishing. "So' called last night. Call her, man."

Silence.

"Oscar. I know your ass heard me."

"Look, I ain't got the time to be worrying about that bitch."

"Why she got to be all that?"

"Fuck it. Next subject. What you doing tonight? Watching me?"

Jack sighed, then went on with the program. "Not. I got a date."

"Oh yeah? I hope you ain't screwing none of my hoes!"

"Not. I'm taking out Djuana, the one I've been telling you about."

"Djuana? What a name. So, now you two are an item?"

"Kinda, sorta. She brought me some soup last night."

Oscar sat up, moving the girl aside, "Get outta town! You finally hit it?"

"Nope."

"You bitch-ass! No, tell me you getting it tonight."

"It ain't like that. I really like her. I plan to see what she's about."

"Spare me. So where you taking her?"

"The movies and then dinner."

"The movies? What, are y'all teenie-boppers?"

"Maybe."

Djuana was dressed and ready by 5:30; a half hour early and a record for her. Seven years of dating the same chronically late man had instilled bad habits. She looked in the full-length mirror for a third time - the more she looked, the more she killed her decision-making skills. The jeans just didn't fit right, she grumbled. The red sweater had too much lint. She changed clothes.

In the kitchen, Emma was smoking a cigarette out of the window; Djuana had told her not to smoke in the apartment because of the baby. She really needed a drink. The thought of her pregnant daughter going out on a date with a baseball player seemed ridiculous to her.

Djuana sprinted in the kitchen. "Do these jeans look too tight?" She asked her mother.

Emma puffed deeply and blew out of the window. "What was wrong with the others?"

"I know you ain't smoking?"

Emma dropped the cigarette on the window seal and blew more smoke out of the window. "Of course not. Come here."

She inspected the jeans, lifting up Djuana's t-shirt. There was little space between the jeans and Djuana's belly. "Do they feel tight?"

"No."

"Well, just don't eat too much or Junior will bust these pants open. Speaking of that, what does this baseball player think of you being with child?"

"Mom, he doesn't know. And I plan to tell him, so please don't mention it."

Emma smirked, "Scandalous. What's the deal here?"

"No deal, Mother. He is just a friend who asked me out on a date. And I feel like I need it." Djuana shook her head at the questions. "I am going to wear the stirrups."

Emma just nodded. When her daughter was gone to change, she relit the cigarette.

Devon was more excited than his sister. He had worshipped the Crowns for as long as he could remember, but never saw one in person; not counting the time Bingo snubbed him and his buddies. They had waited outside of Adkins Stadium for autographs after a day game two years ago. But the players hurried to their cars and left without notice. They picked an expensive car and sat on it, awaiting its owner. Bingo waltzed out with his wife, and pushed them off his ride.

Devon barked to Bingo he loved him and the Crowns, to which Bingo replied, "You should."

Devon understood Jack would just pull up and Djuana would get in and they would leave, yet he was preparing for a quick glimpse. He planned to ask Jack to autograph his poster of the team, so he took it off the wall and raced into the kitchen, where he hunted for a pen.

"Where's the marker, Ma?"

Emma looked him over, "For what? So you can draw a damn mustache on the man's picture?"

"No! Of course not. I'ma get him to sign it."

"Please. I thought you were all crazy about the other Crown, Wango, Pango, whatever the hell his name is."

Devon laughed at his mother's ignorance while tearing up the utility draw. "Bingo. Bingo, Ma. Yeah, he's my favorite, but in the meantime, I'll get J-New's autograph. I mean, it is worth money you know."

"Oh, my. Then you better have him sign this napkin for you poor old mother, too." She chuckled.

"Har-har! You're a riot, Alice," Devon said, mocking his mother.

Jack was trying to speed across town to avoid being late, but he ran into Friday afternoon rush hour traffic. He glanced at his dash board clock and muttered a curse. His impromptu stop to buy roses threw him off time; after buying the roses, Jack took them to Atwater's restaurant, where he planned to take Djuana for dinner.

Jack picked up his cell-phone and called Djuana. As the phone rang he was amazed that he had set the number to memory that quickly. An older sounding woman answered and put Djuana on the phone. Jack apologized for being behind schedule.

Jack said to Djuana, "I should be there in about ten minutes."

"That's fine. Are the directions okay?"

He didn't want to tell her he had already been there, camped out for her like a love-sick teenager. "Sure. It's apartment 3B, right?"

"Yes, but you don't have to come up, I'll met you down stairs."

"No, that wouldn't be right the first time I come by. I'll come up."

He was right, and Djuana was charmed by his thoughtfulness and respect.

Jack slowed his Pathfinder along the parked cars on Tudor. He double parked, removed the key and slid out of the car. Before locking his doors, he went into the rear of the wagon and removed a colorful bouquet of flowers.

He briskly walked to the entrance of the building. He couldn't help but notice the jamming sounds coming from Tudor Park. Hip-hop was being blared from huge speakers. The unusually humid May day had brought out the hibernating for an informal Friday night block party. Many freshly washed automobiles were stationed three deep at the mouth of the park. The sight brought back fond memories to Jack, who had grown up in New York going to 'jams' in concrete parks.

Devon was leaning most of his body out of the window, trying to see into Tudor Park from the living room window. He was really looking for Jack. The window was one of two in the apartment that faced the avenue - the other was being manned by Emma in the kitchen. Devon spotted the Pathfinder pull up, thinking it was another neighborhood drug dealer until he saw the familiar frame.

"He's here! He's here!" Devon bellowed throughout the apartment. The shrieks sent a lump up into Djuana's throat. She was in her bedroom talking to the mirror.

Devon snatched up the poster and fine point pen - he gave up looking for the marker - and ran into Djuana's room.

"Chill! Everybody chill! He'll be up here in a minute!" Devon put on his Crowns baseball cap and ran back through the apartment shouting, "This is not a drill! Repeat! This is not a drill!"

Emma glared at her frantic brat and shook her head, saying, "You want a breath mint?"

She then yelled to her other child to shut up her brother.

Djuana's nerves turned her stomach, or was it the baby? She asked Devon to calm down as she walked through the apartment. She looked into the foyer's mirror and smirked, "Here we go."

She didn't believe so, but she looked radiant. She wore a poly-Lycra black body suit, a hunter green vest adorned with multicolored sequins and bugle beads on the front, and faded blue jeans. The sassy, one-inch gold, fuchsia and green beaded shoes matched the vest. The shoes were also very comfortable.

Then the knock came. Devon first froze, then dove for the front door. Djuana pulled him back, and pushed him into the living room. Djuana opened the door and was greeted by Jack's warm smile and a bright array of flowers. Her nerves ceased. He was unreal, was her first impression. She welcomed him in, and he walked into the living room. Devon was standing, all smiles. Jack noticed the wide entrance to the spotless kitchen on his right. The wall blocked the sight of Emma still seated at the window.

He felt welcomed. Djuana followed him in and introduced Jack to Devon.

"Your my favorite baseball player in the world," the boy said blushing.

Djuana laughed, "Oh really?"

"Dee!"

Jack intervened, "As long as you like the Crowns. Then you're okay by me." He turned to Djuana and offered the flowers. "These are for your mother."

Damn, Djuana thought. Her mother hadn't received flowers in years. She moved past Jack and leaned into the kitchen and whispered to her mother, "Come and say hello."

Emma rolled her eyes. She rose her round body defiantly and waltzed into the living room. He was handsome, was her first impression. She almost smiled, but was too stubborn. She allowed him to shake her hand while her daughter verbally introduced them. "He don't look rich," Emma said.

Djuana fumed, giving her mother the eye.

"Thanks for the flowers," Emma said blankly. "Have a seat."

Jack looked at his watch and said. "I hate to rush us off, but we are a little behind schedule thanks to me."

Djuana took the cue. She said she was ready. Devon kicked her foot, not hard, but the surprise made her jump. "Devo!"

He whispered mumbles and frantically waved the poster. Djuana devilishly glared at her little pain of a sibling.

"Jack, I hope it isn't an inconvenience, but my brother would like you to sign his poster."

"No problem." Jack took the poster to the coffee table, followed by Devon.

"Put 'to my best pal, Devo' who I will see in the majors one day'. No love stuff!" Devon laughed.

Jack smiled, and did as asked. Devon thanked him and aggressively asked about going to a game, Jack said sure. Devon quickly came up with dates.

"Next Sunday is bat day. Then there's ball day - I really don't need a ball - and then helmet day and..."

Djuana shut him off with a shove, "That's enough. You freeloader."

Jack smiled.

Emma had disappeared into the kitchen to put her flowers in a vase. She reappeared and put the vase on the coffee table, shoving Devon poster to the side.

"We have to go," Djuana announced.

Emma retorted, "Have a nice time. And come home. Tonight."

Djuana shuddered. Jack kept his grin. Devon, the comment over his head, raced to the back of the apartment with his poster.

"I gotta call somebody!" the child yelled.

# 19

The date was all Djuana hoped it would be - but was afraid to wish for. The movie theater was crowded, as was expected on an opening Friday night of a movie with African American stars. But when an usher recognized Jack, they were escorted in ahead of many people and seated. Jack offered the young man a $10 bill to cover the tickets, but he declined, only saying, "Just get better and win us a championship, New."

Jack went back into the lobby and got them popcorn, soda and Djuana's favorite: Goobers. It took him a while because he stopped to sign

Neither one had been to the movies since the previous summer. Jack was busy traveling. Djuana just had no desire. The movie was long, an action-thriller with big name stars. Jack wanted to see a comedy that was premiering that night, but Djuana won out.

When the lights went out, and the coming attractions began, Jack warned Djuana not to try anything. That silly statement loosened her up, and was the key to the evening. Jack was playful and in a extraordinarily good mood. His problems, the Crowns, were in Milwaukee.

The first time Jack tried to feed Djuana popcorn, she bristled. She was not accustomed to the playfulness. Usually, with Dexter of course, it was 'watch the movie and be quiet.' Seconds later, feeling like she should loosen up, she put a Goober to his lips. Jack held her hand, kiss it, then took the candy with his tongue.

"All I get is one," he asked.

"They're mine," she replied.

They played through most of the movie. Jack ate popcorn off her shoulder. Djuana fed him Goobers one by one. Neither one could review the movie, all they knew was who played in it, and how it ended.

Jack said dinner would be a special surprise, and it was. They crossed the river into Northeast Portland, and parked on Fifth. Getting out the truck, Djuana scanned the immediate area with a quick turn of her head. She could not remember a restaurant being near this lot. They walked a block toward the pale-pink US. Bancorp Tower. She knew then, and her heart skipped a beat.

In the elevator she asked, starry-eyed, "We're going to Atwater's?"

"Yeah," Jack frowned. "Don't tell me you don't like it."

"Are you kidding? I always wanted to eat here." She did, and each year on her birthday, Valentine's Day and any other couple's holiday, Dexter would promise to take her.

Atwater's was one of the most expensive restaurants in Portland. It featured live jazz and Pacific Northwest cuisine.

The elevator's doors opened on the thirtieth floor and the sight stunned Djuana. A rosy light saturated the hall. Oriental rugs, covering hardwood floors greeted her feet as she walked blindly behind Jack. She looked beyond him, into the elegant eatery. In the middle of the room was a glass-enclosed winery. She was in awe. She felt the diners were eating with class, speaking yet not being heard. Not many of her friends could handle such an atmosphere.

Djuana looked down at her jeans. She tugged Jack's jacket, "I can't go in there," she whispered. "I am under dressed."

"No," he turned to her and kissed her forehead. "You're beautiful."

The Maitre 'D, wearing a bow tie and red jacket, greeted the handsome couple with a sincere smile and handshake.

"Mr. Newhouse, you table is awaiting." He lead them to a table at the base of a window through the silent eaters. None of the women enjoying Atwater's had on pants, Djuana noticed. As soon as they arrived at the table, Djuana took in the view out of the spotless windows. From their seats, the sights were breathtaking. Below them was the Willamette River and all of south Portland. The antique wooden chairs were very comfortable with cushions on the arms as well as back and seat. Everything was white; the table cloths, the china, the paint jobs and the diners.

A short, stern-looking tanned gentleman, came to their table. Jack rose to shake his hand and they hugged.

"My good friend," the man said with a rich French accent between hugs.

"Marcel, I want you to meet a very elegant lady," Jack swooped his hand in the direction of Djuana. "My date, Djuana Pioneer."

Marcel halted the introductions. "Ah, you are a marvelous player of baseball, but you are poor when it comes to descriptions."

Djuana soaked in the sound of Marcel's voice. It reminded her of the tourist who came into Delux's. She wished she had mastered a foreign language. Marcel took Djuana's hand, bent with his legs straight, and kissed it. She could see the other diners stop to watch.

"My name is Marcel Dion. I am the manager. You, my lady, are more beautiful than any woman I have had the privilege of hosting."

Djuana fought a blush. "Thank you very much. You have a wonderful place."

"And you have brightened it. Anything you want, you call me."

Marcel called over the waiter, a young, cheery soul that had been standing by the door. They began conversing in French, Djuana could tell that Marcel was giving precise, stern orders.

The waiter ran through the restaurant and came back with a dozen of roses. He handed them to Marcel, who handed them to Jack.

"These are for you," Jack said as he sat.

Djuana took them into her hands. "Thanks," was all she could say. She marvel at the tight, rich canary yellow bulbs, and flowery stems.

Jack and Marcel again conversed in French.

"You do like salmon?" Jack turned and said across the table.

Djuana just nodded. The manager and the waiter disappeared into the large restaurant.

"Marcel is making sure you have the best meal of your life," Jack said as he leaned on the table.

"And, you have nothing to do with this," Djuana smirked.

"Actually, no. I told him that I was bringing a special date, but I didn't think they would go out of their way like this."

"He likes you."

Djuana felt more pleased with herself than ever. She looked around, and heads were turning away. She shook her head in amazement.

"Everything okay?" Jack asked.

"Are you kidding? This is my dream come true," she stopped herself. "Do I sound ignorant?"

"No. Not at all."

Djuana could not fight off the negative thoughts. "I bet you probably bring a bunch of women here, and they are all treated like this."

Jack straightened. His smile vanished. "I have never brought a date here before."

Djuana felt saddened. From the moment she had gotten into his car that night, she just knew something was going to destroy the date, a night out with a gentleman. And, she knew, more than likely, it would be her.

Jack continued, "What you think, I've been here a million times? Well, I haven't. This is only my second time. Marcel comes to a lot of games. He and the owner of the team are good friends. He loves having ballplayers eat here."

"But," Djuana pointed out, "I can tell he respects you."

Jack nodded in agreement. "I guess so. But," Jack took her hands into his. "Right now, he respects you more. You're better looking than me."

The sudden appearance of a woman cut the moment short. And, Djuana recognized the pale skinned, golden blonde from television and the newspaper. Portland's leading lady, Mayor Ann Meier had a distinctive air of royalty about her, and the respect of an entire state. She had the features of a model - 5 foot 11, rail thin but curved, and always dress in designer skirt suits. And, she was born into a family tree of an heiress. She was also intelligent, approachable and very family and community oriented. There was no woman in Portland, black or white, that hadn't for a second wanted to be Ann Meier.

And, Djuana was among them.

The mayor took Jack's hand, and he rose, smiling. Mayor Meier kissed his cheek.

"Jack, why don't you call me?"

Djuana was flabbergasted.

"Mayor, it has been a long season, already."

Ann Meier smiled. "Yes, Jack. I have heard. And, stop calling me mayor." She looked down at Djuana, still smiling broadly.

Jack crossed between them, "Ann, I want you to meet a wonderful young lady, Djuana Pioneer."

Mayor Meier took Djuana's hand, thumb on her knuckles, and Djuana instinctively began to rise.

"No," the mayor protested with a frown. "Don't get up. I'm sorry I interrupted your dinner. I just had to come over and say hello, and meet the just gorgeous date my favorite baseball player has here."

"Thank you," Djuana blushed.

"You are a lovely lady, and you are blessed with a fine companion in Jack Newhouse."

"Cut it out, Ann. Your kids aren't getting into the clubhouse anymore."

Djuana was again take aback. She couldn't believe Jack was speaking that way to the mayor.

"Listen, Jack. You do want to be able to drive that Pathfinder around the city without problems?"

Djuana selected a CD and put it into the truck's elaborate stereo. She was thrilled to have learned to use it so quickly. She sat back and relaxed. Jack was driving her home from the best date of her life. She took in all of the night's events in one deep, refreshing, breath. It was 1:30 a.m., still early, yet she felt as if she was out all night. She felt nervous, scared and exhilarated all at once.

Jack Newhouse was being the gentleman Djuana wanted a man to be to her. He was also showing her the complete package that she and Tia had said determined the perfect man. He was kind, thoughtful, tall, strong, athletic, assertive and a gentleman. And, importantly, Jack was interested. Perfect.

Jack was winning her heart — and he had no clue — in a way that made her feel she gave her virginity to the wrong man-although she didn't need anyone to point that out. For a second, that night, she wondered if Jack would change after he got some. Probably. Could be that is all he's after. If it was, she decided, so what? He was giving her all she wanted. He was providing a great escape from the Hell of a reality she had to live.

The thought of sex with Jack was a burning desire. She had to fight the urge that night to ask him to take her home. She needed it like never before. It must be the baby, she reasoned; only because she could not remember being so horny. She smiled to herself at the thought. She cuddled in her seat, her head pressed to the window.

Jack tried to keep his attention on the road, but Djuana's sudden movements, and smiling and cooing divided his concentration. He saw that she had folded her arms across her chest.

"You cold?" he asked.

"A little," she answered. The warm day's temperature dropped drastically with the sun. Jack flicked on the heat.

"And attentive," she whispered to herself; finishing off his assets.

Jack heard, but not clearly. "Listen," he said. "If I keep giving you pennies for your thoughts I'd go broke. So, what's up?"

Djuana smiled. "What, you worried I'm thinking something negative?"

"Are you? Did you have a good time tonight?"

"Please. Good time? Yeah, I really enjoyed myself." Djuana sat upright, and turned down Gerald LeVert. "Okay. Let's talk. Can you answer a kinda deep question?"

Ugh, oh. Jack thought. "Yeah, kinda."

"Seriously," her smile evaporated. "A serious topic."

Jack followed her lead and sobered. He pulled the Pathfinder off of Burnside Street, just before the bridge, parking along side of the pier. Djuana looked around, at first apprehensive, and was at ease with the solitude.

"So what do you want to know?" Jack asked.

Djuana hit right in, "What do you want from me. Exactly?"

Jack looked out across the Willamette. The answer was on the tip of his tongue. He just paused before answering to be sure he should say. He thought he should.

"It's you I want," he began. "I have thought about exactly that, 'what do I want from her?' and I feel really good with you. So far, you've been all I want in a woman. I enjoy your smile and I'm crazy about those eyes."

Djuana's eyes had been riveted to Jack's lips while he spoke. She wanted to believe to him, but experience forced her to be skeptical. Still, she felt flattered. When he was through she slowly turned her eyes out to the lights on the other pier.

"Jack," her eyes dimmed suddenly, as if sleep was her foremost thought. She looked him in the face. Her voice was augmented by her frown. "You have been very sweet, and especially nice, to me."

"But?" Jack muttered, thinking he knew what was coming next.

Djuana lightly smiled, "No buts." She sat back, her eyes fixed downward on her fingers tugging her pants' inseam.

She said, "It's just that this has all been a bit overwhelming."

"You want me to slow us down?"

Djuana looked into his eyes, "Not if it means us seeing less of one another."

Jack took her hand and kissed it. "No problem with that."

Djuana sobered. She had suddenly thought of the stories she had heard about all the women he had conquered. She sat up, away from him. It seemed like she was suddenly repelling.

"Jack, answer me this."

Jack put the weight of his body on the steering wheel using his left side. He sat upright.

"What is it?" he asked flatly.

"It not like I want to have sex with you tomorrow or anytime soon, but would you take an AIDS test if I asked you to?"

He flinched. "Yeah. I would. Is that what you want?"

"Yes. For my sake." She almost said for her baby's sake.

Jack had to force his smile to remain on his face. He glanced beyond her head and into the water. All the times he and Oscar had screwed women unprotected flashed before his eyes. He had never taken and AIDS test, and maybe she was right. What if he was affected?

Djuana relaxed. She longed for one of his hugs; to be held deeply into his chest would help ease her guilt — she should be telling him right now that this woman he cared for ain't all that. I'm a hoe! She wanted to blab. A pregnant fool who needs your love more than you know. That's what she wanted to say.

After yet another deep breathe, she went on. "You don't know me, Jack. You don't."

He tried to cut in, but she was on a roll. She looked up at him; he was there, listening. "If I tell you something about me, you wouldn't want me anymore. Something big."

"I know all I need to, all I care about is your present and future." That was not what he wanted to say. He had felt she was more serious with the man she was dating, the one that left her in the rain crying. Left her alone at night. The one that seems to be hurting her. He wanted to ask her what was up with him.

Djuana liked his answer. But the guilt didn't cease. "I'm using you, Jack. I know I am, but you've made me feel so happy and relieved. You've helped me get away, yet still be there. You understand?"

Jack nodded, thinking, all right now, tell me already. He could see the pain of the conversation wearing on Djuana, so he eased off. He did, however, respect her solid attempts at communicating. Vivian, four years older than she, could learn from her.

Djuana continued, "I like you, Jack. But I don't want to mislead you. I need nights like this, but I am not near ready to take us any further than this."

Jack expected as much and felt she was worth working at a relationship with. "Hey, that's cool with me. So. why don't we just enjoy ourselves and each other and go from there. What ever happens, happens."

She smiled, "That would be good for me."

Jack touched her lips lightly with his right pointer finger. "That's what I want. You to smile." He kissed her delicately, and quickly.

Djuana would have let him kiss her for hours. She loved him; she was sure now. She knew he was the man she wanted. She couldn't remember the last man that could make her as content when she felt low.

"You okay?" Jack asked, his face still inches from hers.

She smiled, and licked her wet lips. "Sure."

"Ready to go home?"

"Yes."

Jack ignited the car and resumed to the bridge. "Good. Your mother will kill me if I keep you out too late."

"Please."

# 20

When Vincent Slight called meetings between himself, his general manager and his manager, it was never for pats on the back. Usually, it was because Slight was on edge. This time the Crowns had fallen into last place for the first time in four years. He wanted to make a blockbuster trade, something to shake up his team, something to show the rest of the baseball world he was still the man.

He had to win a championship that year. He dreaded watching Len Canisa drink and waste champagne with his Gamblers team again. Last year they poured the bubbly on Adkins Stadium's infield during their celebration. Never again, he vowed. He promised to spit 40-year-old scotch on Canisa's MoneyDome artificial turf.

But making a mega-trade was difficult for Slight. He may have owned some of the best talent outside of Las Vegas, but no other team in the league respected him as a baseball man. On the other side of the ledger, he had the most respected general manager in the game in Honeywell. When Honeywell called an opposing GM, that person would look deeply into the proposed deal, fearing Honeywell knew something he should.

And, Honeywell was not about to deal anyone from the Crowns roster. He had faith in the team; he had put them together. He told Slight to let them play, citing the rookie, Aponte and the investigations as distractions.

Aponte had become a fan favorite, though, thanks to his quick start in front of the home fans and Slight prodding the media. In the 20-year-old's first three games, all in Portland, he had 10 hits and knocked in 11 runs. Bingo, hitting behind him, also flourished. Aponte received a standing ovation after hitting his first major league home run, a streaking shot that landed in the bleachers seconds after he swung.

But when the Crowns went on the road, 12 games in 14 days, Aponte evaporated. He had no hits on the trip and three errors. The slump prompted Slight's manager, Hal Juris, to say he had seen enough of Aponte.

"The kid is overmatched," he said during the Crowns' meeting of the minds.

During Juris' six years running the Crowns on the field for Slight, he had never questioned any moves by Honeywell or Slight. If they asked him, though, he was then very verbal. Juris, a six-foot-seven ex-terror on the field in his playing days, was now one of the best managers in the game. He was serious and unyielding in his approach to the game. His forte was handling ball players; and to his credit, he had done a great job holding together the cantankerous Crowns. To his credit, also, was his love for drinking and partying. Those qualities made him a peer as well as a mentor to the players.

The more Juris spoke in favor of sending Aponte back to the minors, the more Slight became animated.

"The kid started on fire, but they caught up to his ass real quick," Juris said. "He needs more seasoning."

Slight would look over at Honeywell every so often while Juris ranted. Honeywell was tightlipped. Honeywell had been standing between the two for Slight, and now he was going to let Juris have his say.

Slight first tried reasoning with Juris, explaining his position.

"I'm trying to change the image of this team. We have to do something different if we expect to beat L.V. And, image is a good place to start. The Gamblers are class all the way."

"Gee Moe Christmas!" Juris went ballistic, throwing his Crowns cap to the carpet. "To hell with image! Don't take apart my team and leave me with Bible reading pussies. Don't do it to me!"

Slight's voice elevated. He leaped from behind his desk. "Your team!!" Tact left his posture, "Fuck you! Your image is just as bad! So, maybe that's why the players drink like fish, screw like rabbits and act like heathens, because they are lead by an alcoholic!"

Juris stood to all his six-foot-seven inch frame, towering over Slight. Honeywell covered his face with one hand, he had seen Juris this angry before and he worried for the health of his boss.

"Well, image this," Juris bellowed. "Fuck you and your mighty plans. I quit." He twirled without grace and headed for the door. It slammed behind him; he slammed every door he faced on his way to the clubhouse.

Slight plopped down in his leather seat behind his desk. "Don't look at me like that!" he barked at Honeywell. "That's your boy, you want to join him?"

Honeywell had enough of emotional arguments. He sat calmly, as he had throughout the discussion. When he finally spoke Slight was near frantic. "Why are you so hell-bent on destroying this team?"

"I want to win more than anyone. It's my pie and I want the whipped cream and cherry on top."

"Vinny, I understand that. You know I do." Honeywell pulled out his psychology degree to coax Slight into relaxation. "We have the tools to beat the Gamblers. We just have to use them right."

"We used the tools as right as we could the last two years, and what? Nothing."

"Give me this year. If we don't win the championship, you can dismantle, rip apart - do whatever you please. Just let me see if we can do it. I know this team can."

Slight was exasperated. He wanted to make a splash that night, turn the league on its ear the next morning. He was tired of reading how the Gamblers were winning game after game. He relented.

"You have the final five months of the season to work a miracle. If we don't beat the Gamblers you're fired. Then I will rebuild the team."

"Fine."

Honeywell had planned to get Slight's ultimatum. He left the office with a precise plan, and put it into effect immediately. Juris was easy to get to return, baseball was his life. Aponte was given a one-way ticket to the minors. Jack was given back his starting job. Honeywell dismissed the Courtnall agency, and took all their surveillance files. He read them carefully and acted on them immediately.

He called an emergency team meeting. In it, the players were first allowed to air their feelings. Jack was sitting in the meeting on edge. He was fearful of not being in Portland as a Crown. The rumor mills were now overflowing with trade possibilities. In that morning's newspaper, Kristen wrote that Buffalo had upped its ante for Jack. She quoted Buffalo's general manager as saying they could be a serious contender with Jack in their lineup.

Jack barely listened as his teammates spoke. When Oscar took center stage, he watched his best friend speak, thinking how terrible it would be to play without Oscar.

"We can win this shit," Oscar said. "I know for a fact the Gamblers are scared to death of us. All we got to do is play like we know we can. Shit! Come on, we can't allow anybody, from the manager to the general manager to the media to the ass we have for an owner take us off track. We got the talent."

The other players that spoke basically had said the same thing; except Bingo. All any of them were accustomed to were winning. All they wanted to do was get back to being a winner. All Bingo wanted to do was leave. He announced he wanted to be traded. His words began bitter, and ended analytical.

"This team will never be a winner. Because all of you motherfuckers think like losers. You've all been trained to believe you can never beat Las Vegas. And, you won't. None of you would be able to play for any other team but this one."

"Then break out," Mike said. "If that's the way you feel, split. We don't need you!" Mike stood. "You need help leavin'?"

Danny and Junior, Mike's backup at the catching position, held Mike from getting near Bingo.

"See what I mean?" Bingo continued with a snicker. "You are some ignorant people, let alone a bunch of losers."

Jack finally spoke. "You've got some nerve. Without us, where would you be? You would be no fucking millionaire, I know that much!"

"Look who's talking? You've lost your skills, not that you were ever anything," Bingo turned back to the captive and angering audience. "I'm out 'cause I want a championship before I retire. And you guys will never win one."

With that, Bingo walked out. Mike threw a book Junior was reading. It hit above the door, missing the mega-star's head by inches. Then, Honeywell spoke, almost standing out of the shadows.

"It's up to you guys. And you know it. Forget Bingo. He wants out, then he'll be out. I'm not keeping anybody against their will. Anybody else want out?"

The room fell silent.

"Good," Honeywell went on. "Then that means you are all in it together, like it use to be?"

"Like it always is," O said, his uniform pants wide open and bare-chested.

"Then, just play ball," Honeywell said, winding down. "To hell everything else. Just play ball."

The team arrived in Los Angeles in last place. Every aspect of their game was pitiful; they had the league's worst pitching and hitting. But, to watch them fooling around in LAX, no one could tell these were the deadbeat Crowns from Portland.

Somewhere between the airport and the team's hotel, Bingo broke away from the Crowns. He missed all three games - nobody missed him - and used his agent as his mouthpiece. He again demanded to be traded, but this time in public, feeling Honeywell was taking too long.

Without their best player, the Crowns returned to their close-knit way of playing baseball. But, they were still rocked in L.A. The Los Angeles Trojans beat them by the scores of 18-2, 11-0 and 23-7.

For Jack, though, those games were the start of his season. He began to feel comfortable at the plate and in the outfield during the California trip. In the outfield, Jack and Oscar again became a tandem, swallowing up balls hit anywhere near the two men. Jack was glad to be back to playing, and was having fun, but he missed seeing Djuana during the Crowns week away from Portland. He called her twice a day during the rode trip; once before the game, and again when back in the hotel room afterwards. They would speak for hours about the games, and Jack would steer the conversation to her day at work, and, though she felt pleased that he was interested, she would always keep her stories short.

"You don't want to hear about my day. I sell bedding. You play major league baseball."

"Your my lady," Jack would reply. "I want to know all about the things you do, and how you feel about them. Especially when I can't be by your side to see that beautiful smile of yours."

Djuana couldn't help but feel better no matter what was on her mind when she talked with Jack. But, during almost every conversation while he was in California, Jack would also express an interest to make love to her. Djuana enjoyed the words, often laying in bed while Jack would say all he wanted to do to her body. She would blush, and even imagine his touch, but she never let on that sex was on her mind daily. She wanted him too, but not yet.

Those phone calls put a hamper on Oscar and Jack's relationship. Jack was no longer interested in hang out after games. Instead he was eager to get back to the room and call Djuana. If a game had lasted longer than three hours, he would call her on his cellular phone on the bus from the stadium to the hotel. His teammates would throw kisses, and imitate females clamoring for Jack's attention, but it didn't slow the conversation.

Oscar would leave the hotel room he shared with Jack, return with a woman and sleep with her. Jack, meanwhile, would still be on the phone with Djuana. When the room became too noisy he would go into the hallway or bathroom with the phone. Even when he would sit outside in the hall, Djuana could here the moans.

"He does this all the time, in every city?" Djuana asked, while the team was in San Francisco.

"Don't worry about that," Jack said.

"I do. Don't you want some?"

"Not unless it comes from you."

Djuana almost thanked him, but she stuck to her guns. "How do I know you don't hang up and get in the bed with them?"

"Because I'm telling you. I have no reason to lie to you."

"I don't know, Jack. It's not going to be anytime soon when we do something. That is not what I am looking for right now."

"I know that. You've told me enough."

"What I'm saying is that you can sleep with someone else if you want to."

"I know what I can do. And, I know what I want to do."

"Look, Jack, I'm telling you can sleep with anybody you want to, just don't lie to me about it, okay?"

"Listen, for the last time, I am serious about settling down, and to me, you worth the wait."

Djuana read the back of a fellow Tri-Met bus passenger's newspaper. The headline read: NEWHOUSE BACK ON TRACK. How true, she smiled. Jack was hitting again. He was back to playing regularly, and contented. He claimed that she brought out the best in him and the best of Jack Newhouse was irresistible. She also understood that playing baseball again was a large part of his metamorphosis.

She remembered the day two weeks ago, while they were off for a drive Jack's car phone rang and his agent told him the Crowns were sending Hector Aponte down to the minors. Jack had never been so happy. He spun the car around and stopped at a liquor store and bought them a bottle of champagne to celebrate with - although he was a bit disappointed when Djuana wouldn't drink any.

A month. Where had the time gone? In a little over four weeks Djuana had come to trust Jack, something she never imagined possible. Jack had been surprisingly easy to talk to, and they really did have a lot in common. At first, she had felt insecure and immature, but Jack's sincerity and patience helped build her self-esteem.

Still, telling him about her pregnancy was difficult. The fear of him not being there, of him leaving her, was more terrifying than her fear of him dumping her once he finds out about the deception. These fears were so real to her, that she never thought of their relationship as dating; just two friends healing one another through tough times. And she loved him for his help.

Jack had procured prime seats for Djuana at Adkins Stadium. Sometimes she brought Devon and Tia together, or separately to share the four passes she had. She even brought her Uncle and his friends once. They just got drunk and made fun of Jack not playing.

When he did play, watching him was a delight. She was able to indulge in endless fantasies as he stretched, chased balls, ran the bases and cracked the bat against the ball. When he was doing well, which seemed like every time he played, and the fans cheered him, she took credit. He belonged solely to her.

Djuana was surprised when Jack invited her family to the team's picnic for underprivileged children in Washington Park. She stood side-by-side with Crowns' wives and helped with decoration and served food. She found the players to be a nice, humorous men. Their ladies were just as inviting.

Djuana expected to be drilled by the women, expecting someone to notice her pregnancy. But, it was a pleasant day. Devon probably had more fun than she did, but she felt apart of the socialites. She felt accepted.

Bingo was more like she expected them all to be. He sat away from the awestruck children, and had his wife bring him food. He was rude to Jack, Djuana hated that, and he didn't participate in any picnic games. Still, Djuana had a great time. She exchanged phone numbers with Sondra and Liela, at their request.

When not at games the couple spent a great deal of time at Jack's house. It was there they could be alone;' no fans staring at him or giving her funny looks. They cooked and cleaned together-Emma hated it. Their water fights were classics. He would drench her with a hose, while supposedly washing the pathfinder. She stood on the commode and dumped a pan of cold water on his head while he showered-which resulted in him dragging her in with him, clothes and all.

In Djuana's burning need to prepare for single-motherhood, she'd forgotten that there were such things as teasing, joking and laughter. Jack reminded her what she'd been missing. He taught her how to experience those things.

There were problems.

Emma was the only person close to Djuana that didn't like Jack, and she would let her feelings known often. She cited his scarred past with women, and the incident in Arizona was always her prime example that Jack was no good.

She would say: "He was in bed with the man's wife with that other male-hoe, Oscar Taylor, and had nerve to question the man as he dragged his wife home. He needed his ass kicked."

Despite his rep on and off the field, Djuana had found that there was a gentleness that strengthened her belief in Jack.

Then, Jack met Dexter.

It happen by accident, the only way it would have in Djuana's mind. She was driving Jack's Pathfinder to her mother's apartment from Adkins Stadium after a night game. She didn't notice Dexter sitting on the stoop, she didn't expect anyone to be waiting for her at 11:30 p.m. in front of her building.

The Pathfinder bumped up onto the sidewalk in front of 657. Luckily, there was plenty of room for Djuana to maneuver into the space. Djuana held her face in her hands, trying not to laugh at Jack's uneasiness.

"That was some driving, Miss Pioneer," Jack said as she ceased the engine and lights.

"I'm sorry. I scared you? I tried to tell you that I was a little rusty."

"A little? Let me see that driver's license of yours. You sure it's valid in this decade?"

"Oh please," she laughed. "I wasn't that bad. You see, that's why I told you my uncle won't take me driving. And when he does the fool wears his old high school football helmet. He looks like a nut, the thing barely fits on his head, and he makes me subconscious."

"But, I bet he's safe."

"Forget you and him!"

They laughed and got out of the truck. Jack waited at the front of the Pathfinder until Djuana locked the doors electronically and came around out of the street. She was smiling broadly until she saw Dexter.

Jack looked in the direction of her suddenly serious eyes. Djuana froze, handed Jack his keys.

"So, who's this?" Dexter demanded, hands in his front pants pockets. "Is this the real father?"

Djuana panicked. Her heart raced. She was at a lost for words, but felt she had to say something. "What are you doing here so late, Dexter? What do you want?"

"You jerking him too?" Dexter moved closer. "How long you been fucking him and me?"

Jack moved between them. "Hold up. There's no need for you to talk that way to her."

"Yo," Dexter unzipped his blue, designer wind breaker and held his hand in the jacket's left breast pocket. "Mind you business before I lay you out."

Fear buckled Jack's legs, but he stood his ground. "Don't threaten me."

"Step off, punk. I ain't playing with you," Dexter was still reaching into his jacket. "You ready to die tonight, or what?"

Djuana doubted Dexter had a gun; he had never carried one before. But, she didn't want Jack to get hurt by the fool. She pushed Jack away from Dexter.

Holding his arms, she said, "He's not worth it, Jack. Please just let me handle this."

Jack moved to the back of his truck, watching the two.

Dexter stood face to face with Djuana and shouted at her. "You talk all that righteous bullshit! 'Marry me, Dex! Be with me only, Dex!' And what you doing? Being a hoe!"

"You don't know what you're talking about, Dexter."

"Yeah right! Screw you. Let me tell you something. If I hear from you about that baby I will fuck you up. I promise you!"

Jack had heard enough. He glided between them and pushed Dexter off his feet. When Dexter scrambled up and walked towards them, Jack knocked him down again, this time with a hard right fist to his cheek.

"No, Jack, no!" Djuana cried. She pushed him with all her might. "He's not worth it. Please Jack, just stay out of this. I don't need you hurt over this."

Dexter sat on the ground dazed. He checked his lip for blood. None. He stood slowly, watching Djuana push the man away. She walked over to him and he felt the urge to grab her beautiful face and grind the back of her head into the ground.

"You bitch," he whispered.

"What do you want, Dexter?"

"Whose baby is that?" he pointed at her rounded belly under the light-weight, oversized denim shirt that covered her hips and black stirrups.

"Yours. And you know it!"

"No I don't. You try to pin it on me, and I will take your ass to court."

Djuana shook her head. She took in a deep breathe and exhaled. The tears stopped. "I was a damn fool to have ever loved you," she whispered so just Dexter could hear her. "A damn fool."

She walked away.

"Don't try no shit. I'll telling you," Dexter shouted as she walked to the building. He looked at Jack, who was glaring at him.

Dexter pounded his own chest with an open hand. "No pain, big boy. No pain."

Jack winked at Dexter and followed behind Djuana.

Guilt ate at Djuana like a stomach cancer, biting chunks of her guts, leading to her heart. She stopped at the steps of her building. When Jack got there she couldn't look him in the eye.

"You okay?" he asked.

"I'm fine," she listened to the sound of Dexter's car streaking off. It helped ease her mind. But, the cat was now out of the bag, kicking and clawing.

She looked over at the Pathfinder. "I'm sorry about all of this."

"What's going on, Djuana?"

She sighed. "Ah. A whole bunch of dumbness. I can't talk about this right now."

Jack pulled her into his chest; the warmth, and the loving way in which he held her, his fingers caressing, sent a spray of goose bumps across her skin.

"Oh, Jack. I'm sorry."

"Don't be. Just tell me what's up."

"I can't," she finally looked into his eyes. He was already looking at her. "I can't right now. Can we talk about this tomorrow?"

"Tomorrow? Why not now? I mean, what's up?"

His hand rubbed her stomach gently, "Are you pregnant by him?"

Djuana closed her eyes. The tears were returning. "Please Jack. Tomorrow I'll tell you the whole story. From beginning to end."

Jack separated them to arms length and looked into her eyes. She turned her head, defiantly. Yet, she wanted him to not let go of her.

"Oh, God," she sobbed, closing her eyes. Streams of tears soaked her face.

Jack decided to ease up. He squeezed her arms tightly and allowed her to fall back into his chest.

"Everything will be all right," he said.

Djuana released her body into his, and hoped it would be.

# 21

Djuana left work early and walked in the light drizzle instead of taking the bus, which would have been free to Waterfront Park. She paced herself, not wanting to arrive too soon and have to wait for him.

Jack was there, waiting for her. He was leaning on his truck with a rose in his hand. He sprang up with a smile when he saw her crossing the street. Djuana didn't think she could smile, but she did in answer to his. They exchanged hellos, and Djuana accepted the flower. Jack was cool, he held his questions, instead allowing her to lead him on a walk into the park and near the pier.

Djuana was quiet. She sniffed the flower every so often and looked out at the water. Jack tried not to stare at her, but he watched her. He was used to her prolonged silences. This time, he understood why.

While they strolled Djuana battled with the task of telling him. She remembered that telling Dexter was easier... she expected to lose him.

Then, abruptly, Djuana opened up.

"There is something I need to tell you before we go any further," she inhaled and blew air out toward the river. She stopped walking and faced Jack.

"I'm four months pregnant. That guy last night was the baby's father. My ex."

Jack's smile dimmed. He leaned on the banister and spit into the river. "That's the guy from the night I met you?"

"Yes. That was when I told him."

Jack scolded her. "I don't understand why you didn't tell me this sooner. We talked about everything else."

"I don't know. I wanted to." She repelled from looking at him. "I guess I was selfish."

Jack went silent for a solid minute. He glanced at her, but couldn't look for long without wanting to curse. He turned his back to her, mumbling to himself.

A brisk breeze blew straight through Djuana. She sniffed and shivered. The early evening sun was hidden in the threatening clouds. She rubbed her arms and looked out across the water. She wished she could snap her fingers and Jack would be the father. Or snap them and she wouldn't be pregnant. Or, better yet, she wished for a brand new start on her confused life.

"You lied to me," Jack blurted in anger.

"No," Djuana shook her head. "I didn't lie to you."

"Yes you did. What you call it? Not telling me?"

"Jack listen, It's not something I'm all that proud of. It took me awhile to come to terms with it on my own. I'm not just telling you now because of last night, but I was near telling you because I feel comfortable with you as a friend, and I feel you should know before we go further."

"Fine. " Jack snapped.

"Don't be like that. I'm sorry," Djuana was standing, arms crossed holding herself, speaking in a nervous tone. "Maybe I should have told you sooner," she continued. "But, like I said, I needed some time to be sure for me first. I haven't handled any of this all that well, I guess."

Jack understood. But he felt cheated. "So, what's the deal with you and him?"

"That is how he acts ever time we try to talk. So I really don't know. There's nothing between us besides the baby, though."

Djuana glanced over at a set of benches. She wanted to sit, needed to sit, because her feet felt like swelling grapefruits. But a couple was at one of the benches playing with their toddler. She envied the sight, and didn't want to go over there.

In a blunt manner, she proceeded. "My baby's father is an ex. He's married. I don't think he wants to be a part of the baby's life."

Jack grimaced while she spoke. He wondered would she have ever told him. His head turned and his eyes closed. He was listening, and he really didn't care that she was pregnant - he had an idea before the previous night's fiasco.

During one of their playful nights he felt the tightness of her belly while tackling her onto the bed. From then on he would take notice to the way her clothes fit, her eating habits and her lack of mentioning a period, ever.

He was in love with Djuana, and afraid she may hurt him. He thought of Slight and his penchant to the Crowns image.

Djuana watched him, looking for any sign of his affection. The love she craved and was so close to being spoiled by. She felt the distance between them growing. It was just as Aunt Earline told her - communication is the key.

She had tried communication with Dexter, but they never talked about anything of substance, thus she should have known where she stood with him long ago.

But this man, this angry man in front of her meant more to her than any effort she gave to keep Dexter. She wanted Jack in a way she had never wanted any man. Although she hadn't thought of what to say to him, she was dead-set on letting him know her feelings. She wasn't about to give up.

"Damn," he muttered.

*127*

"Jack," Djuana touched his elbow. "What are you thinking. Talk to me. You have been so talkative, don't stop now."

He heard her. But at that instant he was comparing her with the many woman he had dated in Portland and didn't answer. As he searched his past, Djuana, in just that instant, came out on top of all the others.

She had never asked about his salary, nor looked for a hand out. As a matter of fact, he recalled, she had never let him buy her anything. He did think that if she did want money, she would ask him now. He doubted it, but still asked her a test question.

"What do you expect from me?" His eye brows were glaring.

Djuana didn't hesitate. "Nothing."

Jack just nodded. He was relieved. She's the one, he knew.

"Look, Jack. If your mind has changed about me. I understand. If you don't want to be with me anymore, I understand."

He cut her off, "No. It hasn't. I just need some time to think this over."

A sharp pain, the feeling of a knife slicing her heart, walloped Djuana. He's gone, she deducted.

"I understand." Her voice was somber. "Take all the time you want."

She looked at her watch and fought off the tears. "I need to get home. It's my turn to cook dinner and I don't feel like hearing my mother's mouth tonight."

Djuana didn't want him to, but Jack drove her home. The ride was solemn. When the Pathfinder stopped at her building, she got out and said good night faintly. Jack didn't look at her as he said good-bye.

She closed the car's door quietly.

"Good-bye is forever," she told him.

Jack hit the steering wheel and cursed. "Good night, Djuana," he said while electronically closing the passenger's window.

It seemed to her as if he could not wait to pull off. Actually, he watched her until she reached the building's door.

"I've lost him, Tia." Djuana sobbed.

Tia sat up in her bed and cut off the television. She had expected the call of doom.

"Damn, Dee. He broke up with you?"

"I told him and he burnt rubber outta here," Djuana was well composed then, yet she had been crying from the time she got in the building until she finished cooking dinner.

"Damn," Tia sighed. "I thought he would. I'm sorry."

Djuana ran by her wild ideas to get him back. "I could go to his house and try to explain it. I don't think he really understands. Or maybe you could call him. Or I could call Oscar Taylor's wife. I met her and she seemed nice.

"I just don't want him to think I was trying to pull anything."

Tia sighed. "Forget it. If it was meant to be he would have understood. You know, I think you don't realize what a tough situation you were asking him to be apart of. You're four months pregnant by another man. He's a star baseball player.

"What did you really expect him to do?"

"Understand. And still be there," Djuana sobbed.

Tia shook her head and looked up to the ceiling of her bedroom. The sound of Djuana crying pierced her heart. Her friend did really love the guy and she didn't think she should.

Djuana cried for a long time on the phone. Tia said little things to help soothed her friend's broken heart, but nothing helped.

"Tia, I love him. I really, really love him, and I need him," Djuana said. "I had him, but he's... Shit."

Tia swallowed the hurt. "I don't know what to say."

Djuana watched the Crowns lose their fifth game in a row, a Saturday afternoon game that Devon wanted very dearly to attend. She had to explain that Jack and she had an argument. To which Devon demanded to know what she did.

Jack had one hit, a hard shot that reached the outfield wall. He raced into second base, having to dive head first to beat the tag. Djuana loved it and, at the same time, hated that he wouldn't be calling to tell her what he was thinking while he ran.

She tried calling him late that night, but he did not answer his home phone and she would not leave a message on his machine. If he had answered, though, she would have hung up. She knew he didn't want to talk with her, but she wanted to hear his voice. She was also a tad bit frightened that he wouldn't return the calls, and thus she would really know he didn't want to be bothered any more.

Djuana spent that night alone, her first in weeks. She cooked dinner after the game ended, then watched Emma leave to meet her friends to play bingo. Devon was invisible. He ate, then vanished into Emma's room to watch television. He was highly disturbed about missing hat day at Adkins.

Tia called for a hot second before her first date with a guy from her Art class.

It was then, in the living room alone, Djuana thought of God. He must be testing me, she reasoned. Why else would she finally meet the man of her dreams, and lose him because the man she thought was in love with her was the father of the baby she so dearly wanted months ago. Now that she's pregnant, she doesn't want the baby, nor does she want to abort it.

She opened up the family Bible that sat on the coffee table. The large, crimson old testament, hadn't been open by anyone in two years. The last person to open it was Calvin during and argument about the *Ten Commandments*, the movie. Djuana read a few verses, but her mind was not into it. She put the book down and thought to call the only religious person left in the family, Aunt Earline, Emma's older sister.

Earline, 58 years old, had been married for 32 years before her husband, Steve, passed a year ago. Djuana had always adored their relationship. They seemed happy, of course they fought, but they always seemed to make up. Djuana would love spending weekends with them – even the full Sundays in church. Steve would help pass the time by sharing complaints with her during the long services.

Earline always answered her telephone after the six ring. She only spoke to important callers, or those who knew her habit. When she heard Djuana's voice on the other end, she immediately brightened.

After the usual 'how is everybody?' and 'why haven't you and Devon visited me?' questions, Djuana asked the best question she could have. And she knew it.

"Aunt E, can I come to church with you tomorrow morning."

"Can you? Oh, I'd love it!"

"Good. Then I'll meet you in front of the church at 10."

"Now, don't tease me, Darling. Are you really coming?"

"Yes, I will be there." Damn, Djuana thought. I should visit her more often. "I need to go."

"Is this about Dexter and the baby."

"Sort of." Djuana hadn't told her, but she knew Emma had burnt up the phone lines.

"Everything will work out, the Lord will take care of it. Darling, I'm so glad you've decided to seek His guidance."

## 22

After the loss, Jack drove the streets of Portland. He was going to stop by Djuana's apartment and tell her he loved her. But, he passed by Tudor street twice without turning down her block. He ended up in Cherrywood Heights, where O lived. He drove up their large, u-shaped driveway and parked off the porch. He rang the bell and was surprised to see Sondra open the door.

She smiled brightly at Jack and kissed him. "O didn't mention you were coming by."

"I didn't know I was. It's good to see you. Is he in?"

"He's in his den."

Oscar's house was a mansion. Ten rooms, and all furnished with the best.

The man of the house was in the elaborate den watching the Gamblers destroy New York on a giant screen, projector-style television.

Jack gave Oscar a tight hand shake, and Oscar rose out of his leather recliner to hug him. Sondra came in after Jack.

"What you doing here, fool?" Oscar asked as he sat again.

"I needed to talk."

"Sondra, get Jack a beer."

"No," Jack waved. "Something stronger would be nice."

"Hmm. Well, bring us the vodka." O flopped back into his chair.

Jack sat on one end of the long, white leather sectional and looked him over. O was in his designer house robe, a thick, white terrycloth with Armani embroidered on the right breast, and socks. He searched for the remote to his expensive entertainment console. The combination, stereo, television, VCR wall-unit cost Oscar three thousand dollars and it all has not worked correctly at the same time in the year he has had it.

"What's up?" O asked as Sondra brought in the ice and glasses.

Jack watched her make the drinks with attitude. She slammed the glasses on the glass coffee table and loudly shifted about. There was always tension in the Taylor household. Jack knew, as it always was, because of a woman.

"Djuana is pregnant," Jack flatly said. He was thinking about small talk first, to break the ice, but he skipped the bull.

O erupted into laughter. He fell to his knees on the rug. "And you chased the bitch! Oh, man. Now that's funny. How much she want?"

Watching his friend ridicule him, Jack realized he was talking to the wrong person. He wanted to believe in Djuana. He knew she was not a golddigger, and golddigging hoes were Oscar's specialty. Twice, once in the minors and again the year before he married Sondra, women hit Oscar with maternity suits. Each time he won out in court. Oscar never had to pay a dime.

"It ain't like that," Jack said as he leaned back on the couch. "She told me this afternoon. And she hasn't asked for no money."

"Yet."

Sondra, shaking her head at her husband, crossed by him and handed Jack a drink. "Do you want more orange juice, it's kinda strong?"

"No thanks," he sipped some, all vodka at the top. "I need it this strong"

"Listen, Jack," Oscar paused while Sondra handed him his drink. "Just drop her. She's going to be nothing but problems. It ain't your baby... right?"

Jack nodded between sips.

"Well, then why be bothered?" Oscar asked. "She's gonna need pampers and formula real soon.

"Then Junior will need clothes, pocket change, hair cuts. What? You want to father somebody else's brat?"

Oscar waved his hand at Jack. "Of course you don't. You ain't got to, my friend. Much bitches want to marry you."

Sondra frowned and yelled at Oscar. "Stop using that word! You are not a rapper."

"Oh, what that got to do with anything?" Oscar asked his wife.

"Just watch your mouth in front of me, at least."

Oscar crossed the room and sat next to Jack. Sondra left. "Listen, keep your eyes open, New."

He poked Jack in the chest with a finger. "You still rebounding from Vivian."

Jack shook his head.

Oscar went on, "That's why I know you don't want this chick. You still love Vivian."

"What are you talking about?" Jack said.

"You know what I'm saying. When Viv wakes up and leaves that punk again, you'll take her back a second later."

"That's bullshit," Jack waved at Oscar. "I haven't thought about that bitch, ah..."

"Jack!" Sondra yelled from the kitchen, about three rooms away.

"Sorry!" Jack shouted back. He finished his drink and got up and fixed stiffer one. He sat back down, turned to his friend and lowered his voice.

"Look, all I'm gonna do is give Djuana all the chance in the world to be my lady."

Oscar shook his head. "No. Don't do it."

Sondra broke in, fork in hand, "Just take your time, New. Maybe you should just see what her intentions are. Feel her out. Don't listen to this fool 'cause Vivian was definitely not the one for you."

"Miss Wisdom has spoken," O sneered.

Jack and Sondra ignored Oscar.

"Just see what's up. Maybe date some other women in the meantime," Sondra said.

As she started to leave the room, she playfully popped Oscar in the head with the fork in her hand.

"Now, see if I hit her, she'll have me on Geraldo, and shit."

"You're not classy enough to get on Geraldo," Sondra laughed.

"Yeah, but your mother likes it!"

Sondra reached down to hit him again with the fork, but Oscar pulled her onto the couch and kissed her.

"Now, don't burn the food like usual we've got company." Oscar said, pushing her up. He patted her behind as she scurried away.

The man doesn't know how lucky he is, Jack thought. Jack turned his head up and emptied his glass to the shrunken ice cubes, and stood to fix another. He stumbled on his way to the bar Sondra set up. One day, he vowed, he too would have a wife to play with; a wife like Oscar's. Then Djuana's enchanting smile appeared in his memory.

"I've found my wife," he mumbled with a smile.

Oscar, who was looking at the television, turned and looked over at Jack in bewilderment.

"Why don't you lay your drunk ass down until dinner is ready?" Oscar said. "You alcoholic."

Djuana was in the shower singing along with Miki Howard. Howard's tape was a mellow stream of sad ballads, but the songs combined with the hot water beading down Djuana's back to help ease her mind.

She heard the knock on the bathroom door, and decided to ignore it. She wasn't ready to get out. When the intensity of the knock increased, she cursed the door. Her little brother finally busted in and announced she had a phone call.

"Tell whoever it is I am in the shower, please!" she angrily barked at him from behind the curtain.

"No can do," Devon said, eyes closed and shaking his head. "It's Jack Newhouse. And I think its time you two made up so I can get some more tickets."

Djuana's heart leaped. The thought of him calling at seven-thirty in the morning made her pulse race. "Move. Get outta here. Go tell him I'll be right there, stupid!"

Devon grinned devilishly. "I thought you would hop to it."

She pushed him out of the bathroom, hiding her wet body with a towel.

Djuana raced into her bedroom and picked up the phone, she heard Devon and Jack talking and abruptly cut in; telling her brother to hang up.

The first thing she said when Devon hung up was: "I thought you had dumped me."

"No," Jack's voice was hoarse, and he was hung over. He had gotten up early to catch Djuana before she left for work. He popped two aspirin, and sipped water to chase them down.

"I told you I just needed time to think this over."

"Have you?" Her heart was beating in her chest, and she was wetting the wooden floor. *He still wants me*, she could feel it.

"Yeah, I thought it over, all right. You are the only thing I have been thinking about since we met. Can you and Tia join me and the Crowns at an award ceremony this Saturday? We can talk then."

Djuana almost yelled a yes. She calmed, then said, "I have to ask her, but I think we are free."

Jack parked the Pathfinder in front of 657 and bolted out. He opened both passenger side doors and welcomed his guests. Djuana was lovely in the halter dress Jack picked out for her for the occasion. It was a stretch knit with a ballerina neckline and ended in full flair. She felt her belly looked bloated, but Jack loved the dress and she wore it to please him.

Tia was wearing a busty column dress with sparkled lace and spaghetti straps.

"You ladies look great," Jack gushed.

They thanked him and Tia complimented him on his tuxedo with the African print bow tie and cummerbund. Djuana blushed and proudly proclaimed she had picked them.

LeClair's was a quiet, casual spot in which to dine and hear great jazz. That night the Crowns had rented out the place to give achievement awards to deserving high school seniors in and around Portland. The students receiving awards, and some got scholarships. Their parents and the Crowns executives and players were all that was in attendance that evening.

Jack sat the ladies at a table next to Sondra and Liela Cruz, Don's wife. He introduced all and went backstage where Honeywell was organizing the players. When it was Jack's turn to present an award, Tia and Djuana cheered loudly, their clapping and shouting was the most hearty applause of the evening.

Djuana felt Liela's long stare. She tried not to cut her eyes at one of Jack's friends. But, she felt uneasy. Maybe she needed more makeup. Or, the dress. *It's the dress. I should have worn a maternity dress, that's why she's staring.* Then, Liela smiled at Djuana and said, "Jack has spoken so much about you. He really likes you."

Djuana warmed. She smiled and said the only thing that came to mind, "Thank you."

Sondra added, "Jack mentioned that you work at DeLux's?"

Uh oh, Djuana thought. *They know I'm piss poor.*

"I like that store. I was just telling Liela how we needed to stop by there."

"It's okay," Djuana said. She tapped Tia's thigh under the table. Tia looked away. She wanted no part of this conversation.

Tia was looking out across the sea of millionaires selecting the prime candidates to be hers. Sadly, to her, the best looking member of the Crowns in her eyes, Cris Carpenter, was married. Still, she stared at him as much as she could, fighting boredom. His rich, dark skin and full lips were inviting.

The formalities lasted an hour and a half. Dinner was as quick. Most of the honored guest left after the last award was handed out, none of the Crowns did. At 11 p.m. the band heated up and the liquor moved quicker to the tables. Jack ordered Scotch for himself and virgin coladas for Djuana.

"Make them extra fruity," he demanded.

Djuana felt Jack staring and elbowed him. He would usually stare at her, but she was feeling so out of place among his teammates and their well-dressed women.

"Do I look all right?" she asked.

"Fine. As always."

"Swear?"

"Cross my heart."

"Then stop staring at me, you're drawing attention."

"What? Some dude looking at my woman?" Jack stood and faked anger. Djuana laughed. "Sit down." She held his hand.

The six-piece band began a mellow swing.

"Let's dance," Jack suggested.

"Jack," she whined. "Nobody is dancing. They're all eating."

He rose, still holding her hand, "Dance with me."

Djuana pulled her hand free.

Everyone seated at the table heard him. Tia's heart melted. She beamed, "Yeah, go girl. She loves to dance."

She sure did. And, Djuana was thinking about dancing since the band began to play. She placed her finger tips into Jack's hand and lifted herself up. He lightly guided her to the middle of the small open area in the middle of the cafe, dodging waiters. Djuana put one hand on Jack's shoulder and he held her other hand. He guided her into a soft sway.

She tightened her grip, forced a smile, and said, "Everybody's watching us, Jack."

He grinned, "No. They're watching you."

The sparkle in her eye turned Jack on.

She had to swallow to clear her throat before speaking. "What are you trying to do to me?"

"Give you love."

Oscar turned his chair to face the dance floor and watched the lone couple glide. Sondra, behind him, slid her hand between his legs and kissed his shoulder. "They act like they're newly weds," she said.

O gave a nod in agreement.

"They are a beautiful couple," Liela said.

Her husband replied, "They are, aren't they. I'm happy for him."

Tia listened to them and agreed to herself. Djuana was in love, it showed. Was Jack in love with her? She hoped he was. Tia shared in her friends good feelings, and wished for them to last forever.

Across the club, Honeywell watched the two dance with admiration. "That's what Jack needs," he said above the chatter at the main table. "That woman is going to settle him into a fine man."

Slight nearly choked on his salmon. "Bullshit, J.A.!" The table silenced as Slight shouted. "All he ever does is screw, so what's a little more pussy?" he bellowed a hearty laugh.

Slight's wife elbowed him. She said, "Vinny, that out there is love. Or are you blind?"

"That ain't love! If he is in love, I'll kiss his diminishing-talent ass!"

"Shoot, that's somebody else's baby she's carrying, anyway!"

Slight felt good dropping that bombshell on his table. It was a piece of gossip he had gotten from one of the locker room attendents. But, no one reacted outwardly.

"If that man is in love, and settles down, you should," Honeywell said. "He could carry this team to its first championship."

"Get off it, J.A. You're wrong about him." Slight swallowed the remains of his sixth glass of champagne. "That man couldn't hit water if he I threw him out of a boat and into the Willamette! Let alone carry the Crowns."

No one expressed any feelings while Slight laughed himself into a deep coughing spell.

Djuana whispered to Jack, "I think your boss is talking about us."

"Forget everybody here. Just have a good time. You are here with me. And that's it."

Honeywell stood up, flipped his cloth napkin onto his plate of half eaten food and asked his wife to dance. She put down her purse and they joined Jack and his new love on the dance floor.

O took Sondra's hand and tugged as he rose. Sondra was pleased, she smiled broadly and followed him. Soon the dance floor was filled with couples dancing cheek to cheek.

After three songs Djuana needed a break. Her feet were swelling in the mid-heels. Jack understood, and took her back to the table. She asked Tia to join her in the powder room. Once they were inside, Djuana, blushing, asked, "So, what do you think?"

"He's so nice. And so damn romantic!"

Both ladies laughed. An older woman exited a stall, smiling. She washed quickly, and as she left said, "You're a lucky young woman, most men have forgotten the art of romance."

Tia stared at her best friend in the mirror. Djuana was applying lipstick, talking and blushing. To Tia, the revelation that she had never really seen her best friend in love before that moment was deep.

"Tia! What do you really think? I mean, he seems incredible, but you know my track record."

"Time will tell, but he is lobster compared to the crabs you had caught."

"Thanks. I hope that's a compliment."

"To him, of course!"

They both laughed.

The night ended when Jack's teammates began to leave. He asked his guests if they were ready, and they looked at each other and decided yes. Jack drove Tia home first. She thanked him for the evening, and he offered to walk her into her apartment complex.

She thanked him again as they walked, then Tia said "I don't know if you know it or not, but Djuana has been through a hell of a lot recently. All I want is to see her happy, and I appreciate that you have made her very happy. But please don't hurt her. If all you are after is pussy, then drop her."

Jack was stunned by her frankness. "Is that what you think?"

"Come on? She's very attractive. And, you're a superstar in Portland. We both know you can get just about anybody you want."

Jack forced a smile. His tone of voice was defensive. "Yeah, that's all true. But I don't waste my time. If it I was only after leg, I would have been at it by now."

"I am not going to stand here and promise you anything. But I do care for your friend."

Tia had watched Jack's lips, eyes and hand movements while he talked. He was handsome and intelligent.

"Jack, I ain't trying to be your enemy. Like I said, you have made her very happy. But, I love that woman. She's my heart."

Tia pointed at Jack. "And, I'll tell you, if you hurt her, I will hurt you."

# 23

Jack locked the door to the garage and trotted up the steps. Djuana met him at the top, she had opened the door using his keys. She didn't go far from the door, waiting to greet. He had been such a gallant date. She marveled at how he had included her friend in every conversation, danced with her and made Tia feel more than the third-wheel she felt she was going to be.

Djuana dropped her purse and kicked off her shoes on the rug. She wrapped her arms around his neck and let herself fall into his arms - she wanted to test his strength, knowing he could and would hold her up. He did, squeezing her rib cage.

"My man is soooo strong," she struggled to say.

Jack wrinkled his forehead, "Your man?" he smiled.

"Well? Ain't you?" She stared into his eyes; her smile forcing one to cross his face. He didn't blink.

"I'd love to be."

She held on as he lifted her up by her waist then legs and torso, and carried her into the bedroom. Djuana kissed him with fire as he laid her down. She wanted him to take her, ravish her, make love to her and make her flow like a river - the way she dreamt he could, and Jack picking up her heavy body turned her on all the more.

Jack was up to the task; he had dreamt of this night also. He glided her silken panty hose down her smooth legs. He pawed and kissed the legs from thigh to toes. Djuana panted when her toes were engulfed into Jack's warm mouth. His tongue parted the soft toes and he sucked each one. When all 10 were moist, he climbed on the bed. On his knees, he undressed Djuana. Christening each inch of her body with a kiss as it became exposed.

That was when doubts began to ruin her mood. Is this all he ever wanted? I'll never see him again once he hits it. Does he know I love him, and that is why I'm doing this. Why am I letting him have me? Does he realized I ...

Jack kissed her forehead, nose and when he reached her lips, Djuana invited him in with a warm, exploring kiss. All her thoughts, and fears, were momentarily erased.

After a few seconds, Jack pushed her back down and resumed a kissing trail that led him from her butter-like neck to her soaked vagina. He stopped at her belly to kiss it tenderly and whispered to the baby. Djuana couldn't hear him, but it brought tears to her already wet eyes.

"I wish this were your father," she cried softly. She rubbed his curly, shortcut hair. She ran her nails over his shoulder blades. All the while, one thought, one dreamy image crossed her mind: He was finally making love to her, consummating their love.

Jack planted a peck on her pubic hair, then start licking down. She panted wildly and squeezed his head, digging her nails into his scalp and her hips raised instinctively to meet his mouth. She came violently.

It had been so long. Damn, Dexter! Why hadn't you loved me like this? She panted and experienced the tender lovemaking of a person dedicated to his work. She forced air through her mouth. First her toes spread, then she felt the spasms begin in her legs. Then her thighs were trembling. In the throws of passion, she then punched and grabbed Jack's head.

With every movement of his tongue, Djuana could feel a surge surround her body. She continued to pant to keep from screaming while her body trembled.

"Why are you doing this to me?" She whispered. "Oh, Jack, why?"

The words continued as she came.

Jack held her large, soft buttocks in the palms of his hands; fingers squeezing it. He felt her thighs trembling against his face cheeks. His lips caressed her in a deliberate, caring manner. The way he knew so many other women had asked him to do, but he couldn't give of himself as freely as he now could.

Jack rose to his knees and pulled Djuana by her waist to him, parting her legs at his thighs. This was what he had waited patiently for, not cheating on her when he could have easily. She lay gently tasting her own warm tears. Jack didn't notice she was crying. Jack penetrated, and they both groaned, he much softer than she.

Then Djuana lowered her hands and sobbed, "Go ahead, take it. I know that's all you wanted.

"Just fuck me and get it over with."

Jack stopped. Djuana's words sliced through him like no others had before. He withdrew and stood up. Djuana turned on her side, balling into a fetal position.

Jack stood there a long moment, thinking that probably every guy wanted to pound that wonderful body of hers; and most probably did. That must explain her feelings, her reasoned. He thought he was making love to it. Or was he?

Djuana continued to cry, and told Jack to just leave her alone. He forced himself to move, grabbing his clothes in one swoop and left her in the room. A few doors slammed, alarming Djuana. Jack jumped into the Pathfinder and sped off.

Djuana was watching for him out of the window when the Pathfinder slowly pulled back into the garage two hours later. She had cried so much in that time span, that her eyes and nose were sore.

Djuana met him at the door, holding it open with her arms folded. She was watching for him when the pathfinder pulled into the garage, two hours later. Her face was pale and her nose darkened red from crying. No words were spoken; Jack brushed by her, making no contact, and entered the kitchen. He yanked a glass out of the cabinet, slammed it on the counter. He swung open the icebox and put a couple of ice cubes in the glass. He poured himself a three-finger shot of Scotch.

She told herself to speak; say something, anything. But her heart was clogged in her throat. She followed him to the wine rack, then out to the screen porch at the end of the dining room. She walked out into the nipping air, wearing only his jersey. She stood on the sliding door's track, her feet leaning. She watched him drink, then stared as he nested his face into his hands, leaning his elbows on his knees.

Djuana wanted to kiss him. Hold him. She couldn't stop the tears; she was used to them by now.

"I'm sorry, Jack." she finally had nerve to say. Her hoarse voice made the words sound feeble. "Tonight was the best date I've ever had. I'm sorry I destroyed it."

Jack sat motionless. The drive had relaxed him, but returning to find Djuana's beautiful body attractively wearing one of his baseball jerseys was fanning the fires.

"Do you want me to leave?" She asked. Please say no.

Jack gulped more Scotch. "I don't feel like talking right now. Just leave me alone for awhile." He sounded more bitter than he actually was.

"Are you angry with me?"

"Yep."

She moved into the porch, slowly, and stopped in front of him. He couldn't look, but as she spoke, those soft thighs were eye level.

"Jack, I am not trying to tease you or play games with you. I want you to make love to me. I want you as much as you want me, but I'm not ready. Not yet."

Jack stood up, picked up the Scotch and his glass. "Whatever," he spewed as he brushed by her.

Djuana became angry. She was doing what she had to do. So, why wasn't it working? She darted after him and caught him in the dining room.

She pulled his arm, and he turned to meet her. "No, Jack. Don't be like that. I just need time."

Jack was becoming sympathetic, but he wasn't showing it that well. He couldn't sustain his anger. He face twisted in a smirk, his eyebrows bent and eyes blazing. To Djuana, the look reeked of anger. But, it was confusion. Jack began to realize, by looking Djuana in her eyes, he was more frustrated than upset. He could have used the sex to release some of his frustrations. He backed up and exhaled a breeze.

"I understand," he threw up his hands, still holding the liquor. "It's cool."

She explained, almost pleaded, that, "I've heard so many lies from my baby's father that they have become one long line. How do I know you aren't giving me lies?"

Jack's stare sliced through Djuana.

"I can't hurt you." She attempted to cut him off, but he continued. "I love you. I love you with all my heart."

Djuana turned her body sideways. "Please don't say that. Don't say it."

"It's true," Jack moved closer. His eyes searched hers. "I love you."

She put her hand up to his chest. "You don't love me. How could you? You don't know me that well."

"Doesn't matter. I know the way you make me feel."

"You're just horny, and used to getting it whenever you want it," said Djuana.

Jack had to restrain himself from exploding. He forced his voice into low. "Fuck it. Think what you want to."

She didn't believe he was just horny. But, she wanted to be sure. She stood there, listened to the man, knowing in her soul he wasn't lying. She had seen horny men before, and none of them acted blase about her saying no. None of them gave in, most of them offered love.

But there was Jack's sincerity, which he had always displayed. She was truly sorry to have agitated him again.

She grabbed hold of his buttoned up shirt and slid her hand between the buttons, grabbed the material into a fist. Her eyes spread open and she gritted her teeth.

"You make this so hard!"

Jack shook his head. "Baby, I..." He stopped, glanced at her, then continued.

"Look, if you don't want to do anything, fine. I just want to get some sleep and put this behind me."

"I believe you, Jack. I know you love me. I'm not sure of what kind of love you have for me, and maybe you know and understand it, but all I know to do is protect my heart. If you hurt me it will only be my fault."

She stepped into his chest, "Just hold me."

He did. Crossing his arms around her back, glass in one hand and the bottle in the other.

Djuana's eyes glossed; no more tears, she vowed. His hold was firm. "Just be there, and please, don't give up on me. I need your love," she said.

Jack closed his eyes. He thought getting with her would be difficult, but wow. "I'll be there," he kissed her forehead and whispered.

"It can't get any worse."

# 24

Stacie began calling Jack every night around eleven when he suddenly became unavailable. Used to be, she could depend on him calling her about once every two weeks, and if she needed some sex, he would supply it amply. If Jack was not home, she'd call his car phone. When she got him on the phone it was always the same conversation, she would ask to see him and he would say no. During one of their quick conversations she became confrontational.

"So, what's the deal with this bitch you screwing? You all into it?"

"She's not a bitch. And don't sweat it."

"Oh, she's all that? I see. So, she be the latest flame?"

"Bye, Stace."

"You ain't even hangin' up, boy. You miss this juice too much. Shit, I know your dick still aches from the last time you hit it. What, you bus' six nuts that night? I know she can't hang like that."

"Whatever. I'm tellin' you, I'm keeping this one. So just..."

"Cut the 'nice boy' act. I've had your dick down my throat and up my ass too many times, and you loved it. I know that bitch can't take it like me. She a church girl, right?"

Jack smiled. He wouldn't argue. He wanted sex, especially the rough kind Stacie offered. Still, he knew to avoid her if he wanted to keep Djuana as his woman. At Adkins, he would push her on Oscar, and O would give her to a rookie. Twice, since Jack and Djuana settled, new Crowns spent the night with Stacie, but it wasn't enough. They weren't Jack; they were not as gifted. And, they weren't saying no.

One night, Oscar did become suspicious. "Yo, why won't you bone Stace?" he asked while they sat in the dugout between innings of a home game.

"Why should I?"

"I ain't saying you should," O said as the crowd cheered Mike's high home run.

"Look. I've been trying to tell you that I ain't into that anymore. I want one. The final one."

O shook his head as they rose to greet Mike as he entered back into the dugout.

The last time Stacie ever called Jack's house Djuana answered the phone. Jack was at a team meeting at the stadium, and Djuana asked to be left at the house. She wanted to cook him a healthy meal. They had been eating out often; Portland has the most restaurants per capita than in any other West Coast city - and she felt as though they had tried them all.

In the month of their serious dating, Djuana's waist had thickened and her stomach grew. The skin from her below her breast to the bottom of her stomach felt stretched. No more fatty foods, she vowed. The baby would give her enough fat.

Djuana would not have answered Jack's phone had she not called Tia's place less than an hour before and had given Bernadette the number for Tia to call back. Djuana felt uneasy about the phone. Women never called, at least when she was there, but she expected them to. The stories, all from her mother, about Jack's wild sex life had begun to get to Djuana. She expected women to be driving up to the front door naked.

Stacie knew Jack was not home, and she was hoping to get the woman that was stealing her time. That was why Stacie almost screamed for joy when she heard the soft, feminine voice on the other end. She immediately became treacherous.

"Who is this answering his phone? Where is Jack Newhouse?"

"He's not here, can I take a message for him?"

Stacie said, in her raunchiest dialect, "You must be his sister, 'cause he don't be leaving any hoes in his house."

Djuana remained cool. This is what she expected, she reminded herself. She calmly asked the vile woman on the other end if she wanted to leave a message.

Stacie released an evil chuckle and continued, "Yeah, Ms. Secretary. Tell him he left me sore like a motherfucker! He got ta ease up when he's in the ass. Shit, he knows better. Does he hurt you like that?

"Oh, what am I saying? You the main stain, he wouldn't dare *fuck* you!"

Djuana slammed the phone down, her heart racing with anger. She rubbed her ear, it felt nasty, like if the woman's breath had reach through the phone. She tried not to get angry, but the noxious feelings overflowed. Not again, she worried. Two of Dexter's women had gotten Djuana's home number and called her; claiming 'they' were his women and 'she' was intruding.

Stacie had laughed so hard she titled off her bed and tumbled on the floor. She decided to have fun with the *chosen bitch*. She called twice, and had a crony call also. The final time Stacie called she told Djuana how she was "slobbering on Jack's dick while he was telling you how to get there."

"How did he like the chicken soup you made for him?" She asked Djuana. "I bet he licked the bowl?"

Djuana exploded into the phone, "Who is this! How you know about that?"

"Bitch, wake up? What, you think you the only one in his life? What, he told you him wuv you? Come on! He a famous hoe.

"Fuckin' everybody!"

Djuana wanted to hang up. But, she was frozen still. *This can't be happening.* Djuana tried to sound confrontational, but she sounded feeble when she said, "Why don't you come over here and say this when he's here. Why you got to do it like this?"

Stacie just laughed loudly into the phone and said, "No, why do you come over when I'm there; and I'll teach ya' how to keep him happy!"

Jack sped into his driveway and jumped out of his ride. The scout meeting had lasted longer than he expected. It was the usual gathering before a series began. The advance scouts would tell the players what they learned about the opposing teams. Most veteran players understood who, and what, they were up against. The meeting was extended when Honeywell once again addressed the team on his plans for the remainder of the season, which included trades. The general manager would not disclosed who would be going, or coming, but he said that no one would be exempt as the Crowns were on the road back to the championship games.

Jack didn't care; many of his teammates didn't either. They understood that Honeywell, who loved meetings, would have one every week, and say about the same thing. But, for Jack, his carelessness stemmed from having a woman he loved to come home to. And it showed. Baseball was still very important to him, but now it was a second love; finally.

Jack stopped off and picked up a cheesecake and fresh flowers. His taste buds were exploding; he loved Djuana's cooking as much as he adored her legs.

Djuana heard him come in; he was whistling.

"The bastard," she cursed under her breath. "I told him, damn near begged him, not to ever lie to me. There was no reason for it. I told him if he wanted to screw somebody, all he had to do was tell me. Shit, I told him that."

Jack heard Djuana's voice, but assumed she was on the phone. "Hey, Babe! I got us a cheesecake for desert!" He shouted from the dining room, less than five feet away. He put the flowers on the glass dining room table and entered the kitchen.

The aroma of the food whet his appetite. He entered the refrigerator, put the cake in the freezer and poured himself a glass of iced tea. He started small talk; saying the meeting was the usual talk about the upcoming series against Milwaukee and that Mike fell asleep and was snoring.

Djuana's back was to him. He didn't notice her tears. She was cutting onions, with other ingredients at her side. All four burners were in use, and pots and groceries were all about.

"Your dinner would've been ready sooner," she said between sobs. "But my nerves. They're shot."

Jack wrapped his arms around her and lightly kissed her neck and rubbed her stomach. "You okay? Want some help?"

Djuana closed her eyes. His touch was nauseating. "Where were you, Jack. Where were you this afternoon?"

Jack stepped back. "At Adkins, you knew that."

Djuana's body trembled in anger. Her stomach knotted and her heart leaped into her throat. "Don't lie to me, Jack, I asked you to never lie to me." Her tears flowed evenly.

Jack sobered. "Baby, what are you talking about? You know I would never lie to you."

In one quick motion, she spun and stabbed Jack in the left side of his abdomen. The shock and sudden pain hit him harder than the feel of the kitchen knife. He retreated a few steps before falling. His hands covered the wound, and were soon covered with blood. "What did I do to you?"

Djuana dropped the knife, feel back against the counter, and when she saw his blood she fainted. Jack ignored his pain and sprawled his body to cushion her fall. She landed in what seemed a slow, dramatic drop. He held her, then guided her limp body down as gently as he could on the tile floor, fighting to not let her head thump, and to not bleed on her.

Jack then muscled his way to his knees, picking the phone off its base. He made the call to 911; clearly giving his name, address and both his and her condition. The operator paused, and sounded horrified as she asked his name again, "The Crowns Jack Newhouse?"

The police arrived first, having to break into the house. The ambulance workers were a quick second. Then more cops and plenty of press. A wide-eyed emergency technician leaned in on Jack and said, among the hundreds of questions, "You're bleeding, Mr. Newhouse."

Jack grabbed the woman, his strength abandoning him, and replied, "She's pregnant. Handle her first."

He tightened his grip. "Make sure that baby is okay."

The female medic grinned, a reassuring smile, at the bleeding, famous, baseball player. "Don't worry, J-New, we are here for the three of you."

A moment later, Jack passed out.

# 25

St. Vincent hospital was in a frenzy. Reporters, camera crews and cops were everywhere. As Crowns players arrived they were mobbed. The Pioneer family entered the hospital amid the madness unnoticed, until an orderly told a reporter they were related to Djuana. Then, they too were mobbed. Emma was rude, knowing the media would be against her daughter.

She had her brother take over, and Calvin manhandled the press. He elbowed and shoved them away from the family. The feeble looking reporters were easily scared away; all but the pretty white woman with no badge, no pad, no pen, nor camera.

Kristen approached Calvin with a piece of advise.

"You need to make some kind of statement, or the hounds will bother you forever."

"Thanks, but mind you own fuckin' business lady."

"Listen to me. The woman stabbed a Major League Baseball player. Could have killed him. Don't you think that is news?"

"People want to know what happen."

Before Cal realized it, Kris was with the family, and she got their version of what happen. This was before any person in the family had spoken to Djuana. But, Kris took their claims, mixed them with facts she received from the police, and boom: a front page exclusive and a story run throughout the country. The cover of the Portland paper in the morning read:

"NEWHOUSE STABBED, VICTIM CLAIMS RAPE"

Djuana was being held by the police on the third floor, in maternity. The cops waited for a doctor to run tests - she and the baby were fine - then they officially arrested her. Only her mother was allowed in the room, besides the female officer sitting guard.

When Emma entered the room her knees shook at the sight of her daughter crying and handcuffed to the bed. Djuana had turned her body into the fetal position, her right hand cuffed to the bed board. The cop was seated near the door, without expression. Emma took short, deliberate strides to the bed.

"Are the shackles necessary?" Emma glared at the cop.

"Yes," the officer politely replied.

"She ain't going no fucking where!" Emma tried not to shout, but did.

When she finally put her big, thick arms around her daughter, Djuana's crying became uncontrollable and loud.

"I didn't mean to, Mommy," she sobbed. "I didn't mean to kill him. I love him."

Djuana had said it. Finally. After thinking for weeks she was in love, and enjoying it, she had refused to say so. But, now saying it seemed to matter more than the feelings.

Emma's tears began as two streams; one from each eye leading to her jaw. She squeezed her daughter and the tears flowed evenly.

"He ain't dead, baby," Emma whispered. "I wish he was. Lord, knows, I wish he was."

Jack was in emergency surgery for an hour before taken to the fourth floor in stable condition. Jack's quick reflexes prevented the knife from deeply penetrating his left rib cage; he did suffer a deep, but not serious, cut on his hand. An intern at the hospital had mistakenly believed the stab involved serious internal injury, and said so to the press.

That same doctor wanted to perform a Laparotomy, a thorough examination of the entire abdomen. The Crowns physicians were against it. Jack would be unavailable to the team for at least a month.

Nevertheless, the team's doctors determined he was stabbed in the lower portion of his left rib cage. Djuana sliced into the pleura, the double layer of membranes in spaces between the ribs and encloses the lung. The fluid provides lubrication and thus allows smooth expansion and contraction of the lungs during breathing.

No vital organs were perforated, nor were any major blood vessels severed. The wound was clean and closed with 11 stitches.

Even though everyone involved knew that Jack was in more than stable condition, the media took the intern's comments about how Jack could've died and splattered them tabloid-style on the covers of newspapers and television screens across the country. Djuana's picture was prominently posed opposite Jack's; the photo of her tears-soaked face being lead to the hospital out of the police car and into the hospital was everywhere.

Jack held firm in his story. He told the police that he and Djuana were playing in the kitchen and she accidentally stabbed him. The police didn't believed him, neither did the team doctors nor Slight or Honeywell. But it was the story given to the press. And Djuana was released from custody. The police believed Emma's claim of rape, though. They questioned Jack thoroughly, but he was unaffected.

Jack told Berger, his lawyer as well as his agent, to find Djuana and defend her in any way.

Berger scoffed defiantly.

"Just do it," Jack demanded, springing forward in his bed. "And make sure the baby is okay."

Berger nearly fainted. "What baby?"

"She's pregnant."

"What? Oh, shit. She's having your baby?"

Jack cut him off, "Just do that for me. Please?"

Oscar had been silent through the ordeal, but Jack knew his friend was steaming. When the room was finally emptied, Oscar got up from the window seal shaking his head.

"I'ma get somebody to bust a cap in that bitch. What she trippin' about? Money? Don't give her a damn cent."

Jack edged onto his wound. He was tired of laying on his right side. "Shut up, 'fore I put something in your mouth. Just let it be. I'll handle it."

"How? She's got you so pussy-whipped, you done forgave her before the wound healed. Don't tell me that's your baby. You just started hittin' it."

"Just chill and have a seat. I'm alive, ain't I?"

"Yeah, whatever. Just don't let me see that bitch strolling downtown. I might accidentally break my foot off in her ass."

Berger approached the Pioneer family in haste. He explained who he was, and that Jack sent him to defend Djuana. Calvin stood from the waiting room's sofa and towered over the short, white man with the expensive suit and briefcase.

"You tell Jack Newhouse we don't need shit from him," Cal's voice was strained.

"Fine." Berger spun on his heels and briskly walked away.

Djuana was released from the hospital just before noon the morning after. Hundreds of people had crowded the front of St. Vincent's. Cards and flowers were sent in support of Jack, but for the most part the crowd was there to see first hand the woman that almost killed one of Portland's few stars. As Calvin and his friend Ed shielded Djuana with raincoats, the crowd booed and cursed Djuana. A couple of the people threw objects, but nothing hit any member of the Pioneer family. The police were of no assistance. The District Three Captain, an avid fan of Crowns' baseball, only sent a dozen cops.

Djuana had her eyes closed as the two men all but carried her to Cal's car. Emma was behind her, with her hands supporting Djuana's backside. They squeezed into the large four door Buick, and raced off. The ride home was silent, no radio, no discussion of any topic. Tudor Street was empty, and the family was thankful.

For two days Djuana became a recluse. She did not leave her room for anything but to use the bathroom. And, when she did, she snuck out and back in. Her mother would bring her meals that she would peck over with a fork. Emma would beg her to eat for the baby's health.

Talking to herself had slowly become second nature to Djuana; who was there to tell that you almost killed a man because you love him and didn't want him to hurt you? And, Djuana knew she was wrong. Jack did not do her wrong. She had reasoned it out; she had plenty of time to think while holding herself hostage in her room. She avoided any and everyone. The radio, which she loved, and the television had become deadly enemies. Her face and name were all over the place. Talk shows either defended her or asked for her jailing.

Sources were saying that Jack tried to rape her, and she fended him off with the knife. Who were these sources? Djuana wanted so badly to call those shows, call the newspapers, and tell people the truth. The whole truth. That she was in love and so afraid of being the fool once again. So afraid of giving her heart and having a man crush it with deception that she would kill.

Djuana would rub her round, tight belly and cry for hours. How could she tell people it wasn't Jack's fault? That she just stabbed him. He came in smiling, happy to see her, with flowers, and she just pounced on him. And, how could she tell those same people, Crowns fans, police, Geraldo, Oprah and Donahue, that she loved him dearly? That she had never loved before in her life; and that included Dexter Forns. She knew this because she had never wanted to die during those episodes when Dexter would disappear. But, now, the thought of never being held by Jack Newhouse was driving her to thoughts of suicide.

She did this to herself, she easily realized. Jack Newhouse was not cheating on her. That baseball player was pleasing her without being asked. Thinking, and guilt, helped her understand that whatever that woman said o the phone was said to get her in a rage; and it worked.

"That day with the soup," she recalled, "He wasn't even my man yet. Shit, I didn't even think I wanted him yet? So why could he screw whoever he wanted to?"

Shit, shit, shit.

Djuana began hating herself. Like the way she did when Dexter had her believing she had gotten pregnant on purpose. She would twirl in her bed, tangling herself in the covers. She'd screamed into her pillow, then fling it at the television. It wasn't on, but she could hear still hear the accusations.

Djuana bolted out of the bed, tripping on the covers she had forgotten that were tied around her. She fell to the floor in a thud. She scrambled to her feet, and ripped open her closet and pulled out Jack's Crowns jersey. Jack had given it to her, and she cherished it.

She tossed the jersey on the floor, near where she had fallen, and piled anything else he had bought for her on top of it. A Crowns hat and tee-shirt, the dress she wore to the banquet and all the cards he had sent her from rode trips.

The cards. She stopped, plopped on the bed, her feet inches from the pile and picked the cards up into her lap. She recalled each individual episode when the gifts were given to her. The cards stung her heart. There were six of them, all with Jack's sloppy handwriting in them, each humorous. They had caused her to watch the mailbox whenever the Crowns were out of town.

"Damn."

No one had ever sent her cards just because.

Her body slowly drifted off the bed and onto her knees. She picked up the floral card, her favorite because inside of it was only Jack's handwriting. He wrote like a third-grader in a hurry, still Djuana saw an endearing testament of his desire.

*Dearest Djuana,*

*I just hung up the phone from you, and I miss you already. I knew that by the time you get this card we will be back from the east coast, but I wanted you to understand that I do love you very much and miss you when we are apart.*

*Truly,*
*J-New*

Djuana cried on her knees, card in hand, and feeling very lonely.

"Jack, who is this woman?" Cecila Rivers asked.

"I met her in April," Jack solemnly told his sister.

"What happen? Why did she stab you?"

Jack pressed the remote, and the stations on his television flashed by. "She had been hurt a lot, and she thought I was hurting her."

"What? What kind of shit is that?"

Jack didn't reply.

"What did you do? The news is saying you tried to rape her. I know you didn't."

"Of course not."

"Then, tell me what happen."

"I came home, she was in the kitchen cooking. Everything seemed cool, then she just turned and stabbed me."

"What did she say?"

"Nothing, really. She thinks I cheated on her, I think."

"That's bullshit! There's got to be more to it."

"I told you all I know."

"Why you ain't call me? Why I gotta hear about this on the news with my children? I told you about these women. So, what, she's pregnant? Is it yours?"

"No."

"Don't lie to me, Jack. I love you, and I don't want to see happen to you what so many other professional athletes go through with golddiggers."

"She's not a golddigger."

"Jack?"

"I'm sure."

On her third day back from the hospital, Djuana ventured out of her room and into the kitchen while her mother and Devon were out of the house. Uncle Calvin, Djuana's personal bodyguard, was asleep on the couch. Calvin was staying there, going and coming from work. There had been threatening phone calls and people shouting curses at 657 Tudor from passing cars.

For the first time in 19 years, the Pioneers had a new phone number; unlisted new phone number.

Two reasons brought Djuana out of solitude: (a) she was tired of baked and boiled chicken, her mother's remedy for anything, and (b) the walls in her room were closing in on her. In the kitchen she found Devon had put anything associated with the Crowns into the garbage. She smiled at first, then sobered at the thought of how many times Jack had called in the past two days before the number changed.

Maybe I should talk to him, she thought. He had done no wrong.

Standing there in the kitchen, with the sound of her uncle snoring a distant buzz, she replayed each of the past three days, not able to think about the stabbing without hurt chilling her heart.

She thought about work, imagining how the customers would curse at her, maybe even hit her. Mr. Thompson had called Djuana's first night home. He told Emma that Djuana should take a week off from the department store. Djuana did not want to take any days off, but the thought of dealing with the public swayed her to stay home.

There had been lots of visitors; both friends and family. Djuana refused to see them all, including Tia. The only person she did see or speak with, besides Emma and Devon, was Aunt Earline. She felt she needed the spiritual guidance more than the Jack bashing everyone else offered.

When Aunt Earline entered the room, Djuana felt brighter. She felt the room illuminate, and her spirits lift. They embraced and shared a warm kiss. Earline remained standing and told Djuana to be seated on the bed.

"I prayed for you," were the first words Aunt Earl said, and just that quickly Djuana was engulfed by a sense of relief.

Djuana threw out a question that first startled Earline, then she caught the drift that Djuana was taking the conversation.

"How did you know you loved Uncle Steve?"

"I knew," Earl smiled that broad Pioneer smile, all cheeks. "I knew. That man had my heart the very first day I saw him at the Rose show all those umpteen years ago."

"But, Aunt Earl, how did you know? How did you know it was love?"

"Baby, words don't explain no love," she said as she paced. "And, don't let anybody tell you different. You don't have to explain it. You're either in it, and know it, or you're not. You just have to believe your heart and go with it.

"That's where the help from the man you love comes in. You see, it may be true that I was head over heels over Steve, but if he hadn't been such a good, kind man that loved much as deeply as I loved him, we wouldn't have ever gotten married."

Djuana was at ease while Earline was there. Her aunt's reasoning allowed her to dream of being with Jack again. *He is a good man. He'll forgive me.* As she let the words free her mind, more questions arose. Some answered themselves. She thought about the first time Jack touched her.

Djuana wondered aloud, "Is there a such thing as love at first touch?"

Earline gave Djuana a serious look. Djuana shamefully bowed her head, fiddling with her fingers.

"I'm all confused," the niece confessed.

"Just follow your heart," Earl kissed her forehead. "Let it go."

"I can't. Every time I do let my heart open, something bad happens, and I end up hurt. I am tired of all this hurt."

"These trials and tribulations you are experiencing now are just the Lord's way of testing your will," Aunt Earl preached.

She sat on the bed, and Djuana rose to meet her, but Earl held her at bay with the palm of her hand.

Earl continued, feeling the heart of her pupil listening, "You can never defend yourself alone against Satan. But, my dear, if you go with the spirit of Christ you will be forever armed."

Djuana would not think of religion in the same light again.

Still standing there in the kitchen, as if frozen by the cold linoleum on her bare feet, Djuana's heart and mind zipped back to the first date, and, subsequently, their first kiss. The softness of his touch. The gentle way he her and guided her chin, How she didn't want to stop. She licked her lips, and moaned.

"I love him."

Cal shifted on the couch, smacking his big lips, but did not wake.

Quietly, Djuana fixed herself a sandwich with the steak undoubtedly, Uncle Cal had cooked. Emma was into her 'chicken heals' mood. Djuana put just about everything in the refrigerator into her sandwich; lettuce, tomatoes, onions, mustard, mayonnaise and the last slice of wrapped American cheese. She was in Hog Heaven at the kitchen table when the telephone's steady buzz startled her. She ignored it, it had come easy after three days. But, after four rings she realized her uncle was dead to the world. She picked up the phone, it had to be family, she thought, since the number had been changed, but it wasn't.

Dexter said, "What's up? Are you all right?"

"Dex, how did you get this number?" Her somber mood fell to that of frustration.

"I got my ways, you know that. I was worried about you. Are you feeling all right?"

"I'm fine."

"I've got something for you. Can I bring it over?"

"No, Dex. I don't need anything."

"Look, you know I always loved you. Yeah, I've fucked up plenty, but you know how I feel about you. I just want to see if you're all right."

Djuana stepped into the living and looked over to her sleeping uncle. "Okay. You can come by. But just for a minute or two."

Dexter sped from Front to Tudor, over a mile, in seconds. He had bought a stuffed animal and was planning to give it to his wife if Djuana had said she didn't want him to come by. He scurried into the building oblivious to the chatter among the women on the stoop about Djuana, Jack Newhouse and him.

Djuana answered the door in baggy, gray shorts - they were Jack's - and a black Portland Trail Blazers t-shirt. She had put on the shorts with out thinking, but when she saw the gold crown on the left thigh she shook her head. Jack was deeply entrenched into her life. Dexter, who was in heat because his wife was still angry about the scene in the grocery store, was disappointed to find Djuana wearing a dark colored shirt. He was hoping to get a look at her breasts. He moved forward to kiss her, but she pulled away.

Dexter came into the apartment and saw Calvin sitting up on the couch smoking a cigarette. Dexter spoke, and Calvin just stared at him. Dexter quickly turned back to Djuana.

"How you doing? You better?"

"Fine, Dex. Just fucking fine."

He handed her the stuffed animal. She accepted it, and looked it over. "What is it? A bear?"

Dex laughed. "No. It's an elephant."

Calvin chuckled, then barked with meanness, "A white elephant?"

Dexter became agitated. "Yeah. You never seen a white elephant?"

"Nope. But, what else would I expect from your sorry ass but a cheap-ass gift. The only reason I don't fuckin' whip your ass is because DJ asked me not too.

"You faggot!"

Dexter held his response. He had come to talk, not get killed by her crazy uncle. He told Djuana he needed to talk to her in private.

Calvin said, "So, talk."

Djuana looked at her uncle and told Dexter to come into the kitchen. Once in there, they both forced whispers.

"What you want, Dex?"

"Listen. You know what I want to know. What's up with you and Jack Newhouse?"

"That's not your concern."

"Oh, really. Is that his?" Dexter ran his hand over her stomach.

Djuana shoved him away. "You are really unbelievable."

He pressed on, "Just answer the question. I know you have been seeing him. You stab him because he don't believe it's his child either?"

"Good-bye, Dexter. I am not answering no stupid questions." She walked back into the living room and toward the front door. She went that way to force Dexter to walk past Calvin again. He slowly followed. Throwing questions as he went, being lead out the door. Standing out of the doorway, he said:

"If you think you are gonna try and dog me 'cause you are on some payback mission, forget it. I will sue you and make you have blood tests done. I ain't paying for his baby if he don't want it."

Djuana lost her cool. She wanted to tell Dexter that Jack Newhouse was not the kind of slimy man he was. But, instead she spewed: "Fuck you, Dexter! Fuck, you. You ain't never planned to pay for shit!"

She flung the door all the way to the wall in the apartment then slammed it shut. The force blew papers about the house. The noise scared her. Uncle Calvin shook his head and pulled away from the coffee table as she entered into the living room and flopped down in a chair.

"Why don't you just let me do that faggot?"

Djuana glanced at the small hand gun on the coffee table. She cut her eyes away with a long blink.

# 26

Jack took a deep breath after he heard her voice. He had been dialing and re-dialing the number for two hours. He had each word planned out. He needed to speak with Djuana, and this was the best way. Finally he said: "Hello, Tia. This is Jack Newhouse."

He was sitting at his kitchen table, inches from where he had been stabbed. His blood had been cleaned up, but he could still see the incident clearly in his memory. He waited for the best friend of the woman he loved to answer.

Tia was infuriated instantly by the sound of Jack's voice. He had some nerve calling, she fumed, "Why you calling me? How did you get my number?"

"Tia, I still had your number from the time I called Djuana there. Please, just listen to me. I need you to help me. I need to talk to Djuana."

"Forget it. I warned you not to hurt her. You did and fucked up."

"I didn't do anything to her! I swear it! I love that woman with all my heart."

"Save it. And do me a favor, Mister In-Love. Lose my fucking number before you really get hurt."

"Then, listen, Tia. Tell me what it is I suppose to have done."

"Don't yell at me!"

Jack dropped his elbows into his lap. He knew he hadn't yelled, and he didn't want to whine or beg, but he did.

"I'm sorry," his voice fell to a faint whisper. "I don't mean to yell at you, but this is crazy. She stabbed me, and I don't know what the hell I did to deserve it."

Tia believed he was being sincere, yet Djuana had been hurt enough. She loved him as much as Djuana did. She saw how happy her friend was when with him. She saw the smiles, giggles and tears of joy. It was the thought of the tears of hurt Djuana had shed Tia could not shake at that moment.

Still, she could not hang up on Jack.

Jack continued to plead, tugging at Tia's heart with each word.

"I love her, Tia," he said. "I love that woman more than anything in this world."

Tia blew air into the phone through her nose, a long sigh. "Jack, I don't know," her voice lacked anger. "She doesn't want to speak to you. She says you cheated on her."

"Is that what she thinks? I didn't."

"Jack, don't."
"I didn't."
Tia sighed again.
"So, what do you want me to do?"

Emma tapped the door lightly and entered among the curses. "Baby, Tia is on the phone. Why don't you talk to her? She loves you and you know she has always been there for you."

Djuana snapped, "I know that. You don't need to tell me that!"

Emma continued her walking on egg shells. "Just talk to her, please."

Djuana picked up the phone, and Emma relaxed and left the room.

"Hey, Dee, you all right?"

"As good as I can be right now. Everybody in this lovely city is calling me a criminal."

Tia paused, she wanted to say the right thing. "It ain't like that. Your real friends are still behind you. And, you've still got your family."

Djuana's nerves chilled. "I know. I know. I'm sorry I haven't answered your calls, but I just am not in the talking mood."

Tia fought off second thoughts. "Please meet me downtown? I want us to eat and talk."

"Downtown? Shit. People will be staring at me."

"To hell with them. You can't live in one room for the rest of your life."

Those words sank quickly. Djuana looked around her bedroom. It was a disaster area. Plates on the floor, on her night stand, glasses on the window seal, floor and on top of the dresser. On the floor, with the dishes, was the radio, smashed to bits. She could see she needed to get out, and could use the fresh air.

Every minute of the short drive to the west side, Calvin would ask if Djuana needed anything - more air, a soft drink, a hug, to go back to the solitude of her bedroom. Yet, he did it in a way that was far from the nagging Emma had done.

Calvin stopped the car in front of Alice's Soul Food Joint. He cut off the engine, put his can of beer between his legs, and shifted his body to face Djuana. In a serious tone he said, "DJ, I love you. Do you know that?"

"Of course I do, Uncle Cal." She was taken aback by his sudden grim expression.

Djuana asked her uncle if he wanted to join her and Tia in Alice's; even though she knew his beer-breath would offend Tia.

He shook his head, "No, because I want you to have some time away from me and live again.

"This bodyguard shit has got to be getting on your nerves?"

Calvin squeezed the paper bag around his tall can of malt liquor.

"Girl, you my heart. I love you more than anything. When you were born your mother used to get on me 'cause I used to stare at you so much. Every time I looked at you, I just loved you more."

Calvin looked away, fighting tears. He took a deep swig from the can and licked his lips. Djuana hung on his every word and movement. Her mouth gapped, and her eyes glossed. He had never spoken a serious word with her besides threats about never letting a man touch her in any way she didn't approve of. He may be drunk more often than sober, but he loved his nieces and nephews. Djuana understood this.

"I'd do anything for you, you know that, right?" Calvin continued.

"Yes."

"And, you know that if you needed me, all you have to do is call me and I'd be there. Right?"

"Yes. I know you would."

Calvin looked away again, then said, looking at her eye-to-eye, "Did that baseball player rape you?"

"No. He didn't."

"Baby. This is me. You can tell me. It's just the two of us."

"No, Uncle Calvin. He didn't," tears lightly flowed down Djuana's cheeks. She wiped them and continued. "I stabbed him because I thought he was being like most men, trying to have me and every other woman he could after he told me he loved me and promised he wouldn't."

Cal ignored this explanation. "You know there is such a form of rape that ain't forcible sex? He could have used lines or lies to get you in bed. Is that why y'all had that fight?"

Djuana had thought about just that, as he uncle described it, and she knew in her heart that she was wrong. She should have asked Jack what the deal was with the bitch on the phone. She looked into Calvin's eyes and patted his hands, which were holding the beer between his legs.

"No, he was honest with me. I was the wrong one. I thought he was being like every other man and I wasn't wise enough to realize the man loves me."

Cal reached across his Cutlass and took Djuana's head with his right hand behind her head and planted a kiss on her forehead. "I love you no matter what."

Djuana held on tightly as her uncle squeezed her too hard into a hug. She didn't protest because she felt his tears on her face. She turned her head in his embrace and kissed his cheek.

"I love you too, Uncle Cal," she whispered to him. "I love you too."

When Alice closed the restaurant for Jack to use personally, Salese asked to stay while the other band members gladly took the paid day off. He knew

Jack as a famous baseball player, and saw him eat in Alice's. Everyone told him he had seen Djuana before, Alice showed him her picture in the newspaper, but he couldn't remember the lady. Salese had been working at Alice's for three years and could use a evening to himself and his girlfriend, but he wanted to see the woman that would drive a man to rent a whole restaurant after she had stabbed *him*.

"Hey, man, Jack," Salese said quietly. "You don't mind if I stick around? Do you?"

Jack's stiff expression didn't change. He sipped the warm white wine and shook his head, his eyes on the tall, slender glass.

"Want to hear something? I have been working on a piece, a nice soft piece I call it *Last Impression*."

Jack's eyes remained fixed on the happenings outside of the door. He did not care what Salese did with his horn. Djuana was coming; he was sure of it. Not only because he had a nifty plan of using her best friend to lure her. No, he knew Djuana was a smart lady. She probably did see right through the thin deception, but he felt she wanted to see him.

Jack enjoyed Alice's restaurant. It was one of the few public places he could relax in. Alice's was a down home dining saloon; all of Alice's tables were small and round, with blue and white African print table cloths. On each table, next to the salt and pepper was her house sauce, that was a spicy, hot mixture that she concocted in the kitchen. The bar was long, comfortable and well stocked.

When she first opened the restaurant, four years before, she was the chef, hostess and part-time bar maid. Now, she had an excellent staff. Now, she had people coming to have a drink, and listen to Salese's group, Alice's house band.

Alice took a break from accounting paper work in her small office off the kitchen and sat with her solemn customer. She took a sip of Jack's wine and began questioning him.

"How long I know you, New," the burly woman asked as she emptied the bottle into the glass.

"Long enough for you to give me another glass of wine while you drink mine," he said without a smile.

"Shit," she grumbled. "Like you need another glass."

She yelled into the kitchen to Pedro to bring out another bottle. Pedro, the master chef, Alice, Salese and Jack were the only people still in the joint.

Jack remained solemn, listening to Salese play a soulful, sad horn when Calvin pulled up with Djuana in his four-door ride. He saw the car, but paid no attention. Jack was expecting Djuana to walk up, or arrive in a cab.

Alice took another sip then put the glass on the round table. Pedro came to the table and uncorked another bottle of wine. He was scared to look Jack in the eye because he more fear he would say something stupid, like "How's the wound?" But, he wanted to say something. When he began working at Alice's as a busboy/waiter/prep cook it was Jack Newhouse who was the most polite to him. Other super stars, like the white players on the Crowns and the Portland basketball players, treated him like hired help, but Jack tipped generously, and often struck up conversations. Jack also urged Alice to get Pedro in culinary school, and Pedro believed Jack paid his tuition - Alice was too cheat to have done that much.

Jack thanked him for the service, and took a sip of the fresh wine.

Pedro bowed and slipped away.

Alice put her legs up on one of the empty chairs at their table. "So, is she worth it?"

"She's worth it," Jack answered glumly.

"She stabbed you. Could've ended you life or your career."

Jack didn't answer. He just watched the pedestrian traffic through the glass doors.

"What if she comes in with a gun, or another knife? I ain't as fast as I used to be, you know."

"Don't sweat it. Pedro will take care of it." Again, no smile, but he turned his head in time to see the swinging doors of the kitchen sway closed.

The combination of Jack's solemn mood and Salese's horn depressed Alice. "Can't you play something upbeat? You killing us!"

Just then, the door opened and Djuana peeked in.

"Are you open?" she said to the nearest person, Salese. Her voice barely carried from the door. She stepped in to hear an answer, and that was when she saw Jack.

Salese had stopped playing when she spoke to him, he was impressed. He had seen Jack with plenty of women, all better dressed than Djuana. Wearing more expensive, revealing clothing and jewelry and hugged up on Jack. But, he saw right away that Djuana was Jack's woman.

Jack and Alice rose at the same time; although Alice had to gather herself off of two chairs. Alice was right about how she knew Djuana, she instantly recognized her as the friend of the skinny woman, Tia, who had often come to her eatery. Her first impression was that the photos in the papers had done the child no justice. Then she remembered the handsome light skin man that often accompanied Djuana and Tia.

Djuana entered, frowning. She looked for Tia, but knew it was a set up. She was at first nervous - she actually thought for a second that Jack may retaliate physically. Alice approached her with a smile and locked the door behind her.

"We are open, but just for you and Jack," Alice said as she disappeared into the kitchen, dragging Pedro back in with her. He had slid out to see the fire works.

Salese whispered to Jack, "You want me to stay, Man?"

Jack continued walking to Djuana and shook his head. Salese packed his trumpet, and left via the back door which led to the club's parking area. Jack asked Djuana to come and join him. She stood there, mumbling.

Jack moved within inches from Djuana. She folded her arms across her chest, she was disturbed by the surprise. "Why did you do this? Are you apologizing?"

"Why? Should I be? I just want you to have a seat and talk with me. Tell me what's up."

Djuana remained still. "Tia had never lied to me before. You got her to lie to me. I don't appreciate that."

"Well, I didn't appreciate getting stabbed. You sit down and I'll tell you my motivation behind getting you here. And then you can tell me your motivation in trying to kill me."

Djuana stared. But Jack didn't flinch. She unfolded her arms and allowed Jack to guide her by her right arm to their table. Alice returned from the kitchen with two bowls of soup.

"Clam chowder will be good for the baby's sex drive," she said to Djuana as she placed the steamy bowls in front of them. Jack grinned, Djuana didn't.

Jack noticed this, and decided to get right to the discussion.

"Alice, can you leave us now. Please," Jack said as he shifted his chair so that he sat directly across from Djuana.

Alice's dark skin was beaming. She was glowing, blushing. "Jack loves you, dear. He does. I have never seen him take to someone like this before."

Alice, then, disappeared.

"Your hair looks great, as usual." Jack said, seriously.

Djuana had her hair out with a head band on the top allowing her hair to flow down to her shoulders.

Djuana politely, yet still distant, thanked him.

Jack began, "So, why is your mother telling the press that I tried to rape you?"

Djuana had felt her mother had been behind the start of that rumor. "I didn't tell her that."

"But, is that how you feel?"

"No."

"You want to tell me what happen?"

Djuana fought the urge to explode into profanity. "Like you don't know?"

"If I did, I wouldn't have been racking my brain trying to figure it out the last week."

"Please," Djuana shifted her body to the side, facing the door. She looked out into the street. Her uncle was standing, leaning on the parking meter smoking a cigarette.

"Are you going to tell me or what?"

"You yelling at me?! I should've..."

"Should have what? Killed me? For what? What did I do to you beside try to love you?"

"Like you love Stacie and those others? You ain't fool me! Never did. But, I told your conceited ass that I wasn't the one to lie to or play with. That's why you got what was just deserved!"

Djuana bolted up, knocking the table to a wobble, spilling the soup, and turned to leave. Jack, stunned by her claims, jumped up and chased after her.

"Don't touch me! You got women, why you want me? Why?"

"I don't have anybody but you. I don't. I wouldn't think of hurting you," he felt her attention and knew he'd better unleash all his feelings..

"I love you Djuana."

"Please don't say that," she feebly whispered.

Jack continued, his voice lowered to her soft tone, "And I don't know what you are talking about. Shit, I haven't dealt with Stacie in over a month."

"That ain't what she told me."

"The bitch lied," he whimpered.

Djuana's eyes moistened; but she was too stubborn to cry in front of him. Also, she was angry and confused. She loved Jack, but couldn't give in to him and be hurt again. But she believed him. She tried to pull away, but Jack held onto her arm, trying to get his explanation heard.

"Let me go, Jack. Get off of me."

She pushed him, and he let go. Djuana did not go far. She sidestepped a few paces, but her legs would not lead her body where her mind did not want to go.

"Don't you know I really love you?" Jack pleaded. "That I wouldn't ever want to see you hurt."

Djuana turned to look into Jack's loving eyes. She relented. She could feel her guards dropping and had no power to force them back up. She wanted to back away, turn and run out the door. But her feet were planted.

Jack took center stage, making sure not to approach her. "I hate the man that has hurt you so deeply that you can't realize that I truly care for you. All I want is to see you happy.

"Make you happy."

Djuana folded her arms and leaned on her heels. She sighed, then bowed her head.

Off to the side, at rear of the restaurant, and standing at the entrance of the kitchen, Alice and Pedro were silently rooting for Jack. Pedro was still holding the carving knife he had planned to use to rescue Jack if Djuana had made any move to hurt him again.

Outside, Calvin was sitting on his car with his eyes fixed on Djuana's every move. He was prepared to race in and shoot the place up if his niece needed it. But, he had become relaxed by her mannerisms, even though he could tell she was crying. His pulse raced, but a deeper urge, to let her be, held him in place.

Djuana stood still. Her eyes looked out toward the street and her eyes caught Calvin looking in at her. She quickly looked away. She folded her arms at her waist, then her right hand raced to rubbed her eyes.

"What am I doing to myself," she whispered.

"Hug her you damn fool!" Alice begged in a grumble of a whisper.

"Shhh!" Pedro elbowed his boss.

Jack, with his arms spread, ended the minute long silence.

"Come here," he called to Djuana.

Acting on an impulse that was far removed from her usual analytical forethought, and without stopping to questions where her actions would lead, Djuana scooted nearer and leaned into Jack's chest. As his arms engulfed her into a close, warm embrace, she decided to just let her heart guide her.

Jack's arms closed around her waist to squeeze her in deeper. She rested her hands on his arms. Slowly, her eyes drifted shut. She felt his lips touch the top of her head, then her nose. Her mouth watered in anticipation, and when his warm lips arrived she parted her mouth and kissed him passionately.

"You haven't hurt me," she sighed. "I've been the one doing the hurting because I'm so damn insecure."

"Look, forget all that," Jack said. "It doesn't matter. I understand now where your mind was. We can deal with it."

"Jack, its more than just that."

He took her soft hand, kissed it. "Then, sit down, relax, and tell me about it."

Calvin had watched his niece kiss the baseball player and he knew. He knew at that moment she was no longer his naive niece struggling with wolves interested in her well-developed body. She was a woman in love. He blew cigarette smoke upward and finished his beer, with a smile.

Djuana sat, and began talking before she realized she was opening up. Jack sat across from her. Each eventually moved the soup to their side.

"In a few short months I will be a mother," she began. "A single mother. I can't afford to be making these kinds of mistakes then with a baby depending on me for a stable life."

"I'll be responsible for more than just my life."

Jack was nodding in agreement until she paused. He had the answer, and didn't want to blurt it.

"I can give you that stability," he whispered, leaning across the table.

Djuana took his hand and rubbed his smooth knuckles. No manual labor, she thought. Jack raised their hands and kissed her knuckles.

She said, "I'm just problems for you." Her eyes watered. Her grip tightened.

"No you're not."

"Yes I am. I made you miss games, and the team and the whole city wants to kill me."

"Not even," Jack held her hands tightly. "Forget them. I am the only one you need to worry about. And, I'm here to tell you that we can work this out.

"I love you, Djuana."

Tears streamed down her face. "I know you do. And. I need that love. Please just give me time."

Jack pulled his handkerchief and gently dried her face with soft dabs. Then he kissed her cheek. "You've got all the time you need."

Alice wiped her tears and looked over at her chef. The two were still eavesdropping from the swinging kitchen door. She handed him a dry, cloth napkin off of a service tray.

"Wipe your eyes, you baby," she whispered, adding, "I knew there was a reason why I like that man."

Pedro rubbed his moist eyes and nodded.

# 27

Losing was putting a strain on the cohesiveness of the Portland Crowns. The core of their squad had played together for at least five years, some longer. Reporters and baseball analyst throughout the country seemed to agreed with Slight; maybe it was time to break up the team. The finger pointing among the players began directly after Las Vegas beat them for the third straight year. Had Bingo not struck out 11 times; had Oscar not dropped a fly ball at a crucial time in Game Six; had the bullpen not faltered.

Maybe, had those miscues had not happen, they would have been champions.

Now the Crowns were losing during the regular season, something they hadn't done before. Petty arguments became fist fights in the clubhouse or in hotels. Pugsley and Luis, roommates for four years, and the glue of the team's defense as middle infielders, stopped speaking to one another.

Cris Carpenter, the left fielder, accused Oscar of trying to talk to his new girlfriend. The woman ended up sleeping with Oscar and leaving Cris. Bryant Clark, the third baseman and the second best pure hitter on the team behind Oscar, stopped speaking to his teammates and the press. He asked Honeywell to trade him anywhere. He would never say why he was upset – he would wear tape across his mouth some days in the clubhouse – but it was obvious to most of his teammates that he felt he should be batting third in the lineup instead of Jack.

Then, Bingo Wells walked away from the team when it returned from a road trip. The best power hitter in baseball told the press, before telling Slight or the players, that he had decided he would never play for the Portland Crowns again. He demanded a trade, and shocked the world of baseball when he disclosed the team he wanted to be traded to was the Buffalo Soldiers, one the worst team in the league.

Honeywell and Slight, at the outset, refused to discuss trading Bingo. The team fined him instead, as well as suspending his pay. Bingo took the fines and loss of pay in stride.

When reporters asked why he wanted to leave Portland, Bingo told them, "I don't need money," he told reporters. "I need a championship ring. And, I'll never get one playing in Portland."

Bingo spoke freely about Lee Spencer's $10,000 a week cocaine habit. He gave details about Oscar's robust sex drive and the nights Oscar and Jack had slept with up to four women at one time.

Before he was done he had aired all of the Crowns' dirty laundry. That was his method of making certain Slight would not try to retain him; he knew Slight would take the breach of privacy personally.

Slight had Honeywell trade Bingo to Buffalo for Bruce Leonard, Raul Montanez and minor leaguer Russ Jones. All marginal players, in comparison to Bingo's worth at the time. The next day the trade escalated into a nightmare for the Portland Crowns and their fans. The Las Vegas Gamblers traded six marginal players and two million dollars to Buffalo for Bingo and Lee. The night of the trade, Bingo played for the Gamblers and hit two home runs.

Slight was devastated. He refused comments to the press, and was depressed for a week. He then saw no way to beat Las Vegas and get his hands on the championship trophy. Honeywell demanded an investigation, telling the media that Las Vegas had set up Portland in a quest of their fifth consecutive championship.

Jack lined balls into the nets of Adkins Stadium's under ground batting cage in the wee hours of a quiet Tuesday morning. The batting cage was located between the Crowns' and the visitors' clubhouses. It was a renovated stock room, with a pitching machine in the center of the always damp, well-lighted, cement chamber. The dirt and chalked batter's box was surrounded by nets.

With each hard shot off of the pitching machine his thoughts about turning this season around became attainable dreams. He could see those thuds against the back walls as home runs against Los Angeles, San Francisco and Miami. He could lead the team back into playoff contention, they didn't need Bingo.

As Jack was hitting the balls with authority, he could feel the muscles in his hands and arms tire. But he had so many more thoughts to hammer out. He worried about Djuana and how she was dealing with her pregnancy. He thought about her working everyday, standing on her feet. If the baby were his, no way would she have to work, he imagined.

He thought about her eating habits, how he should call her to see what she had eaten that day. He worried that the father of her baby might still be upsetting her.

Jack didn't notice his teammates start to arrive. A few stood off to the side, stretching and swing their bats.

"You gonna let somebody else hit or what?" an agitated Bryant Clark said. "Shit, can't hit a beach ball if my grandmother lobbed it to you!"

After 100 more balls, Jack gave way to Bryant. Before he did, he confronted him.

"Why don't you be a man and say what's eating you?"

"Fuck you, New. I ain't got words for you."

"Grow up, BC."

"Fuck you. Step off. Mind your fucking business before I *stab* you."

Two other Crowns laughed, but the batting cage fell silent. The old Jack they knew would have strangled Bryant. Jack did grab Bryant. He wrestled the smaller player onto the ground and pinned him down. He kissed him about the face and neck.

"You need some love, motherfucker?" Jack tugged at the back of his uniform pants. "I'll give you some love!"

The Crowns standing around burst into laughter; laughing harder as Bryant struggled to free himself, cursing Jack, and them for not helping him.

Jack walked into the clubhouse where more of his teammates were dressing. Oscar arrived as Jack reached his locker.

"Damn you early," O said, handing Jack one of his extra juices from the training table.

"Yeah, I needed some extra BP," Jack answered.

"How's the wound?"

"It's okay. I didn't even feel it while I was hitting."

O undressed slowly, as he usually did. "We gotta sweep San Diego. We lose to them motherfuckers then we are sorry."

"We'll beat them."

Kristen and another reporter entered the clubhouse and began talking to the pitchers on the Crowns before they came to the outfielders section, where Jack and Oscar reside.

Kristen smiled a hello at Jack and nodded to Oscar.

Oscar immediately barked, "I ain't got shit to say, so don't ask me shit!"

The other reporter, Hank Goldberg from the local sports radio station, asked him a question anyway. He pointed his microphone at Oscar and said, "How are you guys going to manage without Mike Colbert behind the plate?"

"I see you're deaf," Oscar said as he smacked the microphone and recorder to the floor.

Jack shook his head but didn't say anything. Hank glared at Oscar.

"You're an asshole," Hank said.

Oscar replied, "Then, why don't you kick my ass and teach me to be a good citizen?"

Kristen stood over Jack while he put on his cleats. "I guess none of you know that Mike was arrested last night for spousal abuse. Honeywell released him from the team this morning."

"Damn," Jack grumbled. He looked over at Oscar, who was still asking Hank to hit him. "We're falling apart at the seems."

"Can I quote you on that?" She asked with a sly grin, holding her pen at the curve of her lips.

Jack stood and reached into his locker for his cap. "No. I think not."

"Help me out. Say something," Kristen playfully pleaded. "Everybody is claming up."

Oscar, finished with Hank, who wanted no parts of a physical confrontation, sucked his teeth and hissed.

"No," Jack said loudly. "I don't have anything to say either."

"I thought not," she slipped Jack a note and walked away.

He opened it and it read:

Jack,

Please have lunch with me tomorrow. I need to talk to you about something important.

Around 1 p.m. 1811 St. Clair.

Please come.

Kris

Djuana returned to work a week after the incident without fanfare. She had never before missed more than five consecutive days from DeLux's. Each year since she became a manager, she would spread out her 14 vacation days; five days here, a couple of days around Christmas. She never left Portland, though, on a vacation.

Calvin drove Djuana to work, and picked her up in the evening; he was in between jobs. Her work schedule, though, had been sliced down to three days. Djuana didn't mind too much, she didn't want to be out at all. Mr. Thompson had discussed firing her with his supervisors; but they could smell a lawsuit. Mr. Thompson argued that the negative press would harm the store. But, the upper management didn't see it that way. They hoped crowds would come to see the woman that stabbed Jack Newhouse.

And, they did. Fans of Jack Newhouse, especially young women paraded through the linen department; some even bought something. But, the traffic on that floor was as heavy as during white sale days every afternoon. Of the verbal bombs, none hit as hard as the one a white woman in her 40's fired. The woman followed Djuana out of the mall and to Cal's ride.

"Jack Newhouse did not try to rape you, and you know it!" the woman said, walking steps behind Djuana.

Djuana was not afraid, nor was she angry. She just listened.

"That's a good man. You don't know all he has done. I've seen him give food to the hungry and clothe the cold. You can't break that kind of person! Not with what you're saying!"

Djuana absorbed the abuse from anyone that had something to say. It drove her uncle crazy.

"You can't let bitches and motherfuckers just roll up on you berating you and shit!" Cal said as the white woman turned away.

"Fuck her!" Cal moved toward the woman, Djuana caught him.

"Its not a big deal," was all Djuana said as she got into the car.

Djuana felt guilty of attempted murder, as the newspapers were now saying daily. Everywhere she looked there was either a newspaper, billboard advertisement or a T-shirt with Jack's picture or likeness on it. On television, it seemed that now every channel carried his sunflower seeds commercial.

One day, her third day back at work, Djuana walked six blocks to have lunch at Hamburger Mary's on Park Avenue. The waitress recognized her, but was coy. The little diner was crowded as usual, but Djuana, and the baby, had a craving for a Mary burger and a shake. When the waitress brought the thick and juicy burger, piled high with lettuce, tomatoes and sweet fried onions, Djuana's mouth flooded.

The waitress stood there a second, popped a straw, and said, "How are you, honey?"

Djuana looked up, ketchup in hand, and nodded. She took in a good view of the waitress; Anne, her name bar read.

"You keep your head up." Anne smiled and spun away.

In the next booth, Djuana was facing them, three older Black men were eating loudly, and discussing Jack Newhouse's problem. Djuana felt compelled to listen, at the same time hoping they wouldn't turn and see his problem right behind them.

The graying men sitting near the middle of the diner, two booths ahead of Djuana, and across the floor, seemed to know all there was to know about the Crowns. They praised Bingo and Oscar, one man said that O was the best player in the game. Djuana silently disagreed. Then one man, a little older looking and thinner than the other two, with a head full of gray hair under a dusty, old Crowns cap, brought Jack into the conversation. Djuana perked up from her seat, craning to hear them, but hoping not to be seen.

"But, I tell ya," the older man, Harold Grimes, said loudly, drowning out one of his friends. "When J-New gets back on track, that's it. They run away with it."

"Fool, please," the light-skinned man, Petey Knolles, with the tie and sports jacket said. "Jack Newhouse is finished. His mind ain't in the game. They are right to try and trade him. Let that kid Aponte play. He can hit, I hear-tell."

Grimes shook his head slowly and pulled his bottle of beer up to his lips from between his legs. Mary's didn't serve beer.

"No, man. Listen to me," he said after a hearty swig. "I'm telling you that Jack Newhouse is the key. I've been watching him, and if he just lays off the plate a little, like he used to when he was the best hitter in the league..."

"Best hitter in what league? Little league?" Knolles interrupted as the older man passed the beer to the quiet guy. "C'mon! That guy was never the best hitter in *any* league! What the hell are you talking about?"

Then the bigger guy, facing Djuana, and could see her if he turned his head slightly to the left, really pissed Djuana off.

He said, "If he stopped porkin' every piece that is thrown his way, he'd be all right."

"Them young gals throwing leg at him," the capped-guy added. "Hmm. He can give some to me, and he'd still have too many."

Djuana shook her head as the men laughed loudly.

"Fools," she said too loudly. But no one budged.

The older man broke off into another subject, "He didn't rape that girl."

"I know he didn't!" Knolles proclaimed.

Djuana's pulse race.

"Shit, why he got to rape somebody? No reason."

"Then, why she stab him?" Grimes pointed his fork at the light-skinned guy.

Djuana's burger lost it's appeal. She looked at it, half eaten, still fries about the plate. The men went on and on about J-New and the "nut" and "liar" that stabbed him. Djuana covered her face with the cloth napkin. She knew she couldn't snap her fingers and disappear; there was no where to go. Crying wouldn't help, either. She took a deep breath, removing the napkin slowly. She calculated a mad dash to the door.

"I heard the girl lives out by you, Jeff," Djuana heard one of the men say.

"Yeah, Janice said she went to school with her."

*Janice McKnight's father?* Fright brought Djuana to her feet, but they wouldn't guide her legs out of the booth.

A different waitress, tall and very dark skinned, busing a table near Djuana, saw her stand, and knew immediately it was the men's conversation. Other diners were listening, and commenting. Some knew the only person eating alone was the woman that almost killed Jack Newhouse.

"You okay, honey," the older Black woman said, putting her pad down on Djuana's table and touching Djuana to console her.

"I have to go." Djuana said after a second. She wanted to allow herself to be hugged.

"I know, baby. Don't worry about the bill." Then, the woman's voice suddenly lowered, causing Djuana to look deep into her eyes and lips. "And, child, don't worry about what's being said. People ain't living if they ain't gossiping. As long as you walk with God, no words can harm you."

Jack accepted Kristen Eisen's invitation only after he called and she promised not to mention the Crowns nor the stabbing. But then, Jack wondered, what would they talk about? Jack thought about that the whole ride to the Nob Hill section of Portland.

## LOVE'S HOME RUN

Nob Hill was Portland's most happening spot to shop; a small version of New York's Greenwich Village. It was an upscale neighborhood, where you could find antiques stores, boutiques, card shops, design studios, ethnic restaurants, galleries, interior decorators and pubs along its main street, West Burnside, and on adjoining streets.

Jack rang the bell of the brownstone, and saw through the glass doors as Kristen came down the stairs to let him in. Her place was as bright as the smile she greeted Jack with. The walls and high ceilings were painted white and she had a collection of lamps and overhead lights; all of which were on.

"Can you see what you're doing all right?" Jack quipped as he walked into the living room on the first floor.

"Sure," she smiled.

"I mean, do you have enough lights?"

"I like the place well-lit. It gives me a sense of security."

"Really?"

"Have a seat. You want a drink? I have some wine chilling."

"Yeah. I'll take a glass of wine."

In seconds, she handed him a tall wine glass with white wine, and set the table in the dining room, which was off to the kitchen in the loft-like apartment.

"Put on some music," she told Jack.

He did, selecting one of the few rhythm and blues artist she had in her cassette collection. He put the tape in the modest cabinet stereo. He sipped wine, listen to Sade and watched Kristen's slender body dart back and forth, setting the table with their lunch.

Kristen was wearing a Crowns T-shirt that met her spandex shorts in length. She was barefooted and had a perfect pedicure, and hot pink toenail polish. Jack wanted to comment, her toes were attractive, but he choose not to.

She called Jack to the table while lighting two long, scented candles. Then, cut off all the lights. Jack, again said nothing. It was early afternoon, and sun light creased through the shaded windows.

"You comfortable?" Kristen asked, eyes wide.

"Sure," Jack said as he sat.

"How's the wound?"

"A little pain here and there, but I'm living."

Kris finally sat, pulling her chair to the table. "I'm sorry that happen to you. But I wish you'd just stop... stop going out with O like that."

"Kris, I'd rather not talk about it."

"I'm sorry." She was. Upsetting him was not on her mind.

She filled his plate with her homemade linguini and white clam sauce.

"Jack, what's up with your team?"

"Are we off the record?"

"*Very.*"

"Well, it seems like we're dying right now. But, we'll be all right. We kicked San Diego's ass last night, didn't we?"

"Please Jack," Kris laughed, "I ain't a novice anymore. San Diego sucks! Everybody is kicking their ass."

They knocked off two bottles of wine, and cleaned her pots. They talked and laughed, neither mention baseball directly. Kristen reminded Jack of her first year covering the team.

"I was so scared. You guys were intimidating."

"No we weren't. You were beautiful, and we just tested you to see if you knew anything about the sport."

"I did. And, I showed you guys!"

"Yeah, you sure did. But, you know, the best move you made was to not sleep with anybody. That would have caused problems."

"What if I tell you I did?"

"You lying!"

Kristen swallowed her last bit of wine. "No. I did. But just one Crown."

"Who? Who was it?"

"Wouldn't you like to know?"

"Yeah."

"Forget it."

Jack shook his head. "Yeah, I knew it."

"Shut up. Until now you didn't know diddle."

"If you say so." Jack sipped his wine with a devilish smile.

Kristen threw her napkin at him. "I shouldn't have said a thing. Now you think less of me."

"Please, woman! If that is so, then what do you think of me?"

She sobered. "You really want to know?"

Jack was smiling, expecting a cute comeback.

Kristen stood and came around the table slowly until she was standing behind him.

"You are the Crown I always wanted," she said massaging his shoulders. She kissed the top of his head, then the back of his neck.

"Wait, Kris." Jack turned to face her and she dropped to her knees.

"It's true. I always wanted you. But, you never paid me any attention." She forcibly pulled his shirt up. Jack held her hands, but she lunged her head into his chest and began planting kisses on his muscular rib cage.

"You want me, don't you Jack? I know you do."

Jack tried to pull her up, fighting off the kisses. "Let's don't do this."

"Where's the wound?" she tugged at his shirt. "Can I kiss it?" She searched for the slash and stitches that Djuana had caused. She tried to peel the bandage, but Jack pushed her hand away.

"Wait a minute, Kris. Let's take it easy."

"No, Jack. No more waiting," she looked up from between his legs. "I held back my feelings because I thought you and I dating would cause a conflict of interest, but that was a waste of time.

"I am sick of watching you be hurt." She kissed the bandage. "I could never hurt you, Jack."

Within seconds, she was performing oral sex.

Kristen rode Jack in the same chair he had enjoyed her meal. She straddled his neck and pumped her body until she came violently. Her body quivered and her moans grew.

"I'll marry you, Jack... I'll take care of you... Please, yes, please Jack... yes, yes, yes... It's yours."

Jack hung on to keep in motion with her wild body movements, and came with her.

Afterward, Kris bathed Jack, put him to bed and passionately made love to him again. When he fell asleep, she continued kissing his body, thinking she could make love to him forever.

Jack fell into a deep sleep. He hadn't sleep through a night since Djuana stabbed him. He dreamt that it was Djuana giving him oral sex, making love to him. He held and massaged Kristen's head. Caressed her body.

"Yes, Djuana. Yes, baby." he whispered.

He could see Djuana, smell her body. She was right there, in his bed. But, where did the knife come from? What was it for? She's going to cut off his...

Jack jumped up, choking Kristen. He was sweating and panting. He looked around her white room dazed.

"What's the matter?" Kris whispered. She rubbed his right triceps, then kissing them, trying to soothe him. "Lay back down. It was just a nightmare."

"Nothing," Jack said, feeling awkward. "Just a dream. A bad dream."

Jack laid back down. He looked up at the ceiling. When Kristen touched him, he pulled away.

"I've got to go," he rose.

"Why? Stay until game time."

"No. I have to go."

Tia rolled towards her night stand and picked up the ringing phone and unconsciously put it to her ear.

"The baby moved! He moved!"

"Wha?"

Djuana was like an excited child. "Tia, I felt him move! I know it was him this time. It was him!"

Tia finally awoke. "Ah huh."

"I think he finally rolled over."

"Juanny, what time is it?" Tia pulled her covers over her head.

"Who cares? My baby moved!"

Tia angled high enough to see her clock. It read 3:31; a.m.

Djuana continued, "God, I have a human, living, being in me!"

"Yeah," Tia was now disturbed. "I knew that. Can I go back to sleep now?"

Djuana let her best friend go back to sleep, although there was so much more she wanted to talk about. Her stomach had expanded and reddish stretch marks had appeared at the bottom of her belly. The past two visits to the doctor's office had been exciting. Dr. Oppen let her see the baby in a sonogram. She thought the image of the being in her to be tiny.

Djuana also had worries. She was afraid of the pending birth of her child. It was going to hurt. Would the baby be healthy? Would the baby love her? Would she be able to handle the baby day in and day out?

She also missed Jack Newhouse.

After the game Jack drove through and around Portland for hours. He stopped at a bar before 1 a.m. and had two beers. Some guys recognized him and cut his private time short. They approached, saying they would be buying the next round, but Jack stood up, pulled his wallet out and said, "Join me, and we all pay, and get blasted."

They did. Jack drank more that night than he had in three weeks. Jack was feeling guilty. He had done just what Djuana said he would: slept with another woman. But, damn, he sure needed what Kristen offered. And, could use some more.

When his pager beeped, Jack's first instinct was to ignore it. It had to be Oscar, and he didn't feel like any freaks that night. But he checked it anyway.

It was Djuana. Her message read:

*Jack, if you are up, call me please, Djuana. 292-0932.*

Jack called her back quickly, darting to the back of the bar. His drinking buddies told him to hurry back.

"Are you okay?"

"Yes. Just can't sleep. The baby is doing flips."

Jack tried to sober. "Are you okay?"

"Fine. I guess he's just having a bad dream." Djuana flopped back on her bed, eyes to the ceiling. "The other day I had a sonogram. And, they said they could tell the sex of the baby."

"So, it's a boy, right?" Jack smiled.

"Maybe. Maybe not."

"I thought you said they could tell?"

"I don't want to know! I can wait. That takes the thrill out of the remaining four months."

"Yeah, but it also makes it easier for people to select gifts. You won't get a bunch of yellow and white stuff."

"How you know so much?"

"Years of showers for teammates."

"Well, I don't want to know."

"Okay."

A moment of silence brought in the sounds of the bar. The voices of Jack's drinking buddies calling him irritated Jack, and startled Djuana. He wanted to say he was in love with her, deep love.

"You have to go, Jack?"

"No. Hold on a second." He put the phone on his thigh and called to the bartender.

"Give them another round on me."

"Anything you say, J-New."

"I'm back," Jack said into the phone. "I'm just at some bar downtown. I needed a drink before I went home."

Djuana heard him, but didn't.

"Jack," she twirled the phone cord. "I miss you. I'm sorry if I destroyed us. I have never been more happy then when I was with you."

"I miss you too, Djuana. And, you haven't destroyed us."

"Why haven't you called?"

Jack had no reason. He paused, and chose not to lie. "I've wanted to, but I just wanted to give you time. I want you to be a part of my life, but I don't want to push you."

"I've had enough time without you. And, none of it has been exactly pleasant. I miss being with you."

"I love you."

Jack paused. He could never describe his feeling at that moment. Shock, he would think it to be later. But, the sensation was more like contentment. He knew then he would marry Djuana Pioneer.

"Are you sure?"

"As sure as I have ever been. I mean, I thought I loved a man for seven years, and I never once felt so warm, safe and loved with him like I do with you."

"I love you, Jack."

"I do love you too, Djuana. Very much, I do."

# 28

August was Djuana's favorite month for one reason: The Mount Hood Festival of Jazz. It was the highlight of her summers because she could never afford to travel out of Portland. The event was hosted by the Mount Hood Community College in Gresham, thirty miles from Portland. It showcased some of the best professional jazz musicians from all parts of the world. Djuana wasn't a huge fan of jazz, but she loved live performances and she enjoyed the crowds and the vendors.

When she told Jack how much she cared for the event, he immediately made plans to insure she would have a great time this year. His ideas and promises were thrilling to Djuana, usually it would be her and Tia at Mount Hood, now she would be able to enjoy the romantic evening with a man.

Jack had made just about every day since she met him special. And, since he found out she was pregnant, he has been more gallant. After she showered or bathed, he would massage her back, shoulders, legs and feet. He would also care for the rippled, stretch mark rash that, now entering her sixth month, had developed beneath her belly from the growth of the baby. He would soothe it with lotion and then corn starch. The feel of his gentle touch would put her to sleep with a grin.

Jack would cook her healthy meals and bring home various snacks that sometimes did include forbidden treats, like cheese cakes and pies.

When Djuana needed a set of ears for her worries, Jack not only listened intently, he would offer sound advice and constructive criticism. His easygoing, caring manner was like a magnet aimed at Djuana's soul. She found herself staying at his house most nights of the week.

Djuana was often worried about giving birth to the constantly growing human in her stomach.

"This is going to hurt like hell," she would say at least once a day.

Jack's reply would be a nod, and careful words. "It sure will, but hey, women do it everyday all over the world. You'll be fine."

"Sure. But that doesn't mean it won't hurt like hell."

Jack did not let a day go by with out telling Djuana how beautiful she was, and how she would make a wonderful, caring mother. He sincerely believed all he told the lady he loved.

"I am not beautiful," Djuana said. "I am a fat pig. I know you don't find me attractive."

"Yes I do, Baby." Jack would kiss her. "You're gorgeous."

Then, although satisfied that he was thoughtful enough to lie, Djuana would push for more compliments.

"How do you know that I would be a good mother?" she'd frown.

"Because I can see your heart is made of gold." Again he would kiss her, and hold her. "I see how you deal with your brother and the tender way you are when you see a baby.

"You'll be a great mother."

His words would warm Djuana. She was more happy now after four months of knowing Jack than she had ever been in her life. And, still their relationship hadn't evolved from the friendship stage.

Jack had come to the realization that he was not going to make love to Djuana until she felt ready. And, he noticed, that was no time soon. He was content to wait for the arrival of the baby. But, the women he knew continued to offer him sex.

Kristen was in love with Jack, and she could not help but show it. Before and after games she would ask him out. He always said no politely. Kristen hated it. After a game in Miami, Kristen held Jack in the empty clubhouse.

"What is it, Jack? Did I do something wrong?"

"No," Jack flatly answered. "You know what it is. I'm seeing Djuana. And, this time I plan to keep her and make her happy."

"Why you talking to me like this? Would I ever stab you? What does this, this female have over you?"

Jack stared in Kristen eyes. He saw the glossy look, but could not pick up on the fact that she was in love with him. All he saw was the venom of a jealous woman.

"What has gotten into you?"

"You. Jack, you have. I have always cared deeply for you, you know that. That woman is pregnant, she's violent and she can't love you like I can.

"Just give me a chance to show you."

Oscar walked up on them, coming in from outside the stadium, as Kris ran her hand over Jack's groin area.

"I can love you like you need to be, and you know it," she said.

O cleared his throat. Kris jumped back, and Jack snatched up his Crowns travel bag.

"The bus left us," Oscar said. His serious tone startled Jack.

"We'll take a cab then," Jack said.

"Come back to my room," Kris said.

Jack walked briskly passed O and out the clubhouse. Oscar stood there a minute staring at Kristen.

Kris wiped her eyes, and glared at O.

Oscar said to Kris, "You need to stop begging."

She sprang her middle finger up to O's face.

Djuana sat on her side of their bed, refusing to touch his side until he was laying there. She was wearing his gray and burgundy baseball jersey, watching the Crowns play in Miami wishing she was there. Dr. Oppen was against her taking the long flight across country, and when Dr. Oppen was against something Jack enforced his rule.

Djuana had a bowl filled with fruit Jack had bought between her legs on the bed. She nibbled on the green grapes and strawberries, craving a Snickers bar, when Tia phoned from Portland State. Her summer class had just let out for the day and although she was suppose to go and pick up the Mount Hood tickets and take a taxi to Jack's house on Djuana, she wanted Djuana to drive into the city to pick her up.

"How about you meet me at the Square," Tia suggested.

"I don't know," Djuana sounded worried. She rubbed her belly. "It's raining and Jack would hit the roof if he knew I was driving in the rain. He's so protective of me and this baby.

"He's worse than Momma."

"Yeah, and you know you love it."

Djuana blushed between grapes. "I guess I do."

"Come on, Dee," Tia begged. "It's just drizzling. Just get here and I'll drive back and spend the night, if that's okay."

Djuana could use the company. She thought a second, watching the Miami team score another run off the Crowns, then agreed.

Pioneer Courthouse Square was crowded on a misty, foggy Saturday afternoon. The people milling around scared Djuana. She feared some crazy Crowns fan was out there still angry at her for stabbing Jack Newhouse. She felt eyes on her at each step. She thought about Jack telling her that what people thought of her, or them, didn't matter. He said she had to be strong, and she replayed his words with each stride, and her head raised.

Djuana paused to wait for the blue sheron to emerge from the Weather Machine in the square. The mechanical sculpture forecasts the upcoming weather 24 hours each day at noon. Djuana looked at the clock, in seconds a dragon surfaced – meaning a storm was coming – and groans spread through the pedestrians. She was indifferent, now watching the tumbling waterfall, recalling in her mind how her brother had fallen in two summers ago. She giggled, picturing her mother dragging Devon, then six, and crying, out of the two feet of water.

The sight of Tia pleased Djuana more than she expected. They hugged and kissed. Tia looked over her friend. They had not seen in other in a week. A long time for those two not to be together.

"Let me feel the baby," Tia said as she slipped her hand underneath Djuana's maternity blouse. "Girl, you are getting so big! How does that feel?"

"Like a cold hand! Don't you know better than to say something nice or nothing at all?"

Tia laughed and Djuana shook her head.

"I'm sorry. But, hey, that thing is going to burst!"

"Be nice, and I'll let you feel the baby move."

"Really? He's moving a lot now? Where he be going?"

"Give me your hand." Djuana held Tia's long hand against the baby's still body.

Djuana said, "It's sleep now."

Tia was amazed. "Remarkable. I can't believe there is a little human in you."

"Believe it."

After the women picked up the jazz tickets, Djuana had to have French fries. Djuana talked Tia into stopping in McDonald's. She steered into the drive-thru.

"It must feel good to be driving again?" Tia asked.

"Yes it does," Djuana said, carefully guiding the truck. "I haven't driven in years. You know there's only one car in my family and that's Uncle Cal's Olds."

They both chuckled at the thought of Calvin's dirty, but speedy car.

Djuana laughed, "And, you know I ain't getting behind the wheel of that death trap. Bad enough I ride in it time to time."

"It's nice of Jack to let you drive his pride and joy."

"He is a nice guy, you know."

"*Djuana*! I know he is. Believe me, I can tell. He has you smiling more than ever."

"Yeah. He does, doesn't he," she beamed. Djuana leaned on the steering wheel. There were two cars ahead of them on the takeout line.

"I remember the first time he let me drive," she reminisced. "We were coming from the movies and he let me drive back to my building.

"He was flinching, but he was cool. I made some sharp turns, I was kinda rusty. When I parked by my building he got out of the car and kissed the sidewalk."

And Dexter ruined it, she thought but didn't say.

Tia was envious. She looked deeply at Djuana. Her friend's laugh had become so carefree.

"I hope someday I meet a man that loves me that much," she sighed.

"What? That means he loves me to let me drive his car?"

"No. Don't play stupid," Tia slapped Djuana's thigh. "You know exactly what I mean."

The Pathfinder crept in line with the other automobiles to the ordering speaker board. Djuana was thinking about being loved. She was enjoying her turn at it. She remembered how Tia would force the men she dated to include a lonely Djuana on trips to amusement parks, movies and dinner.

Some of Tia's dates would protest, and Djuana did also, but most times Tia won out. Sometimes a guy brought along a friend. That worked once, but both of those guys were dating others. Tia tried her best to ensure Djuana did not have to be a couch potato because Dexter was neglecting her.

Now, Djuana felt she was repaying the kindliness, but, still she felt awkward being the one with a steady. Jack was great when it came to Tia. He was genuine and thoughtful in his attempts to include her.

"Yeah, Tia. I know exactly what you mean," Djuana said in a dead-serious tone of voice. "I love that man for all he has done and all he has been for me."

She turned to Tia, "And, I know you know this, but I haven't given him any yet."

"Shit, I know. Imagine when you do!"

"To tell you the truth, I don't think anything will really change that much."

"You don't think so?" Tia meant Jack was going to tear up her friend because of the long wait, but she didn't push it.

"No. Maybe he might love me more, but he's loving me more now than I could ever have asked for."

At the drive-thru board, Tia and Djuana each ordered fries and a shake, no burgers or sandwiches. They suddenly decided to collaborate on a lasagna dinner.

"So, how are the childbirth classes going?" Tia asked to strike up conversation.

"They suck," Djuana said, sipping her shake. Her eyes were glued to the wet road and crawling traffic. "They teach how to breathe when the pain strikes. I don't know. I think they're going to haveta knock me out."

Tia sucked strawberry shake through her straw. "You can do it, Dee."

"No. I really don't think so," she turned to Tia and dug into the bag for her fries. "I'm really scared. Seriously.

"We saw a movie the first day - I told you about it," Djuana pointed her fry as if to reminded her friend. "And, please, let me tell you, that woman was bigger than me down there, and Lord, did she scream! She hit her husband and fought the bed."

"Nope. Breathing ain't gonna help. I need a little more than that."

Tia was laughing and cramming French fries into her mouth. "You got Jack to hit."

"And what is he gonna do? He got queasy watching the movie. Oh, he'll be loads of help!"

They both giggled.

But after the joke on Jack died down, Djuana gave grave thought to how much help Jack would be. "Tia, I don't know where I would be or what I'd be doing if it weren't for Jack, though."

Tia was still smiling at the thought of the 6-foot-2 Jack wobbling at the site of Djuana spread eagle with a head protruding from her vagina.

"Yeah," she chuckled. "He has been a Godsend. But the doctors might have to hold him up and attend to you at the same time!"

Stacie was sure she saw Jack's Pathfinder go into McDonald's. She was positive. Her best friend since middle school, Kimberly Melendez, never doubted Stacie. But, that time she thought her friend was wrong because it was common knowledge that the Crowns were in Florida.

They sat across the street from the restaurant in Kimberly's husband's car for near 15 minutes. When the black 4X4 eased out of the McDonald's parking lot onto Morrison, Stacie choked up her beer.

"That is Jack's truck!" she announced.

Kimberly looked out in the direction Stacie's head faced. "How can you tell? It's fucking raining."

"Bitch, I know that truck when I see it. You know how many times I got porked in that mother?"

"Not really," Kimberly lost interest. She was tired of Stacie calling her a bitch.

"Follow it! Hurry!"

"You kidding? For what?"

"I want to see who's driving it. I bet it's that bitch who stabbed him. I heard he got back with her. Stupid ass."

"Fuck that, Stace. I got to get home before Ramon. You know how he gets."

"Come on, Kimmie. Do this for me. I just want to scare her. Although, I should bust her ass for stabbin' my man J-New."

Kimberly spun the car into a sharp u-turn and sped after the Pathfinder. In the mist, it took them five blocks before they could tell they were two cars behind Djuana. At each green light they would try to maneuver closer, but traffic was slowly moving along Morrison because of the wet conditions.

In the driver's rear view mirror, Djuana noticed the white Dodge darting in and out of traffic. She said to Tia, "Some nut is in a rush back there."

Tia tried to locate the car, but because of the tinted windows and fog, was unable to.

"I can't see it, but you just stay away from them. I don't want Jack killing us because you banged up his ride," Tia said to Djuana.

"You know it."

The Pathfinder crossed the Burnside Bridge and headed for Interstate 84, the fastest way to Jack's home in Woodland Heights.

Stacie dug into the ashtray near the gears and fingered out all of the coins as Kimberly turned the truck onto the bridge.

"What are you doing?" Kimberly asked Stacie. "Who said you can have our change?"

"Please, ain't nuthin' in here but pennies. I need them to throw at that high-class hoe driving Jack's truck."

Kimberly had second thoughts. "This is stupid. I'm taking my ass and my man's car home. You are losing your damn mind?"

Stacie turned in the seat to face her friend, "Listen, honey dear, I think you better do this little favor for me. Let's not even get into how many favors I've done for you.

"I mean, I ain't gonna mention how many times I've told your loving husband you were with me when you were really out being the happy hooker."

"Shut up."

Stacie laughed. "I thought so. Now speed up so I can bust me some ass."

Djuana sat at a light on Starks Street sipping her shake when she heard something hit the window of her door. She looked down to see a women throw another object.

Tia heard the second penny hit. "What's that?"

"It's that white car," Djuana said. "That woman is throwing something at us."

Djuana rolled down the window before Tia told her to ignore them.

"What's the problem?" Djuana said to Stacie.

"You the problem bitch! I ought to slice that baby outta you!"

Djuana froze. She hadn't heard her right. "What?"

"Forget them," Tia said. "The light's green, let's go."

Djuana did not budge. "I'm not running from those nuts that think they love Jack."

"Who the fuck you staring at?" Stacie said. She held her arms out in a pose. "Take the picture, bitch!"

"You are a joke," Djuana shook her head. The rain drops tapped Djuana's shoulder. She fingered close the window.

"Don't make me get out of this car," Stacie threatened. She moved to open the door, but didn't.

"What is their beef?" Tia leapt to Djuana's window to see what was happening.

Drivers behind them began blowing their horns, but they all missed the light.

"Go fuck her up, Stace," Kimberly said. "She rolled her window up on you like you ain't shit!"

Stacie bolted out of the car. Djuana unhooked her seat belt and opened her door.

"What do you think you're doing?" Tia said as she grabbed Djuana and held her inside the automobile. "That thing at worth you losing my God-daughter."

Stacie grabbed the driver's door of the Pathfinder and swung it open. "What? What you want to do? Come on out here so I can kill you."

The light changed to green again. Djuana yanked the door closed with Tia yelling over her shoulder. The Pathfinder drove off.

Stacie, who was holding onto the Pathfinder's door, slipped and fell onto the doused street. She hit her head on the white car's door. She was left with wet clothes, a headache, and her feelings hurt. She dashed back into the car and ordered Kimberly, who was muffling a laugh, to catch them.

The white car caught up to them coming off of the bridge. Kimberly, now angry that her friend got embarrassed, became more aggressive. She slid in front of the Pathfinder on Burnside Street and their sudden appearance scared Djuana. The white car would stop ahead of them abruptly, then move again.

Djuana tried to be calm, but her nerves were rattled. Tia was telling her to pull over, but she was afraid to get into a fight with those women.

Djuana saw the on-ramp to I-84 ahead on the left and steered toward it. The street continued on after the ramp. The white car allowed her to change lanes, but just before she got to the ramp, the car sped across two lanes and zipped up onto the highway.

Tia never saw the impending danger. She was watching the white car, when she felt Djuana's hand press into her chest a second before total darkness, and the sound of glass shattering.

The Pathfinder hit the side of the on-ramp, crushing the concrete railing, and went off the side. It landed with a thud on its passenger's side. Djuana was tossed in the roll - she had not buckled her seat belt.

Tia listen to the sound of her own heart beat in rhythm with the rain drops, blinking and scared to move. She tried to control her breathing, hoping that would prevent her from panicking. Djuana's limp body had Tia pinned to the passenger's window. Dime-sized drops of blood dripped from Djuana, Tia could not get herself to look up and find out what part of Djuana's body was bleeding.

Tia's legs were mangled, twisted at the knees to her chest, and hurting, but she could move them. She looked down at her legs, the milk shake containers had spilled on her jeans. She wanted to bolt up and run. But, she remained still because fright at the thought of moving the body of her dead friend had engulfed Tia.

# 29

"Help." Tia cried.

The men looking in sideways from the street all said not to move.

She wasn't planning to. The truck was on its passenger's side; Djuana on top of Tia, who was strapped in. She laid still for what seemed like hours. She moved once, turning her head to look at Djuana. Djuana's eyes were closed and blood covered her head. It was dripping onto Tia. The rescue workers were kneeling, looking into the Pathfinder from the cracked windshield.

"We'll get you out of there in a minute," a cop said. "We have to cut you out."

"Help us. Please help us, my friend is dead," Tia thought she was shouting. But her voice did not carry out of the crumbled vehicle.

A fireman came from heaven, Tia thought. He blocked out the sky, and smiled at her from above the wreck. She didn't see his face at first, she had noticed it was no longer raining.

"You'll be okay," he had open the driver's door and was looking in. "Just remain calm."

"She's dead," Tia said. "My best friend in the world."

The fireman did not respond. His and his partners peeled the car open with electric saws and the jaws of life, he reached in and unbuckled Tia.

"Can you move your legs?" he asked.

She said yes without trying. She thought she could, but knew it would hurt to do so.

"Good," the burly, pale-skinned firefighter said. "We are going to stabilize your friend then get you out. Okay?"

"She's dead."

Again, no one replied. The firemen, and suddenly police officers as well, just kept smiling at her, consoling her with encouraging words and working swiftly around her.

Usually the clubhouse phones in stadiums would ring forever during a game. The players were in the dugout, and the clubhouse men would be in other areas of the ballpark or too busy to answer the phone. But Juris had sent a bat boy into the clubhouse for more ice - the players were throwing the ice at each other. As he filled the Gatorade bucket the blare of the phone startled him.

"Joe Robbie Stadium, visitor's clubhouse." he answered.

"Jack Newhouse, please," a female voice said. "This is an emergency."

"There's a game going on, lady." the bat boy said.

"I understand that," the woman controlled her resentment; *Does he think I'm an idiot?* she tried not to say.

"Just get Jack Newhouse to this phone. Please."

"All right. All right, lady, but it will be a couple of minutes. He's on the field now."

The woman looked up at the television. "I can see that. I'll hold."

The bat boy returned to filling the five-gallon bucket, leaving the phone's receiver dangling. He dragged the ice up the stairs into the dugout.

"There's a call for J-New." He said to anyone.

"What? Are you blind *and* stupid?" Juris turned to the kid and asked. "He's on the field, and who asked you to answer the damn phone?"

"But I thought since I was - "

Juris pointed his fat finger at the boy. "Son. Don't think."

Seconds later, Jack and Oscar raced into the right-center field gap chasing a line drive. Jack caught the ball on the warning track, ending an inning in which the opposition scored four runs. Jack and Oscar jogged into the dugout sweating. The bat boy gave Jack a high-five, then told him of the call.

Jack trotted down the dugout steps wiping sweat from his brow, and picked up the dangling receiver and spoke into it.

The woman was now sobbing. Her tears began when she saw Jack trotting off the field. She tried to control her quivering voice.

"Jack, this is Bernadette Williams. I'm Tia's mother. Djuana and my daughter were in an accident."

"Accident? What happened?"

Jack's excitement frightened her.

"They were in a car accident on the interstate. Jack, get here quick, please. Djuana's in a lot of pain and she is calling for you. We're at St. Vincent's."

"What about the baby?"

A few of the Crowns had come bustling into the clubhouse.

"You in the hole, Jack," Scott Wilson said.

Bernadette cried.

Jack forced a calm tone. "What about the baby? Is the baby okay?"

"Oh, God, Jack. Jesus."

Jack's knees buckled.

"Jack!" Scott yelled. "Juris said to get your ass up there, you're on deck now!"

Jack regrouped. He swallowed his heart back into place.

"I'll be right there, " he said into the phone. "Tell Djuana I'll be right there."

Juris barreled his way into the clubhouse, the other players froze as their boss went directly to Jack.

"What's on your fucking mind?"

"It's Djuana," Jack said flatly while taking off his uniform pants. "She was in a car accident. I gotta go to back Portland."

Juris sobered, fidgeting with his uniform's belt loops. His tongue shifted his chewing tobacco in his mouth.

"Is it the baby?" Juris asked.

"Yeah. I haveta go."

Juris yelled to Scott to tell Pappy, Juris' top assistant coach and right hand man, to pinch hit for Jack.

"Shit, Cris has been begging to play, so let his ass get in there for a bit," Juris said. He patted Jack's shoulder as he walked back up to the dugout with his head down.

Jack took a second to marvel at how easily Juris took the news that he was leaving in the middle of a game. He buckled his jeans, buttoned up his wrinkled blue and red button-up shirt, then slipped into a pair of sneakers before racing out of the stadium.

Jack's trip to Portland was a long agonizing venture across country. When he got to the airport in Miami he found he had missed the only flight to Portland that day. He tried every airline, offering to pay any amount, but was told there were no flights that night.

While he sat trying to figure out a way to the west coast, his beeper went off on his belt. It was Honeywell from the stadium. Jack slowly found a pay phone.

"What?" he said as the Crowns general manager answered the phone.

"Where are you, Jack?"

"Still in Miami. There are no flights out tonight."

"I figured such. You heard any more about Djuana?"

"No."

"It's all over the news. She lost the baby. They're calling it your baby."

Jack swallowed. "Shit."

"She's in bad shape," Honeywell continued. "The Pathfinder is totaled. It seems some car cut her off on I-84."

"I got to get back tonight."

"Listen, I'll tell Slight to charter you a flight. Call me back in 10 minutes."

"No, man. You don't have to do that."

"Just let me handle this."

Jack hung up, thinking he should have thanked Honeywell. He looked across the airport. People smiling, others talking. But, nobody caring about his ordeal.

He called back quicker than ten minutes, and was pleased to know the plane was being prepared. While Jack waited his pager filled with messages from Berger, his father and sister, as well as Vivian, among others. He called his father first.

Jack had not spoken to Alvin Newhouse since March, when the elder Newhouse called during spring training to ask for twenty thousand dollars.

"I'm sorry to hear about the accident," Alvin Newhouse began. "So, who is this woman?"

"A close friend," Jack said.

"A close friend? Apparently she was having your baby."

"The news reports are wrong."

"So, then what is the story? She was driving your car? Right?"

"Look Dad, I have to go," Jack spoke with respect, but little patience. "I'm still in Florida. I'll call you when I get back to Portland."

"Fine. But, you know, I'm getting tired of reading dumb shit about my son every other day. You're going to end up blowing what little respect the world has for you over some pussy."

"Good-bye."

His conversation with Cecila was more positive.

"I'm sorry about the baby," his older sister said. "Jack, the wreck looks terrible. Did you hear anymore on her condition?"

"No. No more than what you've probably heard."

"I hope she's okay."

Jack sighed. "Me too."

Cecila held in her disappointment in her brother. "Jack, why is it that you have never mentioned this woman to me?"

"I don't know."

"Is she important to you? I'm sorry. I know she is; or you wouldn't have left in the middle of a game."

"I love her, Ceese. Enough to marry her."

"This is the one that stabbed you?"

"Yeah."

"I'ma fly out there tomorrow."

"No. Don't do that. I'll be okay. But, thanks."

Berger's cellular phone rang and startled the Pioneer family. He got up, flipping the phone, and walked away from the solemn waiting area of the St. Vincent's Hospital intensive care unit.

"She lost the baby. Did you hear?" Berger whispered. "I've been at the hospital since they brought her here. She's got the best doctors available. She's in intensive care. She's got broken ribs."

"Slow down," Jack said. "Did you see her?"

"I said she's in intensive care. Nobody has seen her."

Jack looked at his watch.

"I should be there in the early evening or so. It's about 3:30 in the afternoon here in Florida. Slight is chartering me a flight."

"He *is*?"

"Is her family there?"

"Yes," Berger looked over at them. "The police went and got them."

"Are you near them?"

"Just walked away from them when you called."

"Get them anything they want, you understand? Take care of them. Tell them I'll be there very soon."

"I'm sorry about the baby."

"I am too, Karl. I am too."

The last page Jack answered before Slight's charter was ready was from Kristen. She was in her hotel room in Miami.

"I guess you are going back."

"Yes. I am."

"Well, my paper had a reporter at the scene and now has one at the hospital. But nobody is talking."

"I expect not. You guys were hard on Djuana last time."

"You want to talk to me?"

"I really don't know what's going on, Kris. When I get there and see her, then, maybe."

A solemn pause.

"You love her, don't you?"

Jack wondered if it would matter if he answered.

Kris panted and sniffed. "Don't be a fool, Jack."

"Kris, you don't know - "

"I don't know what? That I love you and she could not possibly love you like I do?"

"Kris, she lost her baby driving my car. I have to go back and see how she is."

"Sure you do. She needs you right? Just tell me one thing. How do you feel about us?"

"Kris, I always respected you. You're a good friend, and I hope you remain a good friend."

"You're a bastard, Jack Newhouse. A stupid bastard. I hope she cuts your heart out and eats it. You deserve better, but you'll never know it. You'll chase behind this... this female until she hurts you for real.

"You know she probably did it on purpose so she wouldn't lose you."

Jack lightly placed the receiver into its cradle.

At the airport in Portland two detectives and two officers on police motorcycles greeted the plane and drove Jack directly from the runway to the hospital. His grim demeanor transferred to his escorts. The sirens were the only sound during the half hour ride.

At the hospital, there were more police and media representatives than when the President of the United States visited St. Vincent's two months earlier. What seemed like hundreds of cops formed a chained circle around Jack and pushed and pulled him into the building. A large throng of reporters and cameramen had awaited Jack. This was the biggest story to hit Portland in years; until Jack and Oscar arrived, there hadn't been any pro sports scandals in the small, quiet city.

The professional basketball team were God's sons compared to the Crowns.

An emergency worker grabbed Jack through the armed guards and apologized for not saving the baby.

"I swear to you, Mr. Newhouse, I did all I could."

"I know you did," Jack said without looking into the woman's eyes.

Mayor Meier raced in front of the convoy of bodies leading Jack to the elevators. The officers halted. The mayor squeezed into Jack's chest, tears in her eyes.

"We will catch that driver," the mayor's thin lips perched in anger. "And he will fry."

Jack mindlessly let the mayor hug him again and kiss him.

"Get him upstairs." She ordered the cops, as she released Jack. And, they again moved swiftly through the lobby.

Jack wiped tears from his face, not knowing if they were his or the mayors'.

Seven cops squeezed into the elevator with Jack. Three stood guard as the doors closed and it went up.

The fourth floor was silent. The whole intensive care unit had been evacuated besides the Pioneer family and hospital workers. The fourth floor seemed smaller than the other six landings. It was designed as a octagon, with three different entrances to ICU. The main entrance was a wide corridor that began at the mouth of the elevators and a waiting area. There had been one patient in ICU before the crash. That person was moved.

Jack looked at everybody, but saw no one. Later he couldn't recall seeing Tia or Emma in the cozy looking waiting area. Some of Djuana's family were at the wide windows, others had moved chairs down the hall to be closer to the ICU. It was all like a dream to Jack. His legs were heavy logs as the police officers held his arms, nearly dragging him to ICU. He did a double take at Berger. His agent, in a tuxedo, had been crying.

Emma cut in between the officers and hugged Jack just before he entered the room. That was when he could no longer hold the tears. He squeezed

Emma as hard as she did him. She believed it was because of him that the police, fire and other emergency workers were as swift as they were.

Emma said, "Not many men would have done what you have for a woman carrying somebody else's baby."

One of the cops flinched, and looked at the others.

Jack was speechless. He forced a thank you up from his dry throat. He couldn't figure what he had done to help.

He wiped his eyes and noticed Tia was sitting in a chair closest to the two large swinging doors that led to Djuana. She was bent over crying, her mother rubbing her back. Jack went to her. Berger tried to get to him as Emma released him, but he waved his agent off.

Bernadette whispered to her daughter and Tia rose slowly. She knew he'd come. She searched the crowd and saw him. She went to Jack, and he instinctively took her into his arms.

"Oh Jack," she embraced him. "She lost the baby."

"I know, I know," Jack let her go to look her over. Tia had a bandage on her left arm and a bruise near her right forearm. She had numerous cuts on her face that seemed like she had fought off a wolverine. He was worried Djuana must be in worse shape.

"It's okay. Everything's all right," Jack repeated as Tia slid back into his arms.

Seconds later, three men in green surgical suits came out of ICU. One stopped at Jack and offered his hand, the other two headed for the elevators. Jack shook the man's hand and he introduced himself as Dr. Harvey White. The family gathered around the doctor, throwing the same questions they had been asking for two hours.

"She should be fine in a few days," Dr. White said in a manner that made everyone feel privy.

"She has a fractured rib," the doctor continued. "And two are badly bruised. At first we feared she might have a collapsed lung or that there was a possibility that the broken bone may be driven inward and damage the heart, which lies behind it, but she was lucky."

"How is she now?" Jack asked.

"When can I see her?" Emma asked.

"Breathing is painful for her," the doctor said looking at Jack. "But we have her on artificial ventilation. She has been injected with a long-acting, local anesthetic drug, so you can see her, but she won't be able to respond until maybe tomorrow afternoon sometime."

The family sighed in relief and slowly dispersed. Jack held onto the doctor's arm as he began walking away.

"Will she be all right?"

## LOVE'S HOME RUN

"I expect her to recover with no problems," Dr. White said as he moved on to the elevators. Jack followed. A cop stood at his side, eavesdropping.

"Her lungs are fine, and by her health history, I think her ribs will mend well."

"How about babies, Doc? Is she going to be okay?"

The doctor smiled. "Try not to get her pregnant for awhile. Until Christmas at least, okay Jack?"

"That means she's okay to have more babies?"

"With your salary, you guys can afford a pitching staff!"

While Jack was thinking, 'what a weird answer,' Berger finally got to him.

"Jack, let me talk to you for a second."

Jack let his agent pull him to the side.

"I know you probably don't want to deal with this right now, but we need to make a statement to the press."

"Yeah, I know. Just handle that for me, please. Make sure to thank everybody. The police, firemen, hospital workers. Everybody."

"No problem. One other thing. Nissan wants to send you a new Pathfinder. They're, er, worried about a lawsuit. What do you want to do?"

"It was an accident. Fuck them. I'll just deal with that later."

Someone he didn't know, a teenage girl standing with Djuana's relatives, offered Jack a soda pop. He accepted out of politeness. He peeled it open and sipped it. He hated orange soda. He looked for a trash can, sipped a bit more, then dumped it. He made his way to a open spot on the couch. There was three club sofas, two had its backs to the high windows. A cop followed him and stood over him.

Before he could get rested, and clear his mind, a member of the hospital's Perinatal Bereavement Team introduced herself. Karen Ross spoke softly and directly. She took Jack into a room on the sixth floor, the PBT office. The police officer waited outside the room.

"Do you know the details of your baby's death?" she began once they both were seated.

Jack was dazed for a second. *My baby?*

Karen Ross did not wait for his reply. She gathered the necessary forms for Jack and Djuana to fill out, and handed them across her desk to him.

"You and the mother have the right to name the baby, dress the baby and to set up your own funeral arrangements. We will have an official death certificate drawn in the name of your choice."

"I don't get it."

"Mr. Newhouse," Karen Ross removed her glasses. She smile lightly, as if explaining something very simple to an adult. "Your baby was stillborn on the way to the hospital."

"Stillborn?" Jack wondered aloud.

"Yes, the mother gave birth, but the fetus was dead."

Jack squirmed in his seat. He wished he had been there. He thought of the immense pain Djuana must have had to endured while he was away playing baseball.

"Would you like to see the baby, Mr. Newhouse?"

Jack looked at Karen Ross. Her round, dark face showed her seriousness. He swallowed, and a sprinkle of goose bumps curdled his arms and face.

"Wait. I," He felt pressed to say yes, but didn't want to see the baby.

Karen Ross reached across her desk and touched Jack's hand.

"It's okay. I know this all may seem a bit overwhelming. You have time."

Djuana was not to have visitors while recovering in ICU, but the hospital was set to accommodate Jack in any way. He was suppose to be in the room with her; a large chair was brought in for him, and a blanket and pillow. But, when Emma asked him if she could stay in the room until Djuana awoke, he couldn't say no. Emma watched her daughter for hours. She was sitting in an uncomfortable chair, leaning her large frame sideways from time to time to even out the body aches. Her family and friends left late in the evening, all planning to attend Earline's church Sunday service the next morning.

Earline had phoned her pastor from the hospital and he came by, said some prayers with the family, and announced to reporters a special service for Djuana and the baby. It was largely attended, as through the night the pastor and his wife made numerous phone calls.

Emma thought it was a nice gesture, but refused to leave her daughter's side to attend. Tia wanted to stay at the hospital also, but her parents insisted she get home to bed and take her pain medication. Emma had not slept since the accident, and she wouldn't until Djuana was taken out of ICU.

Nurse Anna Dodds stood up from her seat at the fourth floor nurses station and looked across the hall at Jack once again. He was sleeping on the couch, the only remaining relative or friend of lone patient in ICU; besides Emma who was sleeping in the room with Djuana.

"See, that's a good man," she said to her co-worker. "Do you see how he sits there and just waits?"

The other nurse just nodded her head and continued her paper work. She had heard this story all evening from her partner.

"Do you know that man up and left the team in Florida, during a game, mind you? And now, he just sits there in a hospital while his woman is in ICU. Damn."

"Arthur, my sister's husband, he works right on the East Side and couldn't even take the day off when she lost her baby."

"Hmm," the second nurse stood and went to the charts.

"You know he let his wife's, or whatever she is - you know the news said they weren't married - mother be in the room. And, the mother won't even let him in."

Jack could hear the woman, but he didn't want to. He wanted to get some sleep in the darkened waiting area, but he was wide awake. He was thinking about what kind of relationship he would have had with Djuana's baby. A boy. He would have enjoyed taking him to the park; he could have taught him how to play baseball.

He wondered what Djuana would have named him. Jack would have been nice for sentimental reasons, he smiled, but he wouldn't have let her do it.

Nurse Dodds stood over Jack a second before he realized she was there.

"Excuse me, Mr. Newhouse, I brought you another blanket." She paused, searching his dazed, yet handsome face.

"Just in case you are not warm enough."

Jack sat up. "Thanks. I'm fine, though."

Nurse Dodds sprang a wide smile, "How about some hot chocolate? Or coffee? I just made a fresh pot."

"Hot chocolate sounds good."

# 30

Djuana's eyes opened slowly. Sleeping had been difficult. With each movement while she slept, the pain from her fractured rib had been streaks of light across her mind. She would later recall them as lightning bolts in her sleep.

Emma rose quickly when she heard her daughter shuffling.

"Baby, don't move. I know it hurts."

"I had the baby."

"I know, I know," Emma bent above Djuana, wiping the sweat from her daughter's brow like she had done throughout the night.

"I want to see the baby," Djuana's voice barely carried. Emma could hear most of the words, and just guessed at the rest.

Emma kissed the spot she had wiped dry. "Baby, do you remember the accident?"

Djuana shut her eyes, the question confused her. She shook her head no.

Emma continued, "You had the baby at the accident, it didn't make it."

Djuana swallowed, and the pain squeezed the air out of her. She panted short breaths of air.

"Where's my baby?"

"The baby was stillborn," Emma didn't hesitate. "Juanny, the baby is dead."

"No, Mommy," Djuana began to weep. The pain forced her to gasp for air and she spit out words. "I saw my baby. I saw it. It was crying for me."

Emma shook her head defiantly. "No, honey. No. The baby died during the crash. It was born dead."

Djuana gave up the fight to speak, the pain was excruciating. She argued in her mind. She had seen her baby cry, knew it was calling for her. She was sure of it.

"You'll be just fine in a few days," Emma smiled. "Everything's for the best."

Djuana cried herself to sleep after a nurse gave her a pain relieving shot. Emma left the room to call family and found Jack with his head bowed in his hands on the waiting room's couch. She had forgotten about him. She observed him from the hallway, soon realizing his eyes were closed and he was asleep. She walked toward him, and like she imaged, he stirred at the sound of her approaching.

"Djuana awoke for a bit," Emma said curtly. "But, I think she's fallen off to sleep again."

Jack bolted up, tossing the blanket onto the couch. He grabbed the giant teddy bear and card he had bought during his many spells of anxiety.

"No!" Emma's shout drew attention. She looked around, then cut Jack's path to the room. "No, you can't see her yet. She's probably resting again. They just gave her a shot."

"Yeah, look, I understand that," Jack tried to add respect to his rushed reply. He called her Miss Pioneer; she had told him not to address her in that manner.

"I just need to see Djuana for a second. I'm going crazy out here."

Jack and the nurses at the station hung on the silence. Emma wanted to say no, to not let him see her ever again. But, she couldn't figure why. She wondered for a second why she despised a man that so sincerely love her daughter. She blamed it on hurt. He would hurt her, she presumed upon first hearing he was a baseball player. Now he had, not mentally but physically.

Jack touched Emma's forearm, "I'm going in there. I'll be a second and a half."

Nurse Dodd smiled broadly, cheering silently. Her partner elbowed her.

The first time Jack entered Djuana's room was the end of any doubts he loved her. He was frozen in his footsteps at the base of the door. The sight of her hooked to the ventilator, ECG and IV and automatic sphygmomanometer. She was on her right side, strapped firmly into a support harness for the flail segment that was damaged. Her eyes were semi-open, and if not for the frown of her eyebrows, she seemed to be in a peaceful sleep.

After a moment of staring, he got up the nerve to approach her. He stopped at her bed side, and continued to stare, not knowing what he should say, if anything. Djuana meekly waved her left hand.

Jack lifted the hand to his lips and kissed it lightly. Then, holding her hand, he kissed her forehead. The frown on her face shifted and her lips parted. Jack heard her say his name, but couldn't make out the rest of her sentence.

"I'm here, Babe," Jack whispered.

Djuana's eyes fluttered open. She panted, and Jack bent down over her ear. Her breathing quickened, she held Jack's hand tighter. She forced the words out in between breaths.

She said, "It was a boy, wasn't it? They won't tell me."

Jack closed his eyes. He wondered about his response. In those drifting seconds he imagined he would want to be lied to or held in suspense.

"Yeah, it was a boy," he flatly said.

Tears gathered, then streamed down her face. "I want to see my baby," she cried.

Jack used his free hand to wipe her face. "It's too late. They had to take care of the body before too long."

"What?"

"I wanted to wait for you, but I really couldn't. And, your family thought it was the best thing to do."

"Where's my baby?"

"Your family buried the baby today."

"No!"

Jack held her. "It had to be done. The baby needed to be put to rest."

Djuana impatiently held her words until the pain subsided. Catching her breath with short, rapid pants. When she felt she could deal with the pain, she spoke in a low, controlled tempo.

"I have to see my baby. You don't understand."

"Yes I do. I understand fully." Jack stood up tall. Djuana's eyes followed him.

He continued, "When the hospital's bereavement people approached me, I didn't know what to do. They wanted me to fill out papers and decide stuff.

"I wanted to wait for you, but realistically, I couldn't. So, I went to your family. Tia and your mother handled it. They dressed the baby and took pictures for you. The death and birth certificates have been held until you name the baby."

"Why didn't my mother tell me?"

"She didn't like any of it. Especially the pictures."

On Monday, Djuana's third day in the hospital, she was moved to a private room on the third floor. There, she was able to sit upright, and lay down in any position, albeit in pain. When the room was assigned, Jack called the florist near his home an ordered $500 worth of flowers.

Elaborate floral arrangements had began arriving at the hospital the day of the accident from just about every city the Crowns played in, and all points of Oregon. Brenda, in Arizona, and still unhappily married, sent a small bouquet with no note. Arrangements from friends and fans of Jack's filled her large private room. It had the smell and feel of a green room. Cards and balloons filled out any other open spaces left on the room's counter tops and night stand.

The gifts and the attention from outsiders did not bring a rise out of Djuana, though. She had not recovered from the abuse Crowns followers heaved upon her just two months before. She believed it was a fan that had done this to her.

She kept the four instant pictures Tia took of the baby under her pillow. He seemed to be in a peaceful sleep; wearing a nice, navy blue baby suit. Djuana was delighted that Jack had gone out and selected the outfit. *He would have made a great daddy.* She wished there were more photos, but understood when Tia explained she just couldn't take anymore. She imagined she could get more photos from family members that had pictures from the funeral.

Djuana would lay in the bed, on her stronger side, and stare out the window when alone. When she had company, other than Jack, they would leave her more miserable. She suffered through the pain of thoughtless remarks and inept attempts at comforting.

"It was God's will... It wasn't meant to be... Thank goodness you never really knew him," she heard from not only health care workers, but from family and friends as well.

Emma was the queen of insensitive statements. During Djuana's third day in the hospital, Emma asked:

"Don't you think you've been depressed about this long enough?"

That comment prompted Djuana to tell her mother that she wanted Jack to stay in the room with her – day and night. He was the only one not just talking to have something to say.

And, Jack was always there. He never left the hospital, having meals at her bedside, sometime sharing them with her. He had a friend drive to his home and bring clean clothes each day. He showered in Djuana's room. Whatever she desired, he got for her. He also refused to let her be depressed.

The Crowns returned to Portland Wednesday evening. The team was to play at home for a short, but very crucial, three-game series versus the West Division's first-place team, the Los Angeles Trojans. Jack was laying next to Djuana watching the late-night news in her hospital bed when a few of his teammates were interviewed before leaving Florida. They talked about playing without Jack against Los Angeles.

"Are you going to play," Djuana whispered.

Jack rose, propping himself on his elbow. "No. I'm not leaving your side."

"You have to play. They need you."

"They don't need me. It takes nine guys to win a game. I need to be with you."

Djuana reached to kiss him, baring the pain. Jack moved in closer.

"Go play, Jack," Djuana said. "The games are only three hours. We still have 21 hours."

That night, her third night in the private room, Djuana experienced the worst nightmares of her life. The baby was coming back to the hospital to kill her, she was certain. She jumped up out of her sleep, causing herself great pain, thoroughly frightened, three times. Each time Jack would be there in seconds from the next bed. He would hold her, kiss her and reassure her the baby was at peace.

"He hates me," she said, sniveling and shaking. "He hates me 'cause he knows I didn't want him."

"Yes you did," Jack would reason. "If you didn't want him you could have aborted him months ago."

Djuana held onto Jack with the little strength she had, ignoring the pain for the terror. "I killed him, he knows it. He knows I killed him. He thinks I did it on purpose."

"No. He doesn't think that. He knows better than that. He knows you will always love him, and he knows you wanted him."

"Don't leave me, Jack. He's coming back."

"I'll be right here," Jack rocked her gently.

Slowly, she eased her grip of his shirt sleeves. When Jack moved to get up, she grabbed him aggressively, "Don't go."

"I just want you to lay back down," he kissed her forehead, but she still cried.

"Don't leave me," she whined. "I'm scared. He will kill me. He hates me."

Djuana wept a deep, hurting cry. She fought to keep her breath, wheezing and exhaling in sharp pants. Jack, embraced her, tried to console her. The crying was afflicting pain to her rib cage.

"Just lay down, I not going anyplace. Just calm down, please stop crying, Baby."

"Sleep with me, please? Please just sleep here in this bed," she said patting the firm mattress.

Jack arched her down. "Sure," he said calmly and evenly. "Just lay down, I'm right here."

Jack laid in the bed, in his jeans. He was as stiff as a board, didn't budge for hours, afraid to cause her any added discomfort. His eyes were wide, watching her. Djuana cuddled into him. She rested her head on his chest and fell into a deep sleep within moments. The feel of Jack rubbing her back and kissing her forehead every so often was the kind of security she had craved.

During the night, Djuana would tighten her hold and moan. The baby came back. With Jack there, she felt safe enough to let him in the bed. All he wanted was an embrace and kiss. Djuana held her baby the rest of the night, while Jack held her.

She never had that nightmare again.

Jack met his teammates at Adkins for practice on Thursday. The three-game series was to begin the next night. He was one of the first players there, the only one in the clubhouse when the Crowns' equipment manager, Carey Shoneholtz approached him.

"Hi, New," the aging, legend of Crowns baseball said. He had been with team for 57 years, beginning as a bat boy.

"We're all sorry about the baby."

"Yeah." Jack nodded as he put on his Crowns warm-up.

"The team voted to wear light blue arm bands on their uniform sleeves to express the loss of your son," Shoneholtz said, jawing tobacco. "It was O's idea and I had my assistant sew them onto all of the home uniforms while we were in Florida."

Jack was speechless. He looked up into his locker, and reached for his jersey. There, on the left sleeve, was the sky blue arm band beneath the Crowns logo.

"I mean, New, it's up to you. Do you want me to take them off?"

"No. No, It's fine with me."

When Oscar arrived, he pulled Jack into a bear hug and kissed his neck.

"You all right, baby? How is she? She feeling better?"

"She'll be okay. Thanks. And, thanks for the bands. I like it."

"Yo, you my man, think nothing of it."

Oscar opened a Federal Express box and tossed Jack some new batting gloves and wrist bands, all light blue. He gave some to Don, Danny and Bryant Clark, as he came over.

"Hey, New, I'm sorry man. I've been acting like an ass lately," Bryant said as he hugged Jack.

"Forget it, we got a lot of baseball to play."

The other players picked up on it, and by season's end they were all wearing something light blue along with the maroon and gold Crowns' uniform.

After practice, Jack went to Honeywell and asked to miss the road trip following the series.

"I can't authorize that," Honeywell told him.

Jack went to Slight's office. Slight flatly said no.

"We can't afford it right now," the team's owner said between forks full of his lunch consisting of an attractive piece of fillet. "We are trying to catch San Fran and LA."

"I know," Jack pleaded, on the edge of his seat across from Slight. It was the first time he had ever asked Slight for something twice. "Just let me miss the Cleveland series."

"You always hated Cleveland, didn't you? No, New. I need you out there. We can't lose any more ground. We need to finish first to have the home field advantage in the playoffs."

"I understand that, Vinny, but I need to stay here a few more days."

"That is not your wife. Is it?" Slight glared at Jack.

"What difference does that make?"

"She's not your wife. I'm just making a point."

"I'll meet the team in Buffalo."

"You want to do what you want to do? Is that it? Then let me give you more freedom."

Slight tossed down his fork, wiped his hands, picking his teeth with his fat tongue and dialed his business manager.

"Bill, get you ass down here right now and bring Newhouse's contract."

Slight, all the while staring at Jack, slammed the phone down. "You're released. Free to do as you please. Like you wanted."

"You're gonna cut me over this?"

"No. You the one making the choice. I am not going to let you tell me what you are going to do while I pay you to perform."

"You ain't some factory worker. You don't work nine to five. You don't get sick days."

Slight became animated, "You get a whole fucking six months off every year."

Jack was paralyzed. He thought for a second of changing his mind, and going on the road trip. But two weeks away from Djuana would be more than he wanted to bear.

"You've let that female take away your livelihood," Slight continued while Jack pondered. "What happen to you? I can't believe a playboy like you let a piece of pussy cloud his judgment. Never thought you'd be whipped of all people."

"So, am I released?"

"If you don't come on this trip you are."

"Fine."

Jack walked out of the office, held Slight's door opened, turned to look him in the eye, but nothing witty came to mind, so he just slammed the door shut. The velocity caused papers to scatter off the desk of Slight's secretary's.

When Jack left St. Vincent's to go to practice Thursday, Dexter entered on his heels. Dexter had been waiting outside of the hospital for three hours. He wanted to catch Djuana alone, or at least without Emma or Jack around. Once he saw Jack leave, he figured then was the best time.

But, then once he got to the information desk, he found he had to wait another hour for the visiting period to begin.

He entered Djuana's room and saw Emma standing over her, propping her pillows. Emma glared at him, but did not speak. Djuana looked around her mother and saw Dexter.

Emma finally said, "What do you want?"

"I just want to see Djuana for a second. I have a pass," Dexter said.

Djuana, who because of the pain could only whisper, tapped her mother and nodded when Emma turned to her.

Emma walked out, not before calling Dexter a weasel in his ear.

Dexter walked over confidently and smiled. "You have a lot of flowers. How are you?"

Djuana nodded.

"I guess everything worked out for the best. You know, like maybe it was God's will."

Djuana's eyes flared. She sighed through her nose.

"It was the baseball player's, right? It's okay, no problem. As long as you're okay.

"My wife says she forgives you, she understands that you just, you know. Look, we ain't got to go into that.

"It's all forgotten."

Djuana reached for him, but couldn't touch him. He noticed and came closer, kneeling over to meet her face to face. She gave his arm a tight pinch, pulling the skin and twisting.

He pulled away. "God damn it! That shit hurt!"

She forced her voice to carry, "I can't believe I never noticed that you were such an inconsiderate bastard."

The Los Angeles Trojans came to Portland a proud ball club; winners of seven games in a row. Four of its starting players were having the best season's of their careers. And, their hated rivals, the Portland Crowns were in disarray.

The Los Angeles ball club was a strong baseball team; in many ways better than the Portland Crowns. They had once owned a streak of 17 straight victories over Portland in the late 1980s. The Trojans had solid pitching, a sound defense and were the finest overall hitting ball club in the majors. The Trojans had a crafty manager in Horace Johnson, who would be their leader for 30 years; with only four seasons of having a losing record.

But, in the past four years, L.A. had not won a game in Portland. In the playoffs, the Crowns had mastered the art of unraveling a better team. The Portland Crowns had something the Los Angeles Trojans lacked, and that was character under fire. And, the Crowns had characters to start a fire.

This season, though, the Trojans looked well on their way to finally getting past Portland and into the World Series. It had been Portland who had knocked the Trojans out of the playoffs in the last three years. The Crowns were bickering among themselves and losing games by the bunches. Daily, it seemed, Portland players were being fined, suspended and traded. But, more importantly, to the Trojans, Jack Newhouse was not having a particularly good summer.

Jack feasted on Los Angeles pitching; arguably the best staff of arms ever assembled. Yearly, the Trojans pitching staff would lead the majors in the least runs and hits allowed, and most strikeouts. But, those stats didn't faze Jack, nor any of his teammates, really. Often, he would single-handedly terrorize that ball club. He saw the ball well in Los Angeles, and, of course, he loved hitting in Portland. He couldn't explain why, but the Los Angeles Trojans brought out the best in him.

Thus, the Los Angeles Trojans were the most delighted team to see J-New struggle on the field and off of it.

Jack sat up on the hospital bed, looking down on his sleeping beauty. He didn't want to leave her, ever. He kissed her forehead, eye brows and then lips. Her eyes opened.

"I have to go to the game, it starts in an hour."

"I know, baby."

"I don't want to go. I hate leaving you."

"I know. It's your job. And, you love it, don't you?"

"I love you."

Djuana took his hand from her side, he allowed her to bring it to her lips. "Go play. Bring me back a win, and I might let you sleep with me."

She patted the bed, beside her revealed thigh out of the covers. "Right here, next to me."

Jack grinned, "LA is getting their asses kick tonight!"

Djuana laughed, and it hurt, and felt good.

Jack kissed her and darted out. O was down stairs in the lobby talking to a nurse when Jack came off the elevator. O kissed the nurse and the two men jogged out.

In the Friday night game, the Crowns scored in every inning to win, 11-2. Jack had three hits, and Oscar hit two home runs. Danny Gross pitched his best game of the season.

Djuana watched a few innings before falling asleep with her mother at her side. The moment of silence before the start of the game made Djuana and Emma teary eyed. Emma, though, didn't like the players wearing light blue accessories.

"What is that all about?" Emma asked her daughter.
"Jack said the team voted to wear them in memory of the baby. I like it."
Emma shook her head in disapproval.
"Ma, just appreciate the thought."

Jack returned directly after the game. Emma left when he arrived, with Djuana still asleep. Jack took of his shirt and sneakers and laid in the bed next to Djuana. Djuana awoke, feeling his presence, as he fell asleep. She, having had plenty of rest, stayed up watching television. She watched him sleeping, listening to him snore. She moved closer to his ear and panted sweet words into his dreams.

"Why do you love me so much? I know you do. God, I know you do. And I love you to. Always have. I feel in love with you right away. I need you, Jack Newhouse and I'm so glad you are here."

She kissed his neck, ear and face until he began to turn to her. Djuana's warm breathe, and tender words, filled Jack's mind with lust. And, she hoped it would. She glided her body on top of his. The embraced and kissed for minutes, with Djuana's passion pinning Jack down.

*No pain*, she told herself. *No pain. It doesn't hurt.*

In the morning, the door to the room opened, and Dr. White stepped in with a nurse. He cleared his throat. Djuana was still on top of Jack. He was holding her, hands under her gown.

"Excuse me, but I'm here to sign you guys out so you two can go home and do that."

Saturday afternoon, LA led the entire ball game until the Crowns rallied in the ninth inning. Russ Jones led off the ninth, the Crowns were losing 5-3, with a bunt singled. Pugsley bunted him to second and Oscar doubled, scoring R.J.

Jack came to the plate in the ninth inning exhausted. Both teams knew he had had only a few hours sleep before taking Djuana home. L.A,'s manager told his pitcher to throw nothing but fastballs at Jack.

Jack, too tired to think, just put his bat on the ball and it bounced down the right-field line scoring Oscar to tie the game. Don came up next and hit a home run to win it.

Sunday's game was held at night for ESPN's national television audience. The announcers talked throughout the subdued game about Jack and Djuana.

The game was a pitching duel, with the Crowns' Floyd Young shutting out LA, 2-0. Oscar stole three bases and scored both runs.

Jack had no hits. He was too tired.

After the game Jack let Oscar take him out for a late dinner at Alice's. Alice made sure he took a plate to Djuana, who was back at her place where her mother was looking after her.

"Man, you need to get some rest," Oscar said as they ate grilled Oregon quail.

"Yeah, I know."

"You going with us on the road, or what?"

"I can't go," Jack said without looking at O.

"Yes you can. She'll be all right. Shit, since they think she done lost your baby they're treating her like the Queen of Lumber out this mother."

"She needs me here. I should be there for her. How would you feel if it, God forbid, but if it was Sondra?"

"Shit. You would tell Slight to kiss your ass."

Oscar chugged his beer, then looked Jack in the face until his friend finished chewing.

"Sondra left me. She found my Hoe Digits' and called them all. Her sisters moved her out while we were in Florida."

"Damn," Jack nearly muttered I told you so. Oscar would leave that huge phone book all around his spacious house as if Sondra was blind.

"So, I guess I won't have to worry about Slight asking me to choose between baseball and Sondra anytime soon."

"I'm sorry, man."

"Don't be. It's for the best. Now I can live my life and she can live hers; the way her sisters and mother want her to, of course. I should have never gotten married. It wasn't for me and I knew it."

# 31

Jack parked the new Pathfinder in a lot on Taylor Street. The brand new model was in the same color as the first one, with all the new features. Nissan installed a phone with the same number and the 4X4 was awaiting Jack when he finally got home. He was going to the Nordstrom department store on Broadway, but couldn't find a legal parking spot on the main thoroughfare. He walked back a block to Broadway and a block north to the store.

The short walk felt good. His short, deliberate strides helped him enjoy the warm sun on a bustling, beautiful afternoon. A few of the many pedestrians recognized Jack, but no one spoke to him. They instead gawked and whispered as he went by.

He was oblivious to the folk on the street; his mind was on baseball. Jack hated to miss games for any reason. He would go nuts during rain delays, and threaten to kill himself if a game was rained out, as often happen in Portland. Jack also played through many injuries. In his rookie season, he broke the pinkie on his glove hand and never said a word. His worst injury was during the stretch run of the Crowns first trip to the championship series. He hurt his knee sliding home, and to this day has never had it checked by doctors out of fear he would have to sit out a number of games.

Telling his teammates that he was not going on the trip was as difficult as dealing with the thoughts of not playing. Jack went to Adkins just as the Crowns were preparing to board their charter bus to the airport. He gathered them around in the clubhouse while Shoneholtz and his crew packed baseball equipment and uniforms in large burgundy bags with *"Property of The Portland Crowns"* in gold block letters. His crew then placed the heavy bags onto huge pushcarts.

"You guys know I love all you, and I love baseball," Jack began. "But right now I feel like my number one priority is to be with Djuana. She needs me and I need to be there for her."

The room was silent. No shock, or stunned faces, though. His teammates had expected him to miss the trip, and they also knew Slight would be furious and retaliate. Jack had Slight in mind as he spoke, looking around the room at the faces and equipment, thinking it would be his last time in a baseball clubhouse as a player.

Shoneholtz lifted Jack's jersey out of the wheeled trunk filled with the rode uniforms. His number 22 and last name were boldly prominent in gold and white on top of the gray button-up.

"You'll be wherever we are, New. Wherever."

Jack turn to the equipment manager and nodded with approval. A couple of players clapped in agreement.

"You know it, Poppa." Don said.

Jack resumed his speech, he wanted to say all he had prepared to say. "I just wanted to tell you guys how I felt before you heard about it in the press, or from Slight."

"You the man, Jack." Mike said. "We gonna destroy people until I you get back. You know, like take shit out on motherfuckers!"

Danny wormed through his now standing teammates to get to Jack in the center of the clubhouse. He said, "We understand, New. You do what you gotta do. It's as simple as that."

Many of Jack's teammates nodded or agreed verbally.

Don added, "Just take care of yours, we'll take care of these few road games."

"Just be ready come playoff time, we'll need you then."

"I'll be there."

Jack took his time in Nordstrom, shopping in a selective manner. If he had been buying for himself, it would have taken a matter of minutes, but not when it came to Djuana. He wanted nothing but the best. He worked the nerves of the salesgirl, one of the few Black workers in the top-of-the-line emporium.

The dark-skinned, quiet salesgirl, a college student, Jack believed at first sight, didn't mind Jack's indecisiveness. She took pride in helping Jack Newhouse pick out clothes for the woman that lost his baby.

Jack purchased over $800 worth of spring and summer clothes for Djuana. He bought dresses, shoes, sandals, sneakers, different styles of shorts; including two pairs of jeans and light weight pants. And, he also bought tee-shirts, pullover tops and cotton button-ups.

Before he left, he walked back into the aisle and found Denise, her name tag read. He reached out his hand, saying thank you, and when she shook it, she felt the folded bill. A twenty.

"No, I can't take..." She looked down at her hand, then up at the baseball player leaving. "Thanks!"

He put the bags into the back of the car, along with his suitcases. He drove quickly over to Djuana's place, and she was there on the stoop waiting. She had been looking up in the clear blue sky hoping Jack would be late so she could enjoy the breeze and outdoors.

Djuana was pleased the Crowns gave Jack two weeks off to spend with her. At first she was hesitant to get back into a car, especially for the amount of time it would take to get to the coast, but Djuana hadn't been to the ocean since she was a child. And, she loved the water.

Jack walked up to Djuana on the stoop and was immediately proud to be her man. She was beautiful, and worth any amount of flack Vincent Slight could dish out. With a little love she could be a true woman and great wife, Jack believed. And he knew he had plenty of love to give.

Djuana was wearing a pair of black jeans she had cut into shorts and his pullover black and gray minor league jersey. The jersey fit below the shorts and her thighs and legs were glistening as if just waxed. She had on black Nikes, no socks; her ankles and legs sent waves of arousement up Jack's spine.

Jack pushed aside thoughts of grabbing her and making love to that body. He had been having vivid dreams about kissing those legs, ankles and feet.

He gave her a hello kiss and slight hug, then said, "I thought I said I'd come upstairs and get you?"

"I just had to come out and get some of this warm, fresh air," she said listlessly. "It's beautiful out here."

"Yeah, it sure is," he said looking up at the cloudless sky. He was hoping the trip would change her mood.

Jack took her travel bag and put it in the back, then helped her sit inside. He had two pillows awaiting her. She used one to prop behind her back, the other against her ribs.

"So, where we going?" she asked when he ignited the car.

"A surprise. Just sit back and enjoy the ride. We'll be there in about two hours or so."

She stared at Jack while they sat through a red light. "You are too good to me," she said without expression.

He turned to her and smiled, "Yeah, I know that."

The new Pathfinder headed west out of Portland on the Sunset Highway. The ride would take under two hours, Jack drove a steady 70 miles per hour. The smooth ride and mellow music knocked Djuana out during the first 30 miles. Jack always enjoyed the drive to the coast. It seemed amazing to him during his years as a Crown, that despite all the water that surrounds Portland, the ocean would be 90 miles away.

Jack looked deep into the various scenes; the far-reaching road ahead of him, the cliffs and mountains, the miles of ocean ahead and thought about being unemployed for the first time since high school.

*What am I going to do for a living? I could open a bar. Or maybe a restaurant. Maybe a chain, one in New York and one here. Shit, I've got money in the bank, I could just pick my nose for two years.*

He looked over at Djuana. She had let her seat back and was laying on her *good* side. Jack wondered what will she think when she finds out he had been released. Then he worried that he should have told her the truth. No. She had enough to worry about, he reassured himself.

Djuana awoke in time to experience the thrilling sights of spectacular vistas, crashing surf, and long quiet beaches along the Oregon coast.

"How do you feel?" Jack asked as she stirred, taking in the sights.

"Fine, I didn't know I was tired until we got moving."

"You need to stop?"

"No. We're about there, aren't we?"

"Just about."

"I haven't been here in years, I forgot how beautiful it is."

The town of Cannon Beach, their destination, was the most used beach of the residents of Portland. Still, it was not a crowded spot, especially during weekdays. When Jack began his major league career he would spend the all-star break in the same rented cottage he reserved for them. That was before he became an perennial invitee to the league's midsummer event, and had played in the last five All-Star games before the season he met Djuana.

Jack would not let Djuana help him bring in the bags. He put most of them in the bedroom, but the new clothing he placed on the couch.

Meanwhile, Djuana was looking over the ocean-side cottage as if they had just bought a new home. She hated the furniture, all colonel wood. The couch and chairs were upholstered in dark plaid. The rug was an old, yet clean, shaggy brown.

She envisioned being in front of the large fire place most of the evening. No television or radio anywhere in the one bedroom cottage. There was an elaborate rack stereo system near the fire place.

The luxurious bedroom featured a queen size, wooden bed. The head and foot boards were solid oak and reached high above the lifted bed. The down comforter, pillow cases and sheets were virgin white. The walls were also white, with wood furniture.

The bedroom and the living room had wide wooden patios with balconies overlooking the beach. While Jack unloaded the car, she watched the sun descend off afar into the dark waters from the bedroom balcony. Goose bumps sprinkled her exposed arms and legs as a stiff breeze blew in from the ocean. She stood there, not relaxed or comfortable, yet at peace.

Jack called to her as he dumped the bags. "I need you to check out this stuff. I bought this without being sure of your size. I hope it all fits. It should, though. I ended up calling Tia for most of the sizes."

Djuana strolled into the living room. Jack watched her intently. Her facial expression seemed to say discontent. She looked over the clothes, not expecting much, but ended up smiling at the great choices Jack had made for her.

"You didn't have to do this," she said, all the time marveling over a sleeveless, blue cotton denim dress. It zipped in the back and had shallow front hip pockets. The same dress she had qawked over at DeLux's, but couldn't afford. This dress, though, was of better quality.

"I know I didn't have to. Maybe I wanted to."

Djuana smiled. How many times had he used that phrase? The linen/rayon trousers with besom pockets and zip front were not an item she would have bought, but something she would wear. The blouses and short sets she couldn't wait to wear.

"Oh, I see you bought something for you," Djuana held up a red teddy. The body of the spaghetti-strap lingerie was sheer, with the bra and hip covers laced.

Jack blushed, "Yeah, I thought I might as well get something for me too."

The market in town had done a great job of stocking the refrigerator and cupboards with the items Jack ordered. The lady that managed the store liked Jack, so she would always take good care of him.

"You need help?" Djuana asked wearing the red silk nightie Jack had bought. He smiled at the sight of her long, large soft legs. The gown was short on her, just as he envisioned it would be, reaching her plump thighs. The v-shaped opening at her chest, she had the strings open, gave way to plenty of cleavage.

Djuana posed as would a model, her left side forward and hands on her thighs. "Say something? Do you like it on me?"

"Of course I do. But, if you don't get out of here, we aren't going to be eating food tonight."

"I'll change, and come back and help you."

"Don't put it away, though," Jack said as she disappeared. "We'll need it later!"

Djuana laughed, "You hope!"

Jack cooked them a spaghetti dinner, with his mother's homemade sauce. A meal he had seen prepared a thousand times. Djuana enjoyed watching him work the kitchen. He sliced and diced like a man would, big chunks, and a large mess. For her part, Djuana set up the table on the patio with candles and they ate in the moon light. The moon, that night, was bright, wide and round. Almost making the candles unnecessary. It was also a bit nippy with the steady breeze off the water, but the mood was set perfectly.

Djuana wanted to dress down, keeping on only the baseball jersey, panties and socks. Jack didn't mind; he wasn't going to change from his cotton polo shirt and jeans. She found a jazz music station on the radio and sat out on the patio until dinner was served. The pain in her rib cage was subtle, thanks to the 800 grams of Ibuprofen.

After dinner, they enjoyed hot tea and brandy inside on the couch with the music. The couch faced the patio, so they still had the stars to gaze at, with the comfort of the crackling flames in the fire place on their left.

Jack was on the floor, his back on the edge of the couch, selecting CD's from his travel case while Djuana sang along with Al Green's *"For The Good Times."* Jack didn't notice, he was more concerned with picking six smooth R&B artist to put on so he didn't have to get up again.

Djuana sipped her tea and the heat spread through her bones; it was laced liberally with brandy. She dangled her feet over Jack's shoulders.

Jack put the CD's in the machine, reaching forward and letting Djuana's feet fall. When he was done, he sat back, and let the feet return to his shoulder. He kissed them lightly. Djuana continued to sing.

When the song changed, Djuana pulled her legs back and laid out across the couch on her good side. Jack rose to his knees and leaned on the cushion, face to face with the woman he loved.

Djuana ran her fingers across Jack's growing beard, and said, "Why do you love me so much?"

"Because you make it easy."

She blushed, kissed his lips, then whispered, "I know you love me, Jack. I can feel it in my heart. But I'm still afraid of you."

She sighed. "I don't know."

"What you don't know?"

"Anything. Nothing." Djuana looked away, out across the moonlit, calm water. The buzz from the brandy was excellent. Why couldn't her life be as peaceful as the Pacific Ocean on that summer night?

She blew air through her nose and scratched her scalp. Her eyes watched her fingers fiddle with a piece of loose material on the front shirt tails of the jersey.

"I want to just give myself to you, let you love me, but," Djuana paused to collect the words in her mind's eye before they came out jumbled.

Jack pulled her closer and planted kisses on her cheek. "Just do it."

She looked into his eyes and saw love, trust and dedication. Her eyes watered. As soon as the tears formed, Jack was wiping them away. At first with his hands then with kisses.

"What If I just get hurt again," she said. "What if you leave me for some model or actress. I'm not as beautiful or glamorous as your teammates wives. I don't even know if I can give you a baby."

"Why you making excuses for me?" Jack whispered. "I ain't going anywhere unless you want me to."

Djuana shook her head, "I'm so sick of crying."

Jack leaned forward and kissed Djuana's forehead. The gentle pecks had been warming Djuana's soul. So, when Jack carefully held her head and kissed her nose, cheeks and neck, Djuana responded. She held onto the back of his neck and kissed him back.

Jack worked down her neck and into the cleavage allowed by the button-up jersey. He pulled it up, planning to kiss her stomach, and maybe her breasts, if she allowed, but Djuana began unbuttoning the jersey. Jack pulled it off her shoulders as the buttons parted.

The sound of Teddy Pendergrass and Harold Melvin filled the background as Jack rubbed and massaged her shoulders while kissing her chest. He slipped her arms out of her bra then worked on her breasts.

Djuana held onto him, giving herself to the man that loved her. The only man that ever, truly did. Jack inflamed her body with oral sex for nearly an hour. He wanted more than just that, but he could hear Dr. White's warnings.

"I want you in me," Djuana finally said.

"No." Jack shook his head. He kissed her lips and whispered. "Baby, not now. We can't."

While he was attempting to reason the idea out of both their minds, Djuana sat up and undid his jeans. Looking him in the eye while unbuckling and unzipping. She slid the jeans down to his thighs. She then straddled him, legs around his hips.

"Take it, Jack," her soul released sensuous whispers. "It's yours."

Jack hoisted her hips to meet his torso. She leaned back and allowed Jack to make love to her in a steady rhythm. Her panting and moaning drove Jack wild. He grunted and quickened the pace, holding the arch of her back with both hands.

"Oh, God, it's so good," Djuana said. "Baby, you're treating it so good."

Her voice raised to an alarming pitch in the thralls of passion. She clawed at him, cursed him, but demanded he didn't stop.

"Don't come in me," she panted, grabbing at him, grasping his shirt. "Please Jack, don't."

He did. Long, hard and strong. He grunted and bent into her chest, breathing hard.

"It's okay," Djuana whispered. It wasn't, but it was.

Djuana's legs trembled uncontrollably as she cooed and running her nails into Jack's back.

After a few minutes, Djuana suggested they go to bed. And, once there, she ordered him to lay down, and she made love to him through the night.

When Djuana awoke in the bright sunshine the next morning, Jack was gone. She laid there a few seconds, fighting panic. But, then she remembering the night before. He must be in the kitchen. Her hand inched over the spot in the bed where they had made love. He was as gentle and loving as she imaged he would be.

She put on the terry cloth robe he bought her on top of her naked body. She smiled at the sight of the night gown across the room on the floor; where Jack had thrown it. She went out onto the deck off the living room and saw him jogging along the shore. The sun was bright, making her think she had slept into afternoon. She watched him from above, some 100 yards away, as he raced towards the house. She expected him to turn, and head for the stairs that led from the beach to the lofty porch, but he evenly pumped his legs past the house and down the shore line.

Djuana leaned on the railing and watched his muscular, sweat-suit clad, body pump away. In that instant, she decided to have breakfast waiting him when he returned from his morning jog.

While she cooked the large meal, consisting of eggs, homemade biscuits, grits, beef sausages and pancakes, she could not resist the urge to call home. Devon answered, letting her know that it was before nine o'clock.

"Thanks for the time check, is mom still there?" she asked her brother.

"Chill, yeah, but you gotta get Jack back here!" he said frantically. "The Crowns cut him and the Gamblers want him. Tell him to sign with them so we can go to the World Series with a winner. Then, when he wins we can go to Disney World with him!"

"What? The Crowns cut him? What does that mean?"

"You with the best player in the league and you don't even know nothing about sports, do you? I don't even know what J-New sees in you!"

The sunny-side up eggs were burning. She flipped them into a mess. Scrabbled, she immediately thought. "Just explain it to me, please?"

"He was released, cut, you know, like fired? He be gone from them, and now he can sign with anyone.

"You wit' 'm, ain't ya?"

"Yeah, yeah. Just put Mom on, please?"

Jack forked his fourth and fifth pancake and fingered them onto his plate. He reached for the syrup and noticed Djuana staring at him, elbows on the table and hands cupping her pretty, yet irritated-looking face.

"What? What's the matter?" Jack eyes circled the table. He smiled. "I didn't say excuse me or something? What?"

"Nothing."

He frowned, "Are you okay?"

"I'm fine. What's with *you*?" she snapped.

"Me? Nuthin'. I'm happy-go-lucky." He cut his pancakes then forked them in his mouth. "You think something's wrong with me?"

She looked at his mouth, full of pancakes, move as he talked, then watched him add milk to it.

"I think we had better wait until after you eat to talk," she concluded.

"Don't do that," he said, trying to speed his swallow. "You started, so let's talk now."

Jack gulped more milk, wipe his mouth with a paper napkin and pushed his plate away.

"Let's hear it? What's up? You've seemed bugged about something since I came out of the shower."

Djuana pushed her spotless plate inches closer to his and erased her slight smile, she began, "Do you still love me, Jack?"

"Where did that come from?"

"Do you? Yes or no?"

Jack sat back and looked her in the eye. "Are you asking me this because of last night?"

"No. This has absolutely nothing to do with last night."

"Yes," he composed himself, sitting in his chair and leaning forward with his elbows on the table. *It had to be about last night, it was our first time making love, now she's being insecure.*

"Djuana, I love you. Still do and will always. I love you more than anything in this world. Anything."

He frightened her with his sudden sober temperament. He stood up and tossed his napkin on his plate. He angled around the table, opposite to her. He refilled his coffee mug, and continued.

"I knew I love you that day when we stood in the street in the rain," he leaned on the counter.

Djuana was mesmerized.

"When I looked at you, with the raindrops glistening on your face, I knew. I knew when I looked into you eyes that you were the one I was supposed to be giving my love to."

He sipped the coffee, frowned - not enough sugar, and looked at Djuana.

"Look Jack," Djuana rolled her eyes away from him... he was erasing her anger with his heartfelt words. "I am not a charity case. I don't need anyone to take care of me. But, I want to be loved and needed, and hopefully by a person that will take care of me without me having to ask."

"What do you think I have been doing?"

"I thought you were loving me, but you lied to me. Why didn't you tell me that the Crowns fired you?"

"They didn't fire me, they released me."

"Oh, big deal! What's the difference?"

"It's not a big deal. I didn't tell you because I just didn't want you to think I had to decide between you and baseball."

"I just didn't want you worried, you've been through enough."

Djuana folded her arms across her chest, "Yes, I have been through enough, and I thank God that you have been there for me. But, I know baseball was your livelihood. You were happy when you were playing. I can't be the cause that you lose your job and happiness."

Djuana pushed her chair from the table, stood and came across the table to him.

"They fired you because you wouldn't go on that trip? Right?"

Jack stood, dropped his napkin, and took her into his arms as she came close, "Don't you understand, I love you and you are what is important to me."

Still, Djuana pouted.

"Let me tell you something," Jack said, holding Djuana's chin. "To hell with baseball, and to hell with Slight and his team. It's not my everything."

"It was, though. Jack, it was your everything until I came along and ruined it. The papers all say this has been your worst year, and I have been the reason."

"That's not how it goes," Jack slipped his hands into the robe, the tie fell open. He held Djuana's soft skin, rubbing her back just above her panty line. "You came along, and now my priorities have changed. You come first. It's as simple as that."

"I feel as though we should go back."

"Why? What's done is done. All I want now is to be with you."

"You are with me," she buried her head into Jack's chest. "I can't help but think of you everyday, every hour, every minute. You've been the best thing to come into my life."

Jack exhaled. "You are the world to me, Djuana."

"I understand that, Jack," she patting his thigh. "But, I also know how much you love baseball. You should be playing. I love the way you are when you are playing baseball. You are happy, relaxed. I want you back that way."

She twirled in Jack's arms and kiss his chin. "I want Jack Newhouse back the way he was when he met me, and made me love him. And, I'm sorry I changed that man."

Jack blinked slowly. He was hung on every word that flowed off the most beautiful set of lips he had ever seen.

"What? You think I don't understand that you playing baseball will have you away from me at times? Sure I understand that, because it's your job. I know you'll be back. And, when you are, it will be you and me."

Jack relaxed. "So, you forgive me?"

"Of course."

# 32

The new Pathfinder raced past Portland toward the eastern suburbs, where Jack had bought his town house after his former house mate, Oscar had married Sondra two years before. Jack liked living alone much more than he imagined he would. He was never one who thought much of privacy, although he was a recognizable figure wherever he went in the country. But, in Portland that didn't matter. The fans in Portland worshipped their professional athletes like any other city would, yet were not the hassling type of people.

In the Woodlands Commons, where Jack lived on Stillwater Drive, most of his neighbors were wealthy; lawyers, doctors, politicians and even players from the Portland's professional basketball team. Jack lived thirty minutes from the city and Adkins Stadium.

Jack let Djuana sit in quiet, only asking her once if she was comfortable. He didn't want to nag her, yet he didn't want her to be sitting in pain. He could tell she was in pain, though. Not the physical pain from the accident, but the usual hardship she seemed to be suffering when silent.

"How about some ice cream?" Jack said as the thought came to mind. "I don't think there is any in the crib, but we can stop and get some."

Djuana sighed into the passenger's window and said no.

"What's up? Talk to me."

During the trip home she had fought off the tears. Now, with Jack's loving eyes upon her she could not prevent her eyes from watering. She pulled her hand away to get tissue out of her handbag.

"I am so fuck-ing sick of crying," she said, wiping her eyes.

Jack gazed into those olive-brown eyes, taking back her hand with the tissue in it.

"Why are you cursing?"

"No reason, all right? I'm a grown woman I can curse."

"Oh, sorry. I forgot."

Jack released her hand and bolted out of the car, slamming the door shut. He went in to the back of the automobile and removed their things, grabbing the baggage with out care. He walked up the steps to the house, dumped everything on the porch and searched for his keys.

He had left them in the trunk's lock.

Djuana watched him raced by her, snatch his keys and run back up to the front door. She got out of the car, and slammed her door also. She walked up the steps slowly, allowing Jack time to get the front door open.

"I'll carry my stuff," she said.

"Then carry it, then. You want to carry shit, carry it."

When Djuana entered the house, the phone was ringing. She saw where Jack had dumped the bags in the living room; he was in the kitchen, in front of her when she came up the stairs in the house, answering the phone.

"You didn't have to curse at me!" Djuana yelled.

"I didn't!" Jack yelled back, turning his head from the receiver.

"Yes, you did!" Djuana said as she made her way down the hall with her clothes.

"Are you guys through fighting?" Jack's agent asked. "Sheez! What happened to the honeymoon? It's over already?"

"What do you want, Karl?" Jack took the kitchen's cordless into the living room and he plopped on his Lay-Z-Boy.

"Teams have been calling like crazy. Offers have been outrageous! This is great, much better than I thought."

"Terrific," Jack said flatly.

"Are you kidding? We could sign with just about any of the 29 other teams. Including the Gamblers. Did you hear?"

Jack winced, covering his eyes with his right hand. He felt guilty for letting Djuana carry her bags in her condition. Then, he heard her crying in the bedroom.

"Karl, I just don't give a fuck right now. Baseball is no longer my everything."

"New, baby, listen. The Gamblers called me and offered us $70 million for six years! Man, we're rich! That's more than they signed Bingo for last week."

Jack sat up. The sight of Djuana returning wearing just his jersey split his thoughts. She walked up to him and stood there, hands on her hips.

"I'm going to lay down, I am not feeling too well," she said, immediately turning to go back into the bedroom.

Berger's voice raised, repeating the offer, "Did you hear me? 70 mil! Woo-who!"

"Hold on a sec, Karl," Jack covered the cordless and chased behind Djuana, calling to her.

Djuana stopped, turning halfway. She said, without expression, "My side hurts a bit. I just want to lay down."

Jack kissed her forehead. "I'm sorry I cursed and yelled at you. I love you."

Djuana didn't say a word. She let Jack hug her.

He released her and kissed her again. "I'm going to get rid of Berger and be right there."

"No, you go ahead a take care of business," she rubbed his face with her right hand, smiling. "You need to get back into baseball."

"Not as much as I need you in my life."

Her smile became a blush. She kissed him softly on his lips.

"I'm sorry about," her voice traced off. "About how I'm acting."

"Forget it."

Djuana's tongue gathered her lips into her mouth as she watched Jack's stare. *He loves me*, she told herself. She allowed him to grabbed her into a stronger, tighter hug. The phone pressed into her back as he squeezed tightly.

"I love you," Jack whispered into her ear.

Djuana's eyes watered, she winced in pain. She tried to reply, but her voice was gone. Nevertheless, Jack heard her.

Jack watched her intently as she went into the bedroom. He felt free to miss baseball, and the feeling overwhelmed him.

Karl Berger pressed his phone into his skull. He tried to hear it all. He considered Jack Newhouse a friend, although Jack kept their relationship businesslike. Berger had 27 clients, Jack was the second highest grossing and one of three that lived in Portland.

"So, what's the deal, exactly?" Jack finally asked.

"It's a beaut!" Berger glowed. "10 mil to sign, 10 mil a year for six years. Guaranteed!"

"Shit."

"Shit is right! Let's do this, New."

"Karl, but what's up with the Crowns?"

"Clean you ears, New! Fuck Slight and his misfits! The Gamblers are willing to build the bakery and supply the dough!"

Jack listened to Berger's devious laugh and thought about the money. Then, he imagined playing for Las Vegas. Winning a lot of games year in and year out. And every year people would be picking his team to win the championship, not lose it. The money would be awesome. He would be making more than Oscar, more than Bingo. More than a lot of players that were said to be better than him.

With the extra millions he could open a business with out financial care. He could then open a large bar, with a restaurant. He imagined Djuana running it with him.

Then, his mind thought about his Crowns teammates. He loved those losers. They would hate him for taking the money and running. There had been players that left the Crowns for the trappings of more money elsewhere, and none of them prospered on the playing field. He recalled all the good times, his first orgy. The first Crowns pool party. The brawls with other teams, where there wouldn't be one Crown who wasn't fighting, or protecting another.

He could not imagine having played his career elsewhere and having as much fun. His teammates were now wearing light blue accessories with their uniforms out of respect for Djuana.

"I don't know,' he told Berger. "I can't do this to O and them. Man, I owe those guys a lot."

"You don't owe them shit. Slight released you, which means you are free to go anywhere you please. And, the money just happens to be in Las Vegas.

"Jack, please. Let's do this. This is a once in a lifetime offer."

"I don't know. Let me make some calls first. I'll get back to you."

"Jack!"

"I'll call you in a couple of hours."

Djuana was laying on the right, unharmed, side of her body, facing the doorway. Her eyes opened when Jack appeared. He walked slowly to her and knelt on the floor, leaning on the bed, on his elbows. He took her hand.

"How do you feel?"

"I took two pain killers, and they should kick in soon."

"It was the ride back, right?" He was hoping it wasn't the love making. Or her carrying the luggage.

"I don't know. I think I just need some rest."

Jack squeezed her hand. "I'm sorry. I'm sorry if I ruined our trip."

"No, I should be the one that's sorry. Like always, you made a dream of mine come true without me telling you about it before hand. I've been wanting to go away for the longest time."

Her eyes darted, glimpsing at each of Jack's eyes and lips. Her slight grin warmed Jack. He listened to her, relaxing more and more as she spoke.

"I'm just so damn insecure sometimes. I sat there in the car and made myself cry because I believed that you would leave me someday. That I don't deserve to have a man treat me as well as you do."

Djuana squeezed his hand, "Silly, ain't it?"

Jack boosted himself forward and kissed her.

"You don't have to worry. I'm with you for the long run."

Djuana shifted backward on the bed, "Here, come lay with me."

Jack laid next to her on his back, and she cuddled into him.

"Are you going to be able to play again?" she asked.

"It seems I have my choice of where I can play," he said, looking into the ceiling. "The Las Vegas Gamblers have offered me $60 million."

"Damn. That's a lot of money."

"They have it to give," Jack took her left hand into his and brought it to his lips. While he kissed her fingers he asked, "How would you like to move to Las Vegas?"

"Las Vegas? Sounds exciting, bright lights and all. But, I don't know. Portland is my home."

Jack looked into the ceiling, thinking it over. He wasn't going without Djuana.

When Djuana fell asleep, Jack left her with a kiss. He eased out of the bed, out of her arms, then tipped out of the room. He tried to call the Crowns at their hotel in Cleveland, but they had left for the game. He cut on the television to the pre-game show.

The host of the show, Burt Mathenson, a former Crowns player, topped his program with the Gamblers offer to Jack. He was glowing as he spoke about the "phenomenal amount of money."

"We can all but squash any hopes of Jack Newhouse ever being a Portland Crown again," Mathenson said.

The show had interviews with the Gamblers' owner and a few of the Crowns; all taped earlier or the evening before. Nobody said much, all waiting to see what Jack would do. And, all expecting him to accept the offer.

Slight took the offer personally, saying:

"The Las Vegas Gamblers want my players. They know we have a team that can challenge them for the next decade unless they break us up.

"The only thing they have over us is an abundance of money. And that's because they rip off their fans with high ticket prices and their owner owns a casino that breaks the legs of big winners."

Len Canisa, owner of the Gamblers, sued Slight over his remarks.

On the show, Oscar was his usual boisterous self. He said Slight was destroying the team, and that he would play out this year and demand a trade elsewhere.

While Jack watched the Crowns beat Cleveland, Bingo telephoned. The Gamblers, in Chicago, had the night off after a day game victory. They had won 31 games in a row after the Bingo trade. Las Vegas had no threats to their throne in the American League. The media, Cansia, and baseball experts were proclaiming them unbeatable.

The stories, as well as the constant phone calls from Cansia, were driving Vincent Slight to an early grave.

"Listen, Vinny, don't bet me," Cansia said one late night after his Gamblers had won by 17 runs. That same night the Crowns had won by two. "First of all, I'm tired of taking your money. Secondly, your boys might not even make the Series."

"Forget it. Don't bet me."

Slight was enlivened, "Really? Is that so? Well, listen to this. Not only will I bet your ugly motherfucking ass triple last year's gift, I will bet you a grand that Bingo won't even get a fucking hit against my boys."

Cansia's laugh grew heartily. "Your funny. Oh, yes, you are a riot. I'll take your money with a smile, you hump!"

Slight broke his phone tossing it against his bedroom wall.

"How nice of you to call," Jack said, his voice reeking of sarcasm. "Let's cut to the chase," Bingo said in his usually hurried tone when addressing mere mortals. "I hate you; fuck you is my mood. But, the Gamblers here, they think you can help them. They want you, so they asked me to call and let you know how much they think of you."

"Really? So, go on."

"The money is straight-up guaranteed. They say you can play right, they'll move Hopson to left and bench Smith. Where you bat in the lineup depends on how your stick clicks."

"Interesting. Do I get to room with you?"

Bingo hissed. "You are not only ignorant, but immature as well."

Jack stiffened. "Yeah, well, whatever," he sat up in his easy chair. "Tell your boss that I have other options that I would like to pursue. And, next time he should call Karl Berger, my agent. And to not have losers call me at my home."

"You son of a bitch. I hope you're stupid enough to turn down the money so I can see you cry again when you don't get a ring. You little bitch."

The phone clicked in Jack's ear before he could return the insult.

Djuana awoke alone in Jack's huge bed. And, she hated it. She leaped out of the bed – her ribs felt better - and she put on her favorite baseball jersey of all Jack possessed. She frowned to herself at the thought that she should wash his baseball jersey soon, but she didn't want to be without it that long.

She found Jack asleep in the living room, and planted a kiss on his forehead. She unpacked their clothes, putting his away and hers on the bed. The dirty clothes she put aside, as Jack had asked. His housekeeper would take care of the laundry.

Housekeeper. Djuana smiled. How would she handle having someone clean house for her? It sounded almost silly. She had spent so many years of being yelled at by Emma to clean up after herself; to become a clean woman, to know how to clean house for her man.

Djuana shrugged the memory of her mother teaching her how to be a wife. She wondered if she would ever be one, despite the training. Jack was there, and she thought he seemed like he would marry her, but would he really? Some days, when she thought about it, it seemed inevitable that she would marry Jack. He was always showing his love with the kind of affection she craved.

Then there were days like today, when she wondered how she would fit into his life.

Djuana undressed and took a long shower. She forced her mind to believe the water felt too good to waste on worries. Under the hot beads of pulsating water she sang happy songs, thinking about hanging out with her best friend when Jack returns to baseball.

Jack had meant to watch one game on video before getting in bed with Djuana. He wanted to make love to her, but knew she wouldn't feel like it. Jack wiped sleep from his face and went into the kitchen and started up the coffee machine.

He went into the bedroom to get some clean clothes and his toothbrush out of his traveling case. He saw Djuana's clothes on the bed, then heard her soft, raspy voice singing from behind the closed master bathroom's door along with the beading water from the shower.

He thought about going into the bathroom to see her body glisten and kiss the warm water off of her soft skin. He daydreamed her accepting him into the shower and them making passionate love. He started for the bathroom door, his heart racing, then, he changed his mind.

Jack used the bathroom off the kitchen and washed up; putting on sweat shorts and a t-shirt. He was sipping a strong cup of coffee, reading the morning paper when a string of steady knocks at the door began. By the time he got to the front door, the person knocking was ringing the doorbell like a madman.

Jack opened the door to find Mike Colbert leaning on the doorway, looking pitiful. Mike had hit his wife once too many times, in the eyes of Honeywell and Slight. They released Mike the day after the team arrived in Cleveland. He was wearing a red and black plaid lumberjack jacket and faded, worn jeans. On his clumped, black hair was a ragged Crowns cap; the old version that the team wore nearly three seasons ago. And, it seemed Mike hadn't washed nor shaved since then.

Mike vaulted into Jack's chest and grabbed him into a bear hug. He hugged and kissed Jack.

"What's up, New?" Mike said as Jack allowed himself to be grabbed.

"Nothing," Jack grimaced. The smell was overpowering. "Besides the fact we both unemployed."

"That's why I came to see you," Mike said as he took off his Crowns cap. "You alone?"

Jack stood aside, back against the open door, and asked Mike in.

"No. Djuana's here," Jack said as Mike made a beeline to the chair Jack had spent the night in. "She's in the back."

I'm sorry to interrupt. But, I need to talk, New."

Jack winced. He loved Mike Colbert. But, Mike was an alcoholic, and was overly talkative. And, usually talks with him lead nowhere. Still, Jack respected him because on the playing field, where he was clearly not the best athlete, he was the heart and soul of the Crowns. Their captain.

"You want a beer or something?" Jack asked.

Mike glared up at his teammate. "I don't drink anymore. You should know that."

Jack nodded. He knew Mike would try some change in his life; the man, whose whole life was baseball and his wife, would be devastated by losing both.

"You're right. I'm sorry," Jack sipped from his mug, then raised it. "How about some coffee. I just made some fresh."

"I can't drink that shit. Naw. Just some water would be enough."

Jack fixed him a glass of iced water and sat across from him on the couch.

Mike gulped the water; some of it streamed down his face. He wiped it off with his sleeve.

"You know," he said. "I miss my wife more than I expected I would. But not as much as I miss baseball and the guys. Shit. I miss baseball something fierce."

Jack was not listening. His mind drifted, trying to recall who told him that Mike's wife had finally left him and moved back to Arkansas. Jack envisioned Jennifer, her bruised face and petite arms dragging suitcases to her sports car.

"The whole league is treating me like I killed her, or something," Mike said. "My agent quit on me. I called around to just about every fuckin' team, even Buffalo who ain't never had a catcher, and they all said no."

Jack looked into Mike's mouth while he spoke. His dull-white teeth, his upper left canine missing from a collision at home plate two years ago, were a reminder of his umpteen years as a smoker. Mike was hard-nosed, built like a spark plug at 5-foot-9, and weighing 178 pounds. (Mike, also sensitive of his size, would force the Crowns to post his height at six feet and weight at 200).

Mike Colbert was the captain of the Crowns, the team's guts. He would lead them, not with his talent, but with his heart and courage.

"I'm the best fucking catcher out there, and you know it! Slight's got me blackballed. He and Honeywell are making sure I kill my-fucking-self."

Jack thought about his reply. He went with honesty: "People aren't eager to sign you because of the drinking and how often you were in the papers getting arrested for beating your wife."

"Yeah," Mike fiddled with his fingernails. He took a deep breath.

"Yeah," he repeated hoarsely, "I know that. But. I've changed. New, I've changed, man."

Jack didn't believe him.

"New, I love my wife. I love Jenny, but she'll start a fucking argument over something stupid, and you know I'll be drunk or getting drunk, and she want to fight."

"That's still no excuse to hit her, Mike."

"I know, I know. And, I am sorry. Deeply sorry."

"Yeah, afterwards," Jack added with disappointment.

Mike frowned at the rug. He looked up at Jack and said: "But, you know I love that woman. You know it."

Jack could not look Mike in the eye after that statement.

# 33

Mike had been to seven other teammates' homes before the Crowns left Portland, and consequently had short stays. He was treated like an outcast by the others, because the players were then very afraid of losing their jobs. They knew then that Vincent Slight was serious about changing the attitude of his baseball club.

Mike hadn't been to his own home in three days, living in his car and barely eating. He listened to his radio, hearing about all the offers Jack Newhouse was getting. He came to his friend, hoping Jack still considered him a friend. He asked Jack to help him get back into baseball.

Jack loved Mike, mainly because Mike was the kind of ballplayer he always wanted to be. Very vocal, and very dedicated to anyone wearing the same uniform as he. Mike was the heart and soul of the Portland Crowns. So, Jack decided to add him to his deal with the Crowns; to demand Honeywell take Mike back also, or Jack wouldn't re-sign.

But, when Jack called Honeywell, he found out neither Mike nor himself were no longer needed on the Crowns.

"I just picked up Howie Roe from New Jersey," Honeywell said matter-of-factly. Roe was New Jersey's top catcher.

"And, Aponte is our right fielder for life."

Those words stung Jack. That was the same sentence Honeywell said to Jack when he was called up from the minors and replaced Don The same thing Honeywell told Jack when he was called up from the minors **six** years before.

"The bottom line is, you guys are no longer in our plans, for whatever reason," the Crown's general manager said. "You can go anywhere, and somebody will pick him up when he lowers his asking price. Did you know he asked Milwaukee for two mil a year?"

"He's worth it," Jack replied with no doubt in his voice.

"Not in the frame of mind he's in now. He's a wife-beater and an alcoholic."

"Yeah, I know that. And you always did know that. The man needs help. He is not the kind of person that can recover on his own. We need to be there for him like he has always been for everybody on the team."

"Fine," Honeywell sounded exasperated. "You spoke up for him, now tell him I said no."

"That's fucked up."

"Yeah. It is, but you made a choice, and a bad one. You choose that woman over us. And, Slight is making you pay for it.

"And, just like you, Mike didn't heed any warnings."

"Wonderful."

Honeywell, pen in one hand at his lips, and the phone to his ear in the other, looked out of his office window on the third level of Adkins Stadium. He watched the grounds crew rake the beautiful, reddish-brown dirt in the infield. Jack was his favorite personality on the team he had built. He wanted Jack back on the team, but he also wanted to keep his job.

Vincent Slight had been good to Honeywell, he thought at that moment. Honeywell had risen in the Boston organization as far as he could, from a minor league nobody, to a fine coach and manager. But, he saw that they were not going to reward his dedication and progress with a front office job. Then, Vincent Slight bought the Crowns and brought Honeywell along.

"Jack," Honeywell snapped. "There's a call on my other line that I have to take."

Jack felt Djuana's presence while he was talking with Honeywell. She was standing at his side, at the arm of the chair with her arms folded. He looked up at her once, but she looked away.

Jack was furious. He had heard Honeywell give many people that same tired line about another call.

"Fine, Mr. Honeywell. You take that call."

Jack pressed the talk button on his cordless and fell back into the chair. He bit on the thick, black antenna. Djuana gazed at him with wondering eyes.

"Are you okay?" she asked.

"Yeah. I guess so?" he said slowly.

Djuana had heard enough to understand that Jack's career in Portland seemed doomed. Her urge to get away from him strengthened.

"I need to get home. Can you take me, Jack?"

"Yeah, I can," he said. "But, I'd rather you stayed. Are you all right?"

"I'm fine."

The phone rang. Jack didn't remove his eyes from his love. It continued to ring. Djuana's eyes lit on the red light blinking on the cordless.

"Answer the phone, Jack," Djuana exhaled and unfolded her arms. "I'll tell you when you have time."

She didn't mean to sound nasty, but her words had bite.

On the phone was Vivian.

"Oh, so you home now?" Jack's ex said.

"Yes."

"Well, then I'm coming over. I need to talk to you."

"That's not necessary. What do you want?"

Djuana, who had been frozen, waiting to mend her curtness, darted into the back of the house. "Shit," she mumbled. "I am fucking this up."

Jack's eyes and attention followed her, then, when she was out of sight, he sat back, exasperated.

"You need to know you deserve better," Vivian went on. "You are a damn good man with a helluva lot to offer. What are you doing with that *girl*? I told you to watch what you're doing with those groupies."

"Vivian, I'll talk to you some other time, I am not in the mood for this."

"What? Is she there? I know she is. Listen, honey sounds like some kind of golddigger. You sure that was your baby? You sure she was even pregnant?"

"Good bye, Vivian."

"Wait! I know she's there and you have to go. You just got back from taking her to our spot, right? That shit ain't right, and you know it. But, let me ask you this before you hang up.

"Did you get her pregnant while we were together?"

Jack shook his head and grinned. "Look, Vivian, I'll talk to you later."

Djuana placed her *bags* at the foot of the staircase leading to the front door. She went in to the kitchen and was pouring a glass of soda when Jack entered.

"You're taking all of your stuff. What's the deal?"

Djuana swallowed the soda eagerly, looking into the glass. But, the glass didn't have the right words at its depths.

Jack moved closer.

"Jack, I just want to go home while you are out of town playing baseball."

"I'm not going anywhere yet."

Djuana sipped more.

"You will be," she muttered, then sighed. She finally looked him in the eye. "I just want to go home, see my family and lay in my own bed tonight."

"All right. Fine." Jack said.

He walked out of the kitchen. He snatched up her two carry-on size bags and the large Crowns duffel bag he gave her – "Leaving me in my own bag," he mumbled – and started down the steps.

Djuana watched him for a second, then refilled her glass.

"Shit."

The phone buzzed twice before she noticed Jack was not back in the house yet. She picked up the kitchen cordless out of its wall cradle. There was an empty pause after Djuana's greeting, then a feminine voice asked for Jack Newhouse.

"Who's calling?" Djuana asked as Jack appeared.

"Tell him its Kristen Eisen, from the Gazette."

Kris was furious. Her whole mindset changed. *How could he have her answering his phone? She's just going to keep hurting him*. Instead of being bubbly like she was while dialing, Kris attacked Jack when he came to the phone.

"I called to see how you are taking unemployment, but I guess you're doing fine."

"Yeah, I'm okay."

Djuana took the last bag down the stairs and into the Pathfinder. She sat in the automobile until Jack was ready.

"That woman has taken you away from your job, you know that right?"

"Kris, if you called to get on my nerves, you are just about there."

"No, no. I'm sorry. But, I can't understand you. You are such a smart man, why are you with that woman?"

"I love her."

The airwaves fell silent. Then Kris began to sob.

"You don't know what love is, Jack," Kris said. "You don't. You will just keep searching for it even though it's right here for you."

"What makes you think you know me that well?"

"Because I do. I love you, Jack. And I can more than some welfare recipient can. I can give you more than she can. Much more."

"Now, why the fuck you say that?"

"Oh, what? You don't know she has been on welfare all her life, and that she lives with her mother in a shady part of town? She has a nowhere job. That woman is about nothing!"

"Don't call me, Kris, all right? I am no longer a Crown, we ain't got shit to talk about."

Jack hung up and tossed the cordless across the kitchen counter and into the sink.

The drive into Portland was quiet. Djuana had her arms folded across her chest, a common sight, but was not frowning now. She whispered along with songs on the radio, allowing Jack to see, if he cared, that she was not upset.

Jack noticed, but he was searching for the right words. The last thing he wanted to do was argue. He wanted Djuana with him, all the time. He did not want to drive her home, he wanted them to be in bed together all that day. But, he dared not say that.

Also, he needed to be home to answer the phone when Honeywell called.

"Damn," he remembered he hadn't called his agent that day, and it was well past noon. Berger could not reach him because Jack had forgotten his pager and cellular phone on the coffee table.

Djuana looked over at him. He was driving with his left hand, rubbing his chin with his right.

"What's wrong?" She asked.

"Nothing. I just forgot to call Berger."

She looked away, out at the other cars as they whisked by. "You've missed another appointment because of me."

Jack yanked the wheel of the 4X4, directing the Pathfinder out of traffic and into the parking lot of a fast food joint. They were blocks from Tudor Street. He ceased the engine, and turned his body to face hers.

Djuana was stunned. She was frightened but his sudden movements. He ignored the horns and curses, and the pedestrians that dove for cover. She allowed him to separate her arms and take her hands into his. She looked into his eyes, and relaxed. She glanced down at their hands, rubbing his long, thick fingers, then back up to the dark eyes of the man who loved her. She loved those dark eyes, they were as soulful as a Motown ballad.

"What's the matter, Baby?"

"Nothing, really," Djuana forced a smile.

Jack wasn't having it.

"Listen, for the last time, baseball is a sport. I made money at it, and I love playing it. But, it was my whole life.

"I can't marry baseball. Baseball can't bring the joy of a family. Of a good woman's love. I need that right now more than I need baseball."

Jack squeezed her hand. "I am not even 30 yet. I can still play. And, I will. But, I am not going to be without you."

Djuana melted. As did her inhibitions. But, her soul felt the need to flush the bad thoughts, to have Jack bat them away like he would a pitcher's fastball.

"But, Jack, I've affected you in the worst way. On TV, in the newspapers and on the street, people are saying you are having the worst year of your career.

"How come you haven't hit a home run this year?"

Jack looked at Djuana puzzled, frowning. "I haven't? So?"

"No, you haven't. And this will be the first time in your career that you won't hit 20."

"So?"

"I am the reason for it, and the reason the Crowns fired you. And, you know it's true."

"I don't give a shit about none of that. Who cares what people say? Fuck them. They think just 'cause they see me on television and at the ballpark, that they know everything about me. They don't

"I'm happy to have met you, and although it seems like this is the worst year of my career, and it probably is," Jack shrugged. "It's not the worst year of my life."

Djuana watched the words flow off Jack's lips and loved that he believed in her, loved her, and that he didn't blame her. She rubbed his chin and lips with both hands.

"Jack, I don't know if I deserve you."

"That's true," Jack smirked. "You deserve better. But, I'm trying."

Djuana blushed and gave her man kiss.

# 34

When one of Karl Berger's professional athletes became a free agent, that was when he was at his best. He was great at being narrow-minded; getting the best for his clients. Most times it was more money than ball clubs were offering, or were set, to pay. Of course, the more millions he garnered for his players, the more his 20% would bulge.

But, in the case of Jack Newhouse, one of the premier players in his stable of thoroughbreds, Berger never really had to work hard. His negotiations with Honeywell were never difficult. Jack wanted no parts of free agency; and, the Crowns, who groomed him into the player that he was, was content on keeping Jack around.

Until the season Jack fell in love.

"Listen, Jack. I'll spell this out for you in plain old English," Berger said over the phone from his office in Los Angeles. "The Crowns don't want you. Las Vegas does."

Jack flopped back into his easy chair, his drink steady in his hand. "I don't care," he said.

"Well, I mean, you don't have to sign with Las Vegas. San Fran has called. Miami, Buffalo and Cincy. Them too. What about Seattle, that's not far from Portland? Come on, New."

"Listen to me, Karl. Portland is my home. I'm not interested in no place else."

"Wake up, New. So, what is it that you want me to do? Even if I drop your price to the league minimum, they aren't going to take you back."

"Then, I guess I won't be playing baseball again."

"Relax, relax. We'll talk more when I get back to Portland."

The team returned from the road for its longest homestand of the season, 16 games with five teams, in two weeks. Jack believed this to be his best chance to get back with the ball club. And, he was right. The Crowns had won six of the seven games on the road, their best stretch of the season by far. The only game they lost, the final game of the three-game set in Cleveland. It was a nationally televised Wednesday-nighter, and it turned out to be big news.

Oscar did not show up for the game. He chose that game to protest the club's treatment of Jack. And, his absence stung deeply. Slight, who loves to see his team on national television, had to sit through a blow out. Aponte was moved to center to cover O's absence, and he had three errors. Two balls sailed over the rookie's head that O would have flagged down easily.

O called the broadcast booth and began a national campaign to get Jack his job back.

"Listen, you know me Joe," O said to Joe Sweet, the color man of the two-man announcing team. Sweet had played for the Arizona Aztecs.

"I take every game seriously. And, Lord knows we need to start winning if we plan to get back into the World Series this year. But, Jack Newhouse is my best friend, we grew up in this organization together and I believe he was released for the worse reason in the world: love."

The announcers seemed, at one point, trying to get Oscar to admit what he was doing was wrong.

"Yeah, but Oscar, by your walking off, you are costing your teammates a game," Joe Sweet said.

"No. They wanted to walk off, and protest, but they can't. They can't afford to. I feel, as one of the veterans on the ball club, it was up to me to lead. To take the front.

"Besides, this one game ain't going to break our season. If anything, now that the whole country knows that Vincent Slight is trying to break up one of the best teams of all time with bogus charges, this game will make our season."

While O was speaking, Cleveland scored four runs, and led at the time 7-1 in the fourth inning.

"See what I mean? We just don't need me out there, Jack needs to be back in right."

"But, Oscar," began Paul Engles, the play-by-play announcer, "From our understanding, Jack Newhouse made a choice. He chose to step down rather than play on this road trip."

"Propaganda. Don't believe that. Paul, would you leave the woman you loved, who just lost y'all's baby, to do a game across the country?

"Be for real. He deserved the time off, all the battles he done fought for Slight."

The backlash on the ball club from Oscar's protest was enormous, much more than O imagined it would be. The Crowns' offices were bombarded with phone calls, and mail from mostly women's groups. The mayor of Portland teamed with the city council, a unison unheard of in Ann Meier's two terms, and held a town meeting. Meier invited Slight, who sent Honeywell back to Portland to attend.

During this battle in the press over Jack's release, Slight stood firm.

"Jack Newhouse quit on us while we were struggling," Slight said to the group of reporters and cameramen outside of his office building in downtown Portland. "We are in last place, fighting to get back to where we belong and he left us for dead. I don't think that is the path of a righteous man."

Honeywell had a tough time with the crowd, and media covering the event. Each time he tried to raise a point in defense of his boss, he was drowned out by the unbelieving council and residents. He eventually gave in, and allowed himself to be shouted at, accused of being a sell out by one Black female on the council. He sat there, ankle on knee, understanding he was debating for the wrong cause.

He saw people in attendance that Jack Newhouse had touched personally. There was the councilwoman that berated him, she had had the luxury of having a famous baseball player at her leisure. Jack had never said no to that woman. He had spoken to her constituents on many occasions; and had campaigned for her.

There were people in the angry crowd that had watched their ailing, or dying children light up whenever Jack Newhouse visited the four hospitals in metro Portland. There was Curt Warner, who ran an after school program. When he needed funding after state cuts, it was Jack Newhouse who hit his teammates for a grand sum of a million dollars, and supplies. Warner now has three facilities spread through out the city.

Honeywell knew all of this well before entering the crowded assembly room in City Hall. But, the boisterous supporters of Jack Newhouse, who knew he had known, pointed it out in detail for him anyway.

Honeywell got home, fixed a soothing mug of tea, and phoned Slight in Buffalo, the Crowns last stop before returning home, with a short version of the meeting.

"I figured as much," his boss said to him.

"I guess that's why you sent me."

"So, what do you think we should do?"

"Re-sign him. I didn't want to let him go anyway."

Silence.

"We need veterans for the stretch run, don't we?" Slight said as if thinking out loud.

"You know we do. We aren't as deep as last year."

"He hasn't hit this year."

"He will in the playoffs."

"How do you know that? His mind is on that Dijona."

"Djuana."

"Whatever. We could pick up somebody else. J.A., the man quit on us."

"Juris wants him back. And so do I."

Slight hissed into the phone. "You know, I don't give a gay fuck anymore. Sign him. I'm breaking this fuckin' team up, win or lose, in January."

Jack glided the Pathfinder in front of Djuana. She got in, kissed her man, and immediately forgot the long day at work.

"How are you?" Jack asked as they merged into traffic.

"Much better now," she smiled warmly.

Jack took her hand into his thigh, she slid over to him. "Why don't you just quit. They have you down to three days, that's no money."

"There aren't that many jobs in Portland, did you know that?"

"Yeah." Jack wanted to say she didn't need to work, but he knew better. "Would you mind if I helped you find a better job."

"Like what?"

"Just trust me."

Djuana gazed out across 10th Avenue. *If I married him, I wouldn't need to work.* The thought had crossed her mind often.

"I've got good news," Jack grinned.

"Are you back on the team?"

"Seems that way." His eyes never left the road.

"So, Oscar's walk out helped."

Jack chuckled. "Walk out. Let me tell you," he looked over at Djuana, her amused countenance held his thoughts hostage for a long second.

"What?" Djuana was hanging on her man's words, listening to him tell her something worthwhile for the first time in too long. And, she understood why he was back to being talkative.

"That fool O," Jack diverted his stare. "He told me this morning that he was at some woman's house, and she forgot to set her alarm clock, so after they did the nasty, he didn't wake up until the game was well under way.

"So, being the friend he is, he did what he always does. Used me as an excuse."

Djuana didn't laugh. "He's really something."

"Yep. That's my boy, though."

"But, at least you're back playing. So when do you play?"

"I have to go to the minors for a week. Vancouver, Canada."

Djuana looked away, out in front of them, at the slowing traffic as the light changed to red. She frowned. *This is how it's supposed to be,* she told herself. *He is supposed to travel. He travels for a living. And, I knew he'd be going back to work soon.*

She bit her lip, recovering from the quick bout with the blues. She took his left arm into her bosom and kissed his shoulder, leaning into him as he drove. "I'm happy for you, and, I know how happy that will make you."

"I just don't want to be away from you."

"Jack. Stop treating me like a basket case. I'll be okay."

"I know you will. Maybe I just don't like missing you."

Djuana's heart warmed, and chills ran along her arms. She rubbed wrist his between her legs, grinding her thighs on his muscular forearm.

"I'll always be here whenever you return." Djuana's voice slipped into a calm, alluring pant.

Jack exhaled, shaking his head. He looked at her deeply, moving his left hand, getting a good grip on the inside of her closer thigh.

"No. I want more than that," he said, with his voice matching hers in volume and tenderness.

The feeling in Djuana's chest was a sharp thud, as if a cannonball had barreled into her torso. She squeezed his right arm with both hands, unconsciously digging her nails into his arm. She thought about beating around the issue; being coy. She didn't want to be wrong, though. Moving in with Jack would be a comfort. She would be out from under Emma, and distanced from being a full-time baby-sitter.

Instead, she held on to him, looking up at the man she so dearly and deeply loved, waiting for the question of her lifetime.

The last time Jack could remember being this nervous was his first at bat in the majors. He came through that tense moment with a lined single off of a good pitcher. But, on that day almost seven years ago, his palms were not as sweaty, nor his mouth as dry. He steered the car in silence, hoping the nerve would come soon.

Djuana sat up, she saw in Jack an uncertainty that through her off. *Just ask me. I want to live with you. Be your lady, forever. We can talk about marriage during the off-season. Relax, baby.*

She stroked his arm.

"Jack, I want to be with you more than anything in this world."

"I want you with me," Jack voice had become hoarse and cracked.

Djuana looked up in to Jack's eyes, his fingers tightened around her thigh. Jack slowed the Pathfinder at another stop light.

Jack near mumbled, "Everyday. I want to see you everyday."

"You can," Djuana's voice fell to a faint whisper. Her heart fluttered, moving with quick, sharp beats. Her breathing quickened.

"Do you know I love you?" Jack blurted, his eyebrows bent and shaped his face into a frown.

"I do. I feel it, see it and I know it. And, I love you too."

She watched Jack's eyes flutter, then his turn back to the traffic as the light changed. She kissed into his shoulder blade.

"I love you more than anyone I've ever known. More than anything."

Djuana smile up at him. "I know you do, Jack." Her voice traced off. Her body squirmed, but she hid it by grinding her legs around Jack's hand, moving closer to him.

"Shit," Jack squeezed her thigh, his hand snuggled tightly. The warm, moist feel of her crotch distracted him. He accelerated down King Boulevard, moving into a open lane.

Djuana could sense the question of a lifetime. It was in the air, in the way Jack could not look her way for any length of time. She wanted to prod and pry the words out of him.

Suddenly, as the Pathfinder moved along MLK, passing the convention center, Jack blurted, "I want you so bad, from the first day I laid eyes on you. I just knew. I knew. You came right into my arms, like it was me you needed."

"We need to pull over," Jack said as the truck hugged the divider and rolled into the left turning lane. He sped across the four-lane street and into the convention center's parking lot.

Jack put the car in park, realizing he had unconsciously taken the streets instead of the highway back to Woodlands. He leaned into the steering wheel. The feel of Djuana's soft palm rubbing his back was a soothing, healing relief. When Djuana first saw the tears on Jack's rich brown skin, she wanted to gently lick them away. Her body inched closer, lips leading the way. But, her heart melted in the heat of her chest. She instead stared at his cheeks.

"I can't be without you anymore," with his head down, his voice barely carried in the cab of the Pathfinder. "I can't sleep unless you're there. Right there with me."

Jack edged up, raising his head halfway, finally looking into Djuana's eyes. She reached up to him and kissed his lips, licking the top, then allowing his tongue to search her mouth.

"I'm yours, Jack," she panted. Her right hand gathered in the material of Jack's polo shirt.

Jack turned his body, clasping his right hand around her neck, searching her mouth for the taste her love gave off from the sweetest tongue he had ever kissed. The feel of the skin on the back of her neck melting between his fingers aroused him. He slid his hand around to her chin. Djuana closed her eyes, licked his lips and awaited on any move Jack wanted to make. She was willing to do anything Jack desired at that moment in the truck, in the empty parking lot, during the late afternoon rush hour.

Djuana had dreamt of millions of ways she wanted a man to propose to her. She knew it would be a man she desired, had to have, but never did her colorful dreams include a man that so enchanted her soul, or filled her heart with love. Mostly, her dream had the scenery darker, and more romantic. Like an expensive restaurant, or a sofa feet away from a crackling fire. Candles and champagne. A beautiful diamond. And, no one around for miles.

But, Djuana would recall that moment, with people milling around less than fifty yards away, and horns angrily blowing in the background, was the most romantic time of her life.

Jack lightly planted a peck on her lips, pulling away as her mouth opened wider. He leaned back, trying to gather his nerve, holding her hands, rubbing the knuckles and staring down at them as if they held the answer to his misplaced courage.

"Djuana," Jack squeezed her hands and focused in on her eyes. "I love you and I want you to..."

"Yes," Djuana panted, vaulting into his chest.

"...marry me."

"Yes. Yes."

Djuana forced her arms around Jack's neck; there was no room, but she swung a leg over his lap, shifting her body into his lap. Her buttocks fell onto the steering wheel, causing their horn to join the others. Jack cradled her body, and Jack sped up his tongue to keep up with the passion steaming from Djuana's jaws.

By the time the Pathfinder had guided into the garage of Jack's home, Djuana had already decided on which teddy she was going to put on once she got out of the shower. It would be her favorite; the black, sheer, body-hugging dotted lace piece with the V-neck and lace trim. Jack had already pictured undressing her, holding her down on the bed and pounding her soft, inviting flesh until he was spent.

They entered he house through the garage to a ringing phone. Jack was doing a great job of ignoring it until Djuana darted into the bathroom. When he did answer it, he had already determined it would be a short call.

The male caller said, "You going back, huh?"

It took Jack a second or two to pick on Mike's voice. He hadn't heard the fiery catcher sound somber too many times.

"Yeah. Honeywell called me a little while ago."

Jack listened to the shower. He imagined that soft body freshly clean, awaiting him in the bed in just a few minutes.

"Hey, Mike, I'm a little busy, man."

"Yeah. I bet."

Shit. "What's wrong, Mike?"

Jack could hear Mike puff and blow. Jack hoped it was a cigarette.

"Everything. Every-fucking-thing. You'd think five years of being on your knees day in and day out for an organization would mean something. But they don't give a fuck."

"Mike, just relax, man. Maybe you should consider playing elsewhere."

"You didn't."

Jack flinched. "Yeah. You're right. But, that was me."

"How many times had I taken hits, had guys run me over. I have had, what three concussions, lost a tooth, and had a broken jaw."

"For what? To have them cut me for arguing with my wife?"

Jack fell silent. Mike was more subdued than Jack had ever heard him.

"It's over for me. I'm finished. I just hope motherfuckers remember that

I cared about them, loved them. It wasn't shit I wouldn't've done for any of you. I loved all of you.

"Loved the games. Wins and losses."

Jack became worried. "Just get yourself together over the winter. And come back in the spring stronger."

"New, man, you know what Honeywell told me? He said, they got a catcher already. That he didn't need me."

"He and Slight are on this image trip. Just take it easy until the spring, and I guarantee you they'll give you a try out. Just stay out of trouble."

"Out of trouble?" Mike mocked a laugh. "My wife won't speak to me. I went to see her and she tells me about some court order. I can't even see my boys.

"I can't see my boys, New."

Jack listened intently. The man the Crowns, and especially opposing players called Psycho was expressing his hurt with little anger, and little profanity.

"Things will come together, Mike."

"I love you, New. Did I ever tell you that?"

Jack listened to Mike's voice crack. Mike Colbert was broken.

"It was you, Jack. The only one who talked to me when I was a rookie. The only one who pulled my coat to things, didn't have me go around like some butthole straight out of Nebraska like I was."

"Man, Mike, I wasn't that much of a vet either." Jack chuckled a bit, but a morbid feeling was overwhelming him.

"Me and you, New. You used ta fire that ball with that rifle arm of yours and I'd hang in there until the last second and we'd nail motherfuckers.

"I loved it. I used to beg batters to hit it to you when men were on base, just so you'd gun they ass, and I get to fuck somebody up."

Mike inhaled deeply, "Man, shit, New. I'm crying like a bitch over here."

It's okay. Where are you? Why don't you come over?"

Jack listened to Mike wipe his nose.

"I gotta go, man. I loved you, Jack."

The click in the phone came too quickly.

Jack didn't hesitate, yet he hoped he was wrong. He raced back down to the garage, keys in hand, noticing Djuana out of the corner of his eye.

"I'll be right back!" he shouted to Djuana.

"What's wrong, Jack?" Djuana was frightened. She couldn't imagined what would make Jack leave at such an inopportune time.

He sped the Pathfinder across town. He phoned the police, and they met him at Mike's cottage up in Wooden Cliffs; a community of expensive, large homes off the beaten path. It was located between Jack's house and the city; usually a 20 minute drive for Jack. He made it in about 10. He and the cops didn't find Mike.

He stood on Mike's porch perplexed. He forced the cops to search the grounds surrounding the house. No Mike. He searched his memory aloud for any hint of where Jenny might have gone with their three sons. Mike was near his children, Jack was suddenly sure of it.

"Mr. Newhouse, are you sure Mike Colbert will attempt suicide?" one of the four cops said after regrouping on the porch.

Jack's memory bank kicked out the answer. "Denver. She went home."

Mike parked his white Porsche on the road, front tire on his in-laws lawn. He walked the good distance across the soft grass to the front door, which was at the left side of the house. The house his money bought. The Lynns were poor when Mike met Jennifer. He saw his wife's red mini van in the driveway. He looked at it most of the way to the door, staring at the two car seats. Mike Junior would sit anywhere he wanted; he was eight. But, Jonathan, two, and Craig, eight months old, needed the protection.

Mike rang the bell twice in succession, then stood back with his arms at his side, hands behind his back. Mrs. Lynn answered the door with a frown. In the house, Mike saw his boys giggling and playing in front of the floor model television his money bought.

Mrs. Lynn didn't open the screen door. She looked out at Mike and said, "You no-good bastard. How dare you darken my doorstep."

Mike sniffed in the early evening air. He stood upright, confident that he looked decent enough. And, he did. He had taken a painstakingly long time grooming himself for this visit.

"I need to see my wife for a minute. That's all."

"Go to hell," Mrs. Lynn slammed the door and locked it. She made a beeline to the phone to call the police. "You lunatic!"

The kids froze on the living room rug, yards away. They knew by their grandmother's reaction it could only be their father.

Jennifer gathered the boys, holding the infant in her arms. Her face had been back to normal a week, the bruises had healed without scars. Still, she refused to go out in the town where she had grown up. Everyone knew her life as a professional athlete's wife was no dream come true.

"What does he want, Mom?" She had seen the Porsche.

"For you to be stupid and go back to him, what else?" she replied, dialing the phone.

"Hang up, Mom. Let me just see what he wants and tell him to go home."

Mrs. Lynn dropped the receiver down in the cradle. "Well, I am going to call your father, and tell him to get right home."

Jenny opened the door, and Mike held his head up at the sight of the woman he married, still upright. He was wearing jeans, a pink polo shirt and sneakers. His hair was clean, and combed back, with a slicked, gel look.

Mike marveled at his wife. She stood in the house, behind the screen door as her mother had. Three kids, and she still seemed like the youthful virgin he had met 10 years ago in college.

"You look wonderful, Jen," Mike said, hands behind his back.

"Mike, why did you come here?" she asked.

"You wouldn't come to the phone. I miss my boys."

His subdued manner eased Jenny; she wanted to get closer to him so the kids didn't have to hear the sure-to-come argument. She opened the screen door and came out onto the small porch.

"You know you lost the right to see us. At least for awhile. You shouldn't 've come." She looked out at the Porsche. It was filthy.

"You drove all the way to Denver? I told you not to."

"I'm sorry I ever hit you."

"You're always sorry afterwards. Go home, Mike. The police are coming. I don't want a scene here, in front of the kids and all."

"I am sorry now. More than ever," Mike inhaled a gust, and exhaled it hard. He felt cleansed. "You're never coming back to me, are you?"

Jenny had thought about that question. No one wanted her to. And, she hadn't listened to them before. She wasn't sure if she would be able to go on with out him. Her lawyer told her she would never be broke.

Jennifer shook her head slowly, her arms holding and consoling herself.

"No, Mike. I'm going to stay here for awhile then get my own place."

Mike's eyes glazed. "I just wanted to see you for one last time. I love you and our kids very much. Always have.

"Good-bye."

Before Jenny could think, react or move, Mike walked away. This scared her more than his appearance.

She called to him, and ran behind him. "You just going to walk away like this?"

"Yeah. I'm done begging like some asshole. From now on, I live my life for me. I am going back to the Crowns, and that's it. Baseball and nothing else."

"Oh, like you have never said that before now?"

"Good-bye."

# 35

The chartered bus carrying the Vancouver Crowns to a game in mid-Canada zipped through the morning. Jack was wide awake among the sleeping 18, 19 and 20 year olds. He watched the farm houses turn in to tiny towns, then become small cities on the land off the two-lane highway. The scenery was familiar to him, yet distant in his memory. He had taken the same road trip with eight years before as a member of Portland's top minor league club.

The manager back then, some eight seasons ago, was a tall, lanky fellow by the name of Leslie Louis. Louis was a straight, mild mannered man who worshipped Slight for giving him his first managing job. Louis believed he would someday manage the Crowns. And, he deserved a shot at the big time because he felt he had transformed 10 of the best prospects in baseball into intelligent ballplayers.

Louis taught Jack the value of hitting to right field; a trait that helped Jack become a feared hitter almost instantly in the majors. Louis worked painstaking hours with Oscar, a man who hated practice of any sorts, on how to study pitchers; how to lean on the basepaths, how to steal a base on any pitcher or any catcher.

O was still a great base runner, but unless the game was on the line, or he just wanted to, he rarely stole a base.

Louis also spent long hours training Mike how to channel his anger and energy into one force on the diamond; how to control a game, player by player, when he was behind the plate. Louis visited Adkins during that season, seeking a job, and besides cool hellos and light handshakes, he didn't utter a word to any of his former players.

Jack hated that Louis blamed the players, along with Slight, for him not getting the Crowns managing job. Hal Juris was a great manager; when he became available Slight and Honeywell jumped on him, signing him two days after New York fired him. Louis, who interviewed with Slight, felt betrayed, and took the snub personally. He quit and made a lateral move to another team. Six years later, and Louis was still not a major league manager.

The sound of his cellular phone was a welcome jerk back to reality. He plucked open the flip-top and answered it.

"Being rich has its rewards, hey big shot?" one of the wannabe major leaguers said, craning his neck over the seat to say.

Jack smirked at the smiling player. Then ignored him. Djuana's voice was it's usual calming, enchanting notes of joy.

"Are you okay?" she asked.

"Yeah." The cracking in her voice caused Jack to check his watch, even though he knew it was only a few minutes past nine.

"You up early? Did you sleep okay?"

"Not really. Don't get upset, but I miss you. Now I understand how married couples get used to having one another in the bed."

"You better believe I miss you too."

"Are you there yet?"

"No. We are still on the bus." Jack looked up and out of the window and saw the bus turn into a Howard Johnson. He couldn't recall the last time he was here, but he instantly remembered the faces and bodies of the girls he and Oscar had slept with there. Two Native Americans.

"I couldn't wait until you called. I've missed you." Djuana shifted herself in their bed. She put her back to pillows and the headboard. "Have you gotten any sleep?"

Jack mumbled an answer. He held the phone to his ear, staring into space. The thought of playing ball was pleasing. The feel of his glove, the model Rawling named after him three years ago. He has been playing with the same glove since then. His mind recalled the feel of his bat in his hands, as if it had been years instead of weeks. He couldn't wait to get back to the majors.

"...and this reporter keeps calling..."

"A reporter?" Jack snapped back.

"Yeah. He wants to ask me a few questions. I told him no twice, but he keeps calling."

"What's his name?"

"Rich Anderson from some paper in Los Angeles."

"I know him, I'll handle him."

"Are you nervous about the game?"

Jack smiled, and Djuana could feel it. "No. Not really. I mean, once it starts, I'll be fine."

"I wish you luck."

"Thanks."

"You don't need it, right?"

"Yeah, I can use anything you got to share."

"Well, then get back here, I got something for you!"

"Don't start that, I won't be back for two weeks."

"It'll be waiting."

"It better be."

"It will be," Djuana blushed. She paused, trying to halt herself from sounding corny or rehearsed.

"I love you, Jack Newhouse."

"I love you too, Djuana Newhouse."

Jack played five games for Portland's top minor league ball club, and he tore up the young, inexperienced pitching in triple A ball. When the games were on, he was extremely focused; more so than he had been all season. During games, he allowed his teammates, and players on other teams, to pick his brain; to ask him anything about the adventures that await the gifted, and/or lucky ones to make it where he was on his way back to.

But, once the games were over, he was a recluse. He gave reporters short answers, and rarely spoke to his teammates. This set off some of his teammates. He was called conceited, spoiled and selfish. It didn't matter to Jack. He did realize he was just like them before he got to the big leagues, curious and eager to taste the big money. But, Jack was focused in on getting back to Portland as soon as he could; on getting back with the Crowns, and getting his arms around Djuana. He spoke with her four and five times a day. When he wasn't on the phone, or in bed, he was taking batting practice.

Jack would arrive at the ballpark five hours before a game, stretch, loosen up, then get in the batting cage and for no less than three hours, he would hit balls off the pitching machine.

Finally, Honeywell visited the team before Jack's eighth game. Honeywell walking through the clubhouse was like God walking on water. The players not in awe reached out to at least touch the man's hand; get him to make eye contact.

That night, he watched the team lose. But, Jack had three hits, all extra base ropes. After the game, Honeywell took Jack aside.

"You could get out of the bed with a fever and get a base hit here," Honeywell said.

Jack just nodded.

"Well, then let's get you back so you can stop wasting your time here."

Honeywell and Jack took the morning flight to the states, then a connecting flight to Cincinnati. They arrived at the home ballpark of the Cincinnati Cougars two hours before game time. When Jack walked into the visitors' clubhouse, the sight of his teammates instantly exhilarated his soul. They were the same rambunctious guys he had lived with, played with, and laughed with for six years.

It was as if he just came from the hotel. Floyd was sitting on a stool facing the inside of his locker reading his Bible, cross in one hand. Two card games were well underway, consisting of four players each. And, they all glared up at Jack before noticing it was him.

"Shit, J-New is back in town!" Juan bellowed. He got up, hugged and kissed Jack on the cheek, all the while hiding his cards. "I thought you were Floyd coming over here to read us sinners a scripture!"

The other players did the same, some hugs longer than others.

When Jack got to his locker he was sure he was back where he belonged; Oscar hadn't arrived yet.

Before he could start undressing, a blur knocked him off his feet and pinned him on the cheap rug.

"Trying to sneak in without speaking, bitch?"

The voice was too familiar to not know. Jack blushed.

"Will you let him up, Mike?" Danny said, disturbed. "You gonna hurt the man before he gets back in the lineup. Sheez!"

Mike squeezed Jack's genitals.

"You faggot!" Mike screamed. He made me hold his schlong!"

Danny helped Jack up. Jack looked over at the smiling captain of the Crowns. Mike had on only his uniform pants.

"What you staring at? You thought I was going to kill myself or something?"

"No, I," Jack held his response. He grabbed Mike's hand, pulled him into a hug.

Floyd came over and asked about Djuana.

"I prayed for her."

Jack thanked him.

"Beat it, Rev, Jack's got to get dressed," Mike said.

Juris emerged from the office and patted Jack on the back. "You ready, I hear."

"Like always, Skip."

"That ain't what I saw. Some kid, not even out of diapers, K'd your ass twice."

"Shit, Skip! I had 17 hits in 23 at bats."

Loudly, over the laughter and chatter, Juris stated, "If I was doing the hitting, I would have had 23 for 23. All line drives."

The laughter and ribbing of Jack continued for a while, until Juris cut it short. "Stop laughing, and giggling like virgins! Get ready to ride some ass!"

Oscar arrived quietly, but soon joined in on the folly. Before Jack could greet his best friend, O called to him, "What, you tellin' jokes on your first day back, sweets?"

Jack just blushed more, thinking he was being the definition of a bitch in the eyes of his homophobic teammates. His eyes were watering, and his heart pumped happiness throughout his body. He could've hugged and kissed each one of them on the lips. And, they would have let him.

Djuana guided the new Pathfinder off of West Burnside and into Washington Park's parking lot. To her surprise, getting behind the wheel was easy; once she got going. She felt like the wife of a soldier, dropping Jack off at the airport - he had driven them there - gave him a long, wet kiss and warm embrace. After watching the plane take off, she shedded tears of happiness.

On her way, many of the people that had been watching them walking hand-in-hand, and then kiss, acknowledged her presence with a wave, light nod and even friendly greetings. Djuana did bristle, though, when a young brown-skinned girl raced from a waiting area. The girl, out of breath, and blushing, asked Djuana for her autograph. Djuana was astonished.

"You don't want my autograph," she told the pre-teenager.

The thin, pretty girl with long braids nodded rapidly. "Yeah, I do," she insisted, pushing a pen and a torn piece of an airline envelope.

Djuana took the paper and pen, a little hesitantly, and looked at the girl. "You sure you don't want Jack Newhouse's autograph?"

"You his wife? Right?"

Djuana nodded with the child.

"My Momma said you a strong woman."

Djuana looked over the child, back to where she had dashed from, a good distance of about 30 yards. In the corner of the cushioned row of connected seats were the little girl's parents. The were standing, the father holding a carry-on bag, and the mother also had a bag and what looked like a child's jacket. The other people were watching while the stewardess began boarding the plane.

"I better sign this in a hurry so you can go," Djuana said as she used her left hand to support the writing.

"I saw you on the news."

"What's you name?" Djuana asked while scribbling.

"Tara Mone Washington," the girl said proudly.

"Oh, how pretty!" Djuana bent down and handed Tara the autograph; her first. She hated it, though. Her name looked nothing like she usually signed it. She marveled at how professionals did it all the time.

"Here, and thank you for asking me for it."

Tara awkwardly grabbed Djuana and kissed her before racing off yelling, "I got it! I got it, Mommy!"

This incident was the first in many inspiring moments for Djuana that first week Jack was gone. It was also the spark that helped calm Djuana and to get her fear of another car crash out of her mind. Still, each time she started the Pathfinder up, she thought about her son, laying still in his little funeral outfit. She would to take a few deep breaths, releasing them slowly, and talk to herself before pulling out. Once on the highway she was fine.

Djuana put the truck as close to the entrance of Washington Park as possible; having to circle the triangle parking lot three times until a prime spot near the mouth of the green, surreal park became available. She then walked in, scanning the area with quick movements of her head and eyes. She felt the few people milling around the entrance watching her, but was at ease; thanks to Tara's mother. She stopped in Lewis & Clark Circle and sat on a shaded bench. She watched the many people entering; looking more closely at the children. They were sure to have more fun than their parents, she imagined.

She shifted her bronzed legs, crossing them under her bright, colorful sun dress and let her mind drift back to when she once enjoyed coming to Washington Park. When she was a child, the image of walking for miles on the winding paths in the deep, mystical greenery of the park would excite her. She would beg to see the hundreds of different roses in the test garden. She would climb the rocky hills, causing Emma to curse because, of course she would scrape and scar her legs. Despite the many signs asking visitors not to pick the flowers; Djuana would pluck anything growing from its safe haven in the ground.

Thinking about how badly she missed those days, caused her to imagined Devon must feel the same way. She vowed to bring him along next time; if all went well that day, though.

The mounted park patrolman spotted Djuana right away. Not because she was the only person seated in Lewis & Clark, nor did it matter the woman was of his flesh, but because he believed once a man was privy to a person that beautiful, they would be able to recognize that person in a dark, crowded room. He steered his horse into a quick gallop, causing the well-rested animal to kick into a speedy trot.

Djuana sat still; she noticed the horseman, but didn't want to seem as excited as she was. He had to never know she missed him, loved him and still worshipped him. The patrolman stopped the horse near the bench Djuana sat on, feet away from her legs. He climbed down and stepped to her.

"Thank you for coming," the dark-skinned, clean shaven man said, holding the reins. He was more handsome than any picture in the family albums.

Djuana stood, hands together in front of her. The sun dress umbrella-ed around her body. "I was surprised you called."

"Well, I had been calling for a while. I went to your job in the mall, but you weren't there."

Djuana felt his eyes absorb her body. She released her hands, spread her arms and let him look.

"You like?"

He stopped his gaze at her eyes, the coloring of his, and his mother's. "Djuana. Of course I do. You're the most beautiful woman I have ever seen in my life."

His seriousness choked Djuana. She sustained her smile. "Well, you did have something to do with it, you know."

"Yeah," Lyle Davis exhaled, fixed in his stance. "Not much, though."

Djuana came to the park wanting to hurt Lyle, but she couldn't. Her father was a pleasant man; he was quick witted, and personable. She wished she had his gift of gab; the man could, and often did, strike up a sensible conversation with any stranger. He was tall and athletic. Strong build, with dark, rich chocolate skin with strong calloused hands. He was tireless, the memory crossed her mind, causing her to search his face. For as long as she could remember, he carried bags beneath his eyes. He would say it was a curse from his never-sleeping through a eight month tour of duty in Vietnam.

Still, she thought as he was approaching, he looked great for 47 years-old; and he was still riding horseback.

During the drive over, Djuana's anger against her father, the man that left her mother to raise two children alone, eased. She could not hate Lyle Davis, even though he had left her, Emma and Devon to fend for themselves. In her mind, there while her father's eyes glowed at her, she recalled the hard times, with little bitterness. The many nights she, or Emma, had to make a "welfare dinner", as Emma called it. It was when whatever was left over was spiced up, or mixed with something else. She thought about her wardrobe in high school; the worst in the school she believed.

Through the years, as she matured, Djuana saw in retrospect that most of her parents arguments were started by Emma. It was as if her mother hated tranquillity, she began to believe. Emma was firing up some controversy daily, pushing Lyle into a verbal battle.

Djuana edged closer to Lyle, feeling his uneasiness. She kissed him on the cheek, and in that instant he pulled her into his arms, squeezing her tightly. The force in which he yanked her frightened Djuana. She gave in, though, letting him squeeze the breath out of her.

"I love you, baby," he began whispering. "I've missed you so much. I am sorry I haven't been coming around."

She listened to him whispering. She panted quickly, regaining her breath. Then, she felt his tears on her cheek. "It's okay, Daddy."

"I'm sorry about your baby. I am sorry I wasn't there for you."

Lyle released her suddenly. He was pleased to see her still smiling. "You still like lemon ice?"

"You remember?"

"I remember everything."

Lyle used up his lunch hour with his daughter. They walked and talked in the park, with the horse in tow.

"I was worried when you hadn't returned any of my calls," he said as they walked. "I called after I read about the stabbing."

"Mom never said anything until I heard you on the answering machine the other day."

"Yeah, well. I expected that. Maybe I should have just come around. I am really sorry I haven't been there. I just can't deal with your mother. I don't need the headache."

"Forget it, Dad."

Lyle blushed a grin. "Dad. It sounds great to hear you say that."

"I can't call you anything else," Djuana said emotionless. "I don't know what really went down between you and Mom. I just wish you two would stop fighting long enough for you to spend time with Devon. He could use a man around."

"I know, I know. Maybe now that I'm back in Portland."

Lyle stopped as they reached a clearing and a fork in the tree lined path. He pulled the horse in the direction of benches to their left.

"Let's sit."

Djuana and the horse followed.

He tied the horse in the grass to some large shrubbery. He removed his hat and gloves. The mid-August heat was getting to him.

"Djuana, how are you? Really."

Djuana sucked lemon ice off of the spoon, and swallowed slowly, savoring the taste. "I'm fine, I'm doing okay."

Lyle gazed at her bruise, cutting his eyes as she looked up. The wound was almost dissolved. He would have not noticed it had he not searched her face so intently.

"I heard your ribs were broken?" he said.

"One was fractured. Two were bruised."

"Are you comfortable?" Lyle began to stand. "We can go someplace else?"

"No, Dad. I'm okay."

Lyle sat. "I should have come to the hospital. I don't know why I let that woman keep me away."

Djuana felt words build, but held them off. She was not looking for her father to come see her, but it would have been a soothing sight.

"What's the deal with you and this baseball player. Between cursing me out and hanging up on me, Emma said something about him abusing you. This guy rape you? Was it him that had you run off the road?"

"No, no, no, no. No. That's not the deal."

Lyle sat up, intently listening to his matured daughter. The last time he had seen her, she was 18 years-old, and a virgin.

Djuana continued, the words flowing, "Jack Newhouse has never done anything but love me. He has been the best thing in my life."

"I don't know. All I know is what your mother said, and what the newspapers say. That guy has been swinger for as long as I can remember."

"I'm telling you it's not like that," Djuana took a deep breath. She paused as a couple with their kids darting out in front of them passed.

"Look, Dad, I stabbed him because I thought he was dogging me out. I thought he was being like my last boyfriend. I was wrong."

"He wasn't?"

"No."

Lyle's head shook rapidly. "I don't know. Don't let this guy hurt you."

Djuana's insecurity resurfaced. She had thought she had it licked.

"He's not going to hurt me," she said, not sounding convinced.

"And, it was his baby?" Lyle asked.

"No. It was Dexter's."

"Not Dexter Forns?! You stayed with that guy that long?"

"Yeah. Stupid, ain't I?"

Lyle chuckled. "No, honey. You loved him. I always knew you did."

"Well, I wasted a lot of years on him."

Lyle shrugged, "No, look at it this way, you got to learn what to look for next time."

"I guess."

"So, then, the stories about you and the baseball player living together are true?"

Lyle's frown disturbed Djuana.

"His name is Jack Newhouse, Dad," Djuana scolded her father. "You sound like Ma. Call him by his name."

"I know. I'm sorry. But, listen, I don't know."

Djuana watched Lyle flip his hands at the subject.

"What? You don't like him do you?"

"Does it matter?" Lyle took his daughter's hand. "You've grown up without me. I haven't been there for you in a long time. How I feel doesn't, or really shouldn't matter.

"You just do what you feel is right."

"I want to know how you feel about it."

"I don't like him. And, I don't want to see this guy hurt you anymore than he already has."

Djuana snatched her hand away, raising both hands in question. "Why you say that?"

Lyle looked into his daughter's eyes. He saw, in those gentle, soft brown pupils that his daughter was deeply in love. He sat up, thinking he needed to break it down for her.

"Since you met him, you have lost your baby, been in an accident, had to stab him and have been the most hated woman in the whole city."

"It's not like that, Dad. Those things happened, but they were not his fault."

"But, when there's smoke there's fire. And, all I hear about is the sexcapades this guy has in about every city. What about that?"

"You talking about that article in *People*? I want you to meet him for yourself."

"I don't know."

Djuana watched her father shake his head for the fifth time since they sat.

"Dad, he asked me to marry him," Djuana said flatly.

"Hmm. Really? You going to marry him?"

"I said yes."

Lyle looked over her tender hands. He picked up her left and held her brown fingers apart.

Djuana noticed what he was looking for, "No, he hasn't given me a ring."

"Baby, this guy is jerking you. He's needs to show the team that he is serious about settling down so he can resign for big bucks. Did he tell you that he's broke?"

"No, I bet he didn't. Him and Oscar Taylor invested most of their money in some bullshit land deal that fell through."

Djuana's heart hurt. She could feel the pain in each throb. Her throat became dry, and her eyes were moistening. She felt the breakdown, and fought it, changing the hurt to anger, then to silence.

She looked off, over her father's shoulder at a couple kissing two benches away.

"Ask him why he's driving a jeep when all his teammates have Benzes or BMWs," Lyle continued. "Look how the man dresses!"

"I'm telling you, he ain't got no money. Don't let him use you to get it. You ain't gonna be happy."

Djuana calmed herself, picking each word as if a fight could be avoided with a proper question. "Why you hate him, Dad?"

"I don't hate him. I don't know him, but -"

"That's right! You don't know him," Djuana nearly jumped up at her father.

Lyle shook his head rapidly, "Yeah, but I care about you, Dee. It bothers me to read and hear about all this with you involved."

"I love him, Dad. And, he loves me. I didn't meet him in some nightclub. He has treated me well since I met him. Very well."

"Okay," Lyle gave in. "As long as your eyes are open."

# 36

The Crowns won all four games in Cincinnati before moving on to Seattle and three weekend games there. The team instantly reverted back to the festive atmosphere before Slight lowered the boom. Lots of fooling around in and out of the clubhouse. During one game in Cincy, Juan Santos, the Crowns shortstop and a master of practical jokes after being the butt of them for his first two seasons in the majors, set the laces of Jack's cleats on fire during the game. Jack didn't take it kindly; he stalked Juan the remainder of the inning, with Juan chuckling and keeping his distance.

Jack got his revenge with the help of Oscar. Before the start of the bottom of the fifth, two innings after the mini-blaze, They jumped Juan at his shortstop position and pulled his pants down; taking his belt and throwing it into the outfield.

Honeywell nearly fell out of his seat in the skybox. "What the hell are they doing!!!"

Slight sipped wine into his mouthful of lobster. "Let 'em have fun," he grumbled. "They ain't going to be playing in October this year, so let them show their asses."

Slight laughed at his own pun, choking on the soft, tasty seafood.

Juan was pissed; his best friend on the team, Pugsley at second, hid his laughter in his glove the whole inning. So, when the Crowns came to bat, Juan, cursing in Spanish vanished into the clubhouse where he tied all his teammates street clothes into a wide circle.

And, of course, the team began hanging out and drinking after games. After the second night game in Seattle, a 5-1 win in the mist of humid Saturday evening, 17 Crowns skipped the team bus back to the hotel and club hopped. Mike was the obvious exception. He stood by his vow to remain sober.

The players hung out, never having to spend a dime. Danny, though, would gather money from his teammates to take care of the bartender or waitress. As the night continued, the number of players began to dwindle until only Don, Jack and O were left. All three were feeling no pain.

Oscar talked them into finishing the night at Herc's, the club they had began the night at. It was a predominately Black nightclub, owned by a muscular, dark-skinned man with two gold teeth and a gold chain with a tiny scoop pendent. Herc was an avid Seattle Monarchs fan, but he liked Oscar anyway. Back then, there weren't many Seattle fans that liked Portland players.

Before Slight, Portland was the easiest team to defeat in the majors. Get a lead on them, and watch them give up. And, Seattle would do it often. When Slight bought the team, that April, Portland opened its season in Seattle, and the Monarchs' players, fans and ownership laughed at the Crowns all through a three-game slaughter. Slight vowed Seattle would never beat his team again. And, they haven't. The Monarchs, a team to never finish first in a season, were in last place each year the Crowns went to the World Series.

Herc's club was emptying out, still there was a crowd on the dance floor for the mellow swing the DJ caused with a string of love ballads. Oscar was glad they returned; he wanted to find a bed warmer. Jack, on the other hand, had been checking the time most of the night. He was supposed to have called Djuana after the game. It was nearing two a.m. when Djuana beeped him. The buzz of his beeper on his belt startled him, he jumped in his seat, causing his inebriated teammates to crack up.

"You jumped like a bitch!" O said, laughing so hard his ribs hurt.

Don knocked over his and Oscar's drinks mocking Jack.

"You guys are dicks," Jack said over the loud music.

"You should know," Don said, fighting his chuckles to get in the punchline. "How many have you seen again?"

"Jesus," Jack watched them laughing at him. "You got your phone, Don? I left mine in Portland."

"No, you crazy?" he said, eyes watering. "So Liela can call my ass? Get the fuck outta here, stupid."

Oscar sobered, a little, "I've got mine in the rental." He tossed his keys at Jack.

"I'll be right back," Jack said as he stood. "Order me another when you morons get refills."

"Right, boss," Oscar nodded.

"You calling Djuana?" Don asked. "Tell her I said hi, and give her my love and shit."

Jack couldn't tell if he was serious.

"Me too. Tell her we gotta go out when I get back. Just me and her!"

"Will you remember?" Jack quipped as he walked away.

"Oh, snap, Poppy! He saying you fucking drunk!"

"I'ma show him drunk when he gets back. I'ma whip his whipped ass!"

Jack came back in the club with the phone at his ear. The music, and the people partying, were loud but he felt more comfortable in the club, than out in the dark parking lot.

"Djuana? You okay?" Jack could hear in her voice she had been sleeping.

"Hi, baby. I'm fine," Djuana smiled, letting the phone rest on her face; her head deep in the pillow. "I'm sorry. I didn't realize it was so late when I beeped you. I must have fallen asleep."

"Yeah, that was my fault. I should have called. I had left my phone in the hotel, thinking I would be right back after the game, but O wanted to hang."

"Oh, that's all that noise?"

"Yeah, I didn't want to sit out in the parking lot and deal with no knuckle heads. Can you hear me?"

"Yes. I should let you go, you're out with your friends."

"No. I miss you, and I'm glad you called."

Oscar's sudden movement caught Jack's attention. O bolted up, after saying something to Don, and joined a table of five women closer to the dance floor. Jack watched him, noticing that all of the women were attractive. The two O slid his tall, slender frame between had enlightening smiles; Jack could see as they turned to allow O in. Jack's eyes lit on the woman on O's left. She had on a deep v-cut blouse revealing plenty of flesh from a large set of breasts.

"Jack can you hear me?"

Jack instinctively said yes.

"So, what time should I pick you up from the airport?"

"We should be in between seven and eight," Jack tried to bring his attention back to his woman, but he spotted O pointed back at the table and the women were laughing.

Jack felt Don looking at him. He looked over at Don and the elder Crown stood.

"Yo, I'm out, Poppy," Don said.

Jack put his hand up to halt Don.

Then, Oscar began calling them over. "Don, get that whipped motherfucker off the phone! These ladies need company!"

The table of women giggled.

Don gulped the remains of his scotch and angrily glared at Jack. "I gotta go, that fool is trying to get us in trouble. The fucking game is at one, and now he thinks of pussy! Man, that young shit will wear my old ass out!"

"Do you have to go?" Djuana asked.

"No. Not at all." Jack was hoping with all his heart that she couldn't hear all the nonsense.

Jack glared at O as he returned to their table. Don sat back in his chair, folding his arms across his chest.

"Get off the phone," Oscar tried to whisper, but he could not control his voice. "The bitch knows you out and shit, tell her to let you breathe!"

Jack's glare was penetrating O's drunken state. Djuana's voice in his ear cooled his anger.

"Jack, maybe I should let you go," her voice lacked feeling; no displeasure or distress.

"No, we're talking. I want to talk to you."

Djuana had made up her mind to hang up. "No, you're out with the guys. I'll let you go. Call me before the game tomorrow."

Oscar waved a disrespectful hand at Jack, "Whipped motherfucker."

He turned to Don, "You hanging, or what?"

"Nope, I'm cutting out. I need some fucking sleep."

Oscar waved at Don, "Step then, and take this ass with you."

Jack held the phone to his chin, minutes after his conversation with Djuana ended in what he felt was a sour tone, listening to O curse out Don. O darted back to the table of women, who were now standing. Jack gave the car keys and phone to Don, who was glad to wait outside. Oscar, helping the ladies prepare to leave, introduced Jack around the table. All the women were smiles. Jack forgot the names as quickly as he was told.

"O, let me talk at you for a minute," Jack said without a hint of pleasantry.

As soon as they we away from the table, Jack said, "What you did was wrong, man."

"What?"

"You see me on the phone with Djuana and you say some dumb shit like that?"

"Relax," O sobered. "Look, you want me to call her and smooth it out?"

"No! Just think sometimes. Show some fucking respect."

"What, you gonna cry now?" O fixed his clothes, looking back at the table licking his lips. "Forget it, I'm sorry. Okay? Now, you ready to get laid and sprayed?"

"Nope. Me and Don are out."

"No, man, hang."

"I'm not hanging like that."

"Shit." O stared at the women, already knowing which one he was going to lay. He cut his eyes back to Jack. "You and Don are acting like little girls. Go on. I'll catch y'all later."

"Wear a cap or two on woody."

"Shut up."

In the morning, as the team prepared to board the bus for the final game of the road trip, loud arguing was the last thing the players who hung out needed. The rude wake-up calls were enough. But, Cris Carpenter was pissed. He slung his luggage off the bellboy's cart and about the lobby of the Hilton.

"Fuck all you motherfucker's. All y'all!"

Jack sipping coffee, avoided the suitcase heading for his shins with a light sidestep.

"What's C's problem? They catch him stealing towels again?" Jack asked a few of his teammates that were watching the tirade.

Juan laughed.

Pugsley, with his short, thick arms folded across his barreled chest, bluntly said, "Honeywell just told CC that his was traded to LA. Now he's putting on a show."

"Shit," Jack whispered, just before taking another sip of his coffee. "Damn, they traded his ass?"

"Yep," Juan said. "And good riddance."

"That's fucked up, Juan," Pugs laughed. "When you got traded here from St. Louis you cried 'cause you didn't want to come here."

"Yeah, but I wasn't being an ass to my teammates to cause me to be traded. St. Louis was my home."

Cris continued cursing his teammates, "Y'all ain't gonna win shit, anyway! Fuck y'all. Shit, I promise you motherfuckers that I'ma bust y'all asses in the playoffs, if y'all can make it."

Oscar came off the elevator with his voice as loud as Cris'.

"Shut the fuck up with all that screamin' like some lunatic bitch out here!" O said, appearing out of the far elevator. He was holding a ice pack on his head drinking a Bloody Mary disguised in a styrofoam cup. "I can hear you on the 30th floor!"

"Fuck you, O! Who you? You ain't the man on this team, although you ack like it!"

"Yo, C, man, you don't want to fuck with me," O was shaking his head, holding his fingers out toward Cris from the cup. "Don and New had my ass drinking scotch last night. I ain't in the mood. I will hurt you."

Oscar moved through the lobby. "You better tell 'im," he said to Jack as he walked through the lobby and got on the bus.

CC, like so many of his teammates was not having his usual good year playing the game of baseball. He wasn't hitting, and without Jack in right field to cover more ground, allowing Oscar to cheat and help Cris in left, he was suffering on the field as well. Jack's return landed the switch-hitter on the bench. Juris gave left field to Russ Jones, a short, always hustling 20 year-old rookie; one of the players the team received from Buffalo for Bingo. CC complained each of the two days the rookie started in place of him.

Most of the teams in the league knew it would be a matter of time before CC would be available. Los Angeles had been trying to pry him away from

Portland for two years. He is, when playing well, just what the Los Angeles outfield needed, their general manager assumed when he called Honeywell and offered a young, solid pitcher; the one thing LA has an abundance of. Honeywell didn't hesitate.

Honeywell's statement to the press on CC's trade read: "If we are going to catch Los Angeles, we have to have more pitching. Cris Carpenter was unhappy, and I will not go into the stretch run with ballplayers that don't want to be Portland Crowns."

Jack stood there a while, sipping his coffee, watching Cris going bananas, cursing guys he had been living with, traveling with, and playing with for five years. Jack knew that could have easily been him departing to play elsewhere; he hoped he would handle being traded with more class. And, he was glad it wasn't him, but sad it was CC. Jack thought of Cris as a good player, who had been in many battles with him. Now he was going to a rival; and from all the shit he was talking then, Jack could see he was not going to be a pleasant opponent.

The players' bus was loaded and ready. The bellhops had to find Cris' luggage and remove it from the bus. Jack, standing outside until he finished his coffee, was not surprised when Cris approached him instead of the three other players smoking cigarettes.

"Man, they trying to turn this team white," Cris said. "Just like the city we play in."

An eavesdropping reporter reached into his bag.

"Shut up, C," Jack whispered. "Just take your ass to LA and do work."

Jack turned away from the reporter. Cris followed. "Listen, they are going to break up this team after the season anyway. So just go play. All this whining is unnecessary."

Djuana walked into the terminal and was surprised at the crowd awaiting the Crowns plane. When she saw that most were fans she understood, but there were also a great deal of women. No way they were just fans. She stood off to the side, away from the boisterous crowd, and watched the plane land. She kept her eyes on the taxiing plane as one of the women attempted to wave at her.

Jack emerged from the ramp in the middle of the pack. He stopped at a family, and the mother kissed him. Djuana thought she wouldn't smile but, when his eyes met hers, she beamed. And, Jack took her into a long embrace, hugging and kissing her.

"I missed you," he said, smiling broadly.

Djuana didn't reply, she just held onto him. Other players came by, some with their wives, and spoke to Djuana. She was not warm, but she was cordial. They grabbed his luggage on the lower level, and made their way to the Pathfinder. Djuana took the driver's seat.

"I'm glad to be back," Jack said, looking out the window as the truck hit the highway.

"Hmm," Djuana grunted.

Her sour mood returned. But, Jack could not sense it. His mind was still glowing over the fine game he had had hours before. He had four hits, and knocked in all of the Crowns seven runs. And, that was all the press asked him about afterwards.

"I saw my father."

The words were said so nonchalantly, that Jack was afraid he had heard wrong.

"You what," he asked, puzzled.

"My father has been transferred back to Portland. I saw him the other day."

"I didn't know you had contact with your father."

"I really hadn't."

"How did it go," Jack mood swung in the direction of Djuana's bleak expression.

"It went okay."

"Don't seem that way."

Djuana exhaled, eyes riveted on the road. "He said some things to disturb me."

"Really?" Jack searched for the best questions to get her mood off her chest. "How long has it been since you seen him?"

"A long time. He left us when I was about 17; just getting ready to graduate high school."

"Oh."

"Jack," Djuana turned to him. "We need to talk, seriously."

"Yeah, sure. What's up?"

"Never mind."

"What?"

"It's not important."

"It was a minute ago."

"Forget it."

"I can't! Now, you started this, finish it."

"Do I give you all you want?"

"Yeah. Of course you do."

"I mean, are you satisfied?"

Jack threw up his hands and shoulders. "Yes. Why?"

"Because if I am not satisfying you, you need to tell me. I'll give you anything you want. You don't have to go anywhere else."

"Wait a minute, is this about last night?"

"Yeah, in particular."

"Nothing happened."

"Jack, I don't care. But, from now on, I want you to know that I will fulfill any need you have. Any."

"Djuana..." Jack watched her eyes become glossy.

"No, I'm serious. Dead serious. Because if you cheat on me I might just kill you."

Before Jack could react, she continued, "I love you deeply. And, if you don't feel the same, like you want a commitment, just leave me. I don't need to be hurt anymore."

"What are you talking about? I want you to be my wife. To be in my life as long as I live."

"Right."

"Djuana? What do you want me to say?"

"That if you ever feel the urge to be with a groupie or some hoe on the road, that you call me and tell me. And leave me. Just break us up. Don't do this to me."

"You talkin' crazy."

"Don't call me crazy! I know what I'm saying! You making love to me, oh, I'm so delicate! And, then you go out and fuck them hoes, getting your frustration out on them! Make them do all kinds of shit for you, putting them in all kinds of positions, but you just make love to me, right?"

"Djuana, what are you talking about?"

She just hit the steering wheel, and let the tears flow. The Pathfinder sped into the middle lane of the highway, sprinting ahead of traffic.

"Djuana, baby. Listen to me. I have had a lot of pussy. A lot. I'm tired of that shit. I don't even be thinking about none of that. When I'm with you, or even on the road, all I think about is how lucky I am to have found you."

Djuana heard him, but she didn't reply. Her mind sped across her father's accusations, and in an instant she was angrier. Mad at herself for letting that man come out of nowhere and cause her to doubt the man of her dreams. But, still she had to know; for sure.

Djuana's head slowly faced Jack in the passenger's seat. "Why don't I have a ring?"

"Is that what this is all about?"

"You're broke, aren't you? It doesn't matter. I love you, Jack. I just want you to be truthful."

"What? You gotta be kidding me?"

"Jack, it's all right."

"Get this exit! Turn here."

Djuana looked up at the sign. "Why? Jack, I said forget it."

"Just get off here."

They were two exits from his home. Jack directed her to a bank's parking lot. He got out.

"Come with me."

Djuana felt both guilty and relieved as she stepped down and out of the truck. She followed behind Jack to the ATM on the side of the banks entrance. Jack pulled his wallet out of his hip pocket and pushed his bank card angrily into the machine and yanked it out. He pushed the buttons with quick pokes. Djuana came up from behind and grabbed his arm.

"Forget it Jack, I'm sorry. Let's just go home."

"Take a look, then we can go," he said calmly.

Djuana glanced defiantly at first, then feel into a deep stare.

"That's over a million dollars," Djuana gasped.

"Yeah, and that's just one bank. You want to go to the other three?"

Djuana continued to stare at the screen. "No," was all she could muster to say.

"Now, as for your ring. I'm sorry you don't have it yet. It's being made. I was hoping to surprise you with it."

Djuana reached onto the screen and cleared it. She thought about saying something smart, something to get herself off the hook. But, nothing would come off her tongue.

"Djuana, you want to tell me what this was all about?"

"I just made the mistake of listening to jealous people." She finally looked at Jack. Her forehead wrinkled in a frown and her voice was hoarse.

"Fine. But, just remember, if there is anything you want to know, ask me. And, there will be plenty more jealous people out there trying to break us up."

"I don't want to lose you," she almost whispered.

"I am not going to let you lose me."

She moved to him and he grabbed her into on of his strong, warm hugs.

# 37

"Yo, you stupid," Oscar bellowed into the phone.

"Thanks, genius," Jack said, falling back in his easy chair.

"Why the hell you tell her you having the ring made, when you ain't even been to a jewelry store?"

"You gonna help me or what?"

"Where is she?"

"In the shower."

"Can you get out, or does she have your ass on lock down?"

"You're funny. I gotta take her to work."

"Just meet me at Gene's in about two hours."

"Two hours?! Come on, man! I want to get this done, be in and out."

"Yo! Hol' up," O swung his legs out from under his silk sheets and his feet planted on the rug. "I'm still in bed, and I got to take my hoe home."

"Excuse me," Jack heard a female voice say in the background. "I ain't no hoe!"

"Shut up, bitch."

Jack shook his head. "Forget it, I'll just go myself."

"Shut up. Two hours. And, bring cash. They don't deal in plastic."

Jack guided his truck along the slowing, heavy midday traffic on West Burnside Street. He was early, so he had plenty of time to find a parking space. He slid into a spot on the corner of 20th Place, two blocks north of the shop. He gradually made his way to the jewelers, doing a bit of window shopping at a art gallery and a women's boutique.

When he entered Gene's shop, Oscar was sitting behind the counter speaking with a blonde.

"Here's the man about to complicate his life!" Oscar announced.

"Don't say that," the blonde said. She approached Jack and shook his hand.

"Don't listen to him. I bet you'll be happy."

The short, attractive woman had an alluring smile. Jack grinned at her, wondering if Oscar had slept with her yet, or was trying to.

A short, well-dressed man, with identical wavy hair as the woman's, came out from behind the curtains which hid his small office from the one-aisle shop. He made his way around the blonde and down the left side of his glass counters. He stuck out his hand to Jack.

"Jack Newhouse, good to see you again," he gave Jack a very business-like grin.

Jack returned the greeting.

"So, you're sure you want to do this, eh?"

"Yes."

"Fine. You have a particular diamond in mind?"

Oscar butted in, "He's in love," he said as he neared the two men. "Price is no object! Give him the best you got!"

Jack glared at his friend. "You as smart as you look."

"Shit, then I'm brilliant."

Gene had a large, navy blue cloth in his left hand that Jack hadn't noticed. He brought it up to the counter and laid it out.

"You're in luck," he said as he opened the cloth and revealed two round diamonds that sparkled in the dimly lit shop. "I had these cut for a pair of earrings, and it seems that I won't be making them."

"Shit," O whispered, leaning on the counter face close to the gems.

The blonde came over, "Oh, my God! They're gorgeous, Gene."

"Aren't they?"

Jack was a believing person, by nature. But, this ring had to be the best purchase of his life. He wanted it to be perfect, a great gem was what he wanted. But, he wasn't sure how to pick a diamond. The more he looked down at the gems, the more he couldn't look away. They were round, a tad bit smaller than a pebble, deep and crystal clear.

"They are three karats a piece," Gene said. He used a tweezer to separate the gems. "They are very clear and of great quality."

"Damn." O looked up to Jack, pointing at the diamonds. "These are bad. Much better than what he gave me for Sondra."

Gene raised his eyebrows at O. Then, after giving it some thought, he nodded at Jack in agreement.

"I don't know," Jack just stared at them. He was thinking that they looked great, but wasn't sure how to tell if they were really three karats.

Gene looked at Oscar again, then back at Jack. "I wouldn't bullshit you,

Jack. These are by far the best diamonds I have. If it wasn't you, I wouldn't even think of splitting them up."

"You got a band to go with it?"

"Anything you want. But, I'll tell you, with gems like these, a simple, traditional band is all you need."

"That's good enough for me. I don't want anything fancy."

Oscar sprang up. "You crazy? Get some diamonds on the side, and shit. Maybe cut the diamond into a pear or-"

"I don't think so," Jack cut off O.

Gene laughed. "You don't want to cut these."

Jack asked, "Do you think maybe I should get a bigger one?"

"No, not really. Let me tell you, I have some larger stones, but they are not half the quality of these."

"No, these are lovely," the blonde said.

Oscar slid in closer to the woman, "How would you feel if a handsome guy gave you the other one?"

"Hmm," she playfully gave it thought, beaming a bright smile. "I'd be so grateful."

"How grateful?"

Gene glared at the blonde. Jack kicked O's nearest ankle.

"How much?" Jack said loudly.

"With a band, let's say three five?"

"Three thousand, five hundred?" Jack asked.

"Yes," Gene bristled. "I can't do no better than that."

"No, that's great. Good looking out."

Jack was expecting to pay a lot more, and would have to get the best he could for Djuana. He went into his wallet and removed a gang of brand new hundreds he had gotten from the bank. He counted out the money, placing it in front of Gene.

"How soon can you have it ready?"

"Give me two hours, say about five?"

"Cool. I have to pick up Djuana around that time, but I can be late."

"No, she won't mind," Gene smiled.

Jack looked around the shop, Oscar followed him.

Gene asked, "You want wedding bands?"

"No," Jack said, stopping in front of the showcase with bracelets. "Do you have any nice anklets?"

"Sure. I got one you may like," Gene walked around the shop, and slid open the case Jack and Oscar were in front of. He removed a gold link.

"She has a normal ankle?"

"No. It's beautiful," Jack said.

Oscar sucked his teeth. "Oh, boy."

Gene shook his head, and grinned slightly. "I meant ankle size."

"Yeah, I think she does."

"This is a nice one," Gene looked at the tag, it read $190. "Give me a $100 and we're clear."

Jack did, and the blonde boxed and wrapped it.

"Let's go to Alice's and grab a bite to eat?" Oscar said as they walked along West Burnside.

Jack looked down at his watch. He had plenty of time. "Sure. I'm hungry myself."

"Djuana still working at the mall?" Oscar said while his eyes and head followed every pair of hips on the block. "You ain't tell her to quit yet?"

"No. But, she will. That job is getting on her nerves."

Djuana sat in front of Mr. Thompson's desk half listening to him, and half wondering how she could quit and be done with this foolishness. She watched him tap his pen on his lip, then bit it as he scolded her yet again. This was her second written reprimand.

"Djuana, I don't know," he widened the distance between his hands. "What is it that you want me to do for you? Since I transferred you up here to the executive offices I have heard nothing but negative reports on your work."

Djuana sat defiantly, her legs crossed under her peach umbrella skirt, both hands at her knee, biting her bottom lip.

"You have nothing to say?"

"Mr. Thompson, what is it that you want me to say?"

"Tell me what's the problem."

"I didn't think there was a problem."

"Well," he sat up and edged closer. "Linda says you refuse to do anything she asks you to do. Paul said you were late twice last week."

"None of that is true."

"So, they're lying on you?"

"All I'm saying is that Linda never has liked me, and you can check my time card to see I haven't been late."

Mr. Thompson lifted the reprimand off his desk. He read it quickly. "Paul says he told you to be in an hour earlier and you ignored him."

"I don't remember him asking me to come in earlier."

Djuana watched her boss shake his head and look away. He pulled a cigarette from his shirt's breast pocket. He lit it, and inhaled deeply.

"I hear that you are living with that baseball player."

"Excuse me," Djuana unfolded her legs and leaned forward.

"You living with him, ain't you? It is common knowledge, isn't it?"

"Wait," she put the palm of her hand up toward her boss. "What does that have to do with work?"

"Everything. Everybody knows you don't care about this job anymore. They have pools going on when you're going to quit."

The anger began to boil in Djuana's skin. "So, that's why everybody has been fucking with me?"

Thompson became defensive, "There's nobody fucking with you. You just have this Holier than Thou attitude."

"This is bullshit!"

"Look at that, still ain't got no class."

"What?" Djuana stood.

"You can go now. But, this will be put in your records. One more written complaint and you will be fired."

"You know something, fuck you and this whole bullshit store. I quit. To hell with all of you."

Djuana quit her job with seven hours left in her shift; seven hours before Jack would be picking her up. She jumped on a bus and rode to Tudor. There, she found the apartment empty, her brother was in summer day camp, and her mother was at work.

The apartment felt comfortable, yet distant; as if she had been on a long vacation. She put her bag down on the chair near the door, and slowly inspected the apartment. Nothing had changed, but it seemed different. She couldn't place the smell, nor the feeling, but it was as if she no longer lived there. And, she didn't. She made her way to her bedroom, and it was spotless. Her bed was made with her spread on it. There was nothing on the floor, no clothes hanging on the back of the door, or bulging out of the closet.

She sat on her bed and picked up her phone. She kicked off her shoes and fell back onto the pillows as Tia's phone rang.

"I did it," Djuana exhaled into the phone.

"Did what?" Tia asked, standing in the kitchen completely puzzled. She was in the middle of making a sandwich for breakfast.

"Kicked that pain in-the-neck-job to the curb."

"Now what," Tia said, quietly biting into her tuna salad sandwich.

"I have to tell Jack," Djuana sighed.

Tia swallowed. "That shouldn't be a big deal. He wanted you to quit."

"Yeah, but I don't want him to think I will be dependent on him."

"Please. Y'all talking about getting married, so then, it will be the two of you from now on. And, the kind of guy that he is, he will always take care of you, and he won't be worried about how much you add to the pot."

"Yeah, I guess." Djuana knew Tia was right, but she just couldn't get herself to agree.

Jack allowed Oscar to drive him to Alice's in his BMW. When they arrived, some time between three and four in the afternoon, the restaurant was empty. Salese came through the glass doors directly after them, patting the ballplayers on their backs.

"You guys are having an early supper," he said, his horn case strapped to his left shoulder.

Jack shook Salese's hand and hugged him. Oscar's attention was at the bar, where to women were fingering spicy wings.

"You kinda early yourself," Jack said.

"Kinda. My band doesn't go on until six, but I usually get her early and grub up. Let me sit with you guy's and break bread."

Alice greeted them after the hostess sat them. "My favorite men. And, you too Oscar."

"Alice, get off my back." Oscar replied.

"That ain't what you said last night."

Jack laughed. Salese was oblivious. He looked over the menu which he knew by heart. "I know what I want."

"Jack's treating," O declared. "He's ready to jump the broom, so he might as well learn what it feels like to be broke."

Jack playfully glared at his friend.

Alice snatched a chair from the next table, which was occupied by a couple, and squeezed her way in between Jack and Oscar. She lowered herself near Jack's lap and whispered:

"You marrying Djuana?"

"Yeah," Jack answered in his normal voice level. "I just bought the ring."

"That's so sweet. That girl loves you."

Salese patted his shoulder, "That's great man, you two make a great couple."

Oscar jumped up, digging in his pockets he said, "I'm going to play some tunes on the box."

He went over to the CD jukebox, where two women were selecting tunes.

"Let me see the ring," Alice beamed.

"It'll be ready at five."

"That bad boy is smokin', right," Alice sat up, not concealing any teeth. "I know you went all out."

"Of course."

"That's so nice. Does she know?"

"Nope. I'm gonna surprise her at the game."

"That's wonderful. You make sure you bring her here, I'll make something nice for you two."

A waitress came to the table, and Alice grabbed her down to her face level. She whispered some orders below the music, pointing at each man individually.

"I've got some champagne in the back. This calls for a celebration."
"No!" Jack protested. "Nothing loud."
"Calm down! You know me better than that."
"If you need a band," Salese said. "I'm quite sure we're available."
"I haven't gotten that far yet," Jack replied.
Alice reached over and touched his thigh, "You guys set a date?"
"No. For the most part, I think she's going to be totally surprised."
"Damn, she's so lucky, "Alice squeezed Jack's thigh.
"Yeah, she is, isn't she?" Jack grinned.

While Jack, Oscar and Salese ate, the eatery began to crowd. Suddenly, like most days after four p.m. at Alice's, there was a wait as long as 10 minutes for a table. The growing chatter around the men caused Jack to check his watch; he still had plenty time to enjoy his food.

Dexter Forns pushed open the glass doors, holding them for his wife, Sahmara. She waited inside for him, then he led her to the bar. There he ordered drinks for them. He kissed her cheek and went to put them on the waiting list for a table before the drinks arrived. That's when he noticed Jack. He played it off, at first. But, he would look around for Djuana every chance he could.

Sahmara looked good. She had lost 10 pounds in the month since giving birth to their second boy. She had turned into a workout freak, building a collection of exercise tapes and gadgets, and a health food nut, forsaking red meat. Dexter ignored most of his wife's new habits. He bought his own food, usually some sort of fast food. Sahmara was also a homebody which attracted Dexter to her when they first met. He could date her, and many others, and not worry about seeing her when out with the others.

Sahmara gave in to Dexter and allowed him to take her out to dinner because she really wanted to hear some jazz, and he bought her a new dress and shoes for the occasion.

"This place is kinda crowded for a Tuesday," Sahmara commented when her husband returned to the bar.

"It gets worse than this later in the week," Dexter said. "But, we won't have that long of a wait, Babe."

"I wish you could get weekends off sometime," Sahmara commented.

"Why? You never want to go anywhere anyway?"

Dexter picked up his drink, sipping the Tom Collins and surveying the scene. *Djuana's here somewhere*, he assured himself. He just wanted to look at her, hoping she would be wearing a tight dress, showing those legs.

The hostess lightly touched Dexter and he jumped out of his skin, spilling his drink on the floor in front of him. She apologized, and the bartender swiftly mixed him another.

"What's wrong with you?" Sahmara asked him.

"Nothing! The bitch gonna roll up on me like a cop and shit. She scared the shit out of me!"

"I'm sorry, Mister," the girl said.

"It's okay," Sahmara assured her.

The hostess led them to their table, further in the back. Jack, and Oscar, saw them go by. Jack looked up from his plate, mouth full, but didn't recognize Dexter.

"Mutherfucker," Dexter whispered. His wife heard him.

"What's the matter?"

"That motherfucker staring at you and shit."

"So?" his wife was agitated. "Take it as a compliment for once."

Jack looked behind him, "What that guy say?"

O was laughing, "Talking about me. I was staring at his girl's ass. She need to take off that dress, it's too small for her BIG ass."

"You have to start some shit?" Jack asked him.

Oscar laughed harder, "I ain't do nothing!"

"Well, you could at least show some couth and whisper."

Salese continued to savor his steak. But, his eyebrows raised when Dexter reappeared standing over Jack.

"Something funny?" Dexter asked in a menacing tone.

Jack sobered immediately. He wiped his face with his hand cloth. "Yo, hold up, don't stand over me."

Jack moved to rise, planting one hand on the table, the other on his thigh.

Salese and Oscar sprang up. Oscar's thigh hit the table, tilting it.

Salese made his way around the table, and slipped between Jack and Dexter. Oscar was already there. All eyes were on Jack and Dexter.

"We don't want no trouble, baby," Oscar said.

"I know. Y'all don't want to get fucked up in here."

Salese pulled Jack by his arm, then pushed him by the waist. "Come on, Jack let's go."

Something clicked in Jack's mind, and his memory revealed a vivid picture of Dexter patting his stomach after Jack laid him out.

Dexter pointed at Jack while Salese stood between them. "You a fucking punk," he said.

The commotion drew big attention. Sahmara, though, tried to ignore it. Still sitting at the table, she held her head in her hands.

O massaged his thin mustache, and moved closer to Dexter. "Listen, I'm gon' save you a beat down. I'll apologize. I'm sorry your girl has a nice ass, and I'm sorry I was looking at it."

"How's that?"

Sahmara arrived at that instant. "Come on, Dexter, please can we just have dinner?"

"I oughta bust your ass," Dexter near muttered to Oscar.

O separated his arms, "Go for yours."

"Oscar!" Jack yelled.

Salese stayed between Jack and the argument.

Dexter allowed his wife to pull him away, then as they reached their table, he spun around and busted into a sprint and leaped into Oscar. O quickly backpedaled and tagged Dexter's face with two quick punches. Dexter went down and Oscar was on top, his elbows flying up and down and he rained punches on Dexter's head.

Jack and Salese were there in seconds, pulling O up. Dexter's body was in a protective ball; the fetal position on the ground. His wife had to squeeze through the crowd to get to him.

Alice came barreling through the towering crowd. "Oh no. Oh no. Cut the shit out. Don't wreck my place!"

Jack and Salese yanked and pulled Oscar away. He was smiling, with a devilish grin, not resisting.

"Oooo, boy!" O sneered. "I busted that skull! You see that?"

"Shut up, O," Jack scolded him. "What got into you?"

"Ah, man, relax. I just needed to kick some ass."

Salese shook his head. "Man, that was stupid. You know that ass hole is going to sue you?"

"Fuck him."

"That guy is Djuana's ex," Jack explained. "He was looking for a fight."

"More reason to bust his ass," Oscar checked his knuckles. The one on his right hand's middle finger was cut. "And, I bet he ain't proud he found a fight."

Alice zipped through the crowded restaurant to Dexter's table, as the food arrived.

"You have to leave," she said, just as the couple had regained their bearings.

The bus boy froze. She motioned him to take the food back.

"Excuse me," Dexter said. "Those guys were rude to my wife."

"I'm sorry. Please leave, or else I will have to call the cops."

"Call the fucking cops, I ain't done shit."

Alice raised her head about the silent restaurant. Salese was there before she could call for help.

"Yo, rise up, Brother," Salese said.

"Oh, so those baseball players get much respect here?"

"You don't," Alice didn't hesitate.

The anger was evident in Sahmara's mannerism as she rose quietly and gathered her hand bag. Dexter followed her lead, and they walked out. But, as soon as they were outside, Dexter removed his suit's jacket.

"Fuck this," he was furious, "I'ma kick some ass. Baseball players can't fight."

Inside, Salese and Jack watched him undo his tie and curse at the window, stalking back and forth, while his wife picked up his clothes and tried to reason with him.

"Look at this fool," Salese chuckled, then he looked at Jack. "Don't go out there, please."

"I gotta go get Djuana soon. And, shit, we got a game tonight."

Oscar went to the bar, ordered a drink, and began a conversation with a pretty lady who was waiting for a table with her two friends. In a matter of seconds he had her clean his cut knuckle with a wet napkin and kiss it.

Jack double parked the Pathfinder in front of Djuana's building, and Djuana briskly walked to the truck with her arms folded across her chest and a steady frown. She smiled at him as she got in and gave him a wet hello kiss.

"How did you get here from work? I'ma have to get you a car."

"You don't have to do that," she said feebly.

"I know I don't have to. Maybe I want to so you can get around easier when I'm in town."

Djuana looked out of her window as the truck drove off.

"I thought you might bring Devon to the game."

"No."

She was going to give short answers, let her anger simmer until she could get the questions out with out bitterness. But, her heart knew better than her mind that Jack was the man she loved, and there was no reason to be angry with him.

"I was going to bring him," she opened up, "but he had plans to spend the night with a friend down the street."

Jack did a double-take at Djuana. She was frowning, one hand rubbing her forehead. "What's wrong?"

She looked over at him, "What happened at Alice's."

Jack looked forward into traffic. Then, as if he found the answer, "Your ex tried to pick a fight with me and O."

"Were you going to mention it?"

"No. I wasn't."

Djuana shook her head. "Why not?"

"Djuana, I hate how that man hurt you. I don't ever want you to have to hear about him, think about him or see him."

"That's not realistic. I dated him for seven years."

"Yeah, I know, but. I don't want to talk about him."

"Did y'all fight?"

"I didn't," Jack sighed. "He was upset because O was looking at his wife and they got into it."

Although the friend that called and told Djuana of the fight had mention that Dexter was there with a woman, the word wife sliced through Djuana's soul like a sharp saber.

"She was there," she whispered.

"Yep."

"You had them thrown out?"

"No. He asked for it himself."

Djuana again returned her sights and thoughts out her window. *That motherfucker is married and I'm not.*

The truck stopped at a red light on 20th Avenue and Sandy Boulevard, and Jack figured this was the best time for a pleasant surprise.

"I got something for you, today."

"What?"

"First, are you going to let me put it on you right now?"

Djuana smiled. "Wait. What is it?"

"No, am I going to be able to put it on you? Yes or no?"

Djuana sat up. "Okay. Sure," she said confidently.

Jack reached across and under her seat, and Djuana's eyes followed the long, wrapped box and his hand go from under her to before her eyes. He handed it to her.

"Open it."

She did, slowly. The gold, link ankle bracelet glittered in the darkening cab of the Pathfinder.

"It's beautiful," Djuana gasped.

Jack gently took it from her soft hands. "Give me your left ankle."

Djuana turned her body, sliding up her long skirt and lifting her leg over the gear console. Jack flipped her strapless shoes onto the floor at her other foot. While horns angrily honked in the background Jack clipped the jewelry onto her soft, wide leg. The feel of his strong hands, although only touching her foot for a second, excited Djuana.

"I love you, Jack," she said.

Jack lifted her foot to meet his lowering lips, and planted a soft kiss on the top of her toes, then licked up to her ankle. He kissed the chain, then released her foot.

"I know you love me, that's why I'd do anything to keep you smiling."

Take away the first inning, and the game that night was relatively a boring one. The Crowns exploded for seven runs in the first inning. Oscar hit a mammoth home run into the third tier of the right field upper decks. Jack doubled after him, and Don hit another long home run, this one to left. But, that was it for excitement. The Crowns defeated New York, 7-0.

Jack couldn't wait for the game to end. He had come up with a perfect plan to pop the question that night. After the game, reporters kept him busy for an half an hour with questions about his first game back in Portland since being released. They surrounded his stall, forming a semicircle around him as he sat, slowly undressing, fielding questions.

Oscar came to his stall, next to Jack's and couldn't reach his possessions.

"You motherfuckers have to move. Y'all all in my shit."

They moved over, huddling closer to Jack. O wasn't satisfied.

"Yo, keep moving, get the fuck away from me."

Jack patiently answered the steady stream of repetitious questions. Then, as the other reporters inquires died down, Kristen began grilling him.

"So, I hear you going to ask Djuana Pioneer to marry you tonight?" went Kris' first question.

The other reporters feel silent, yet perked up. The television cameras were clicked back on and aimed at Jack again, and microphones edged closer.

"Yes. I bought the ring this afternoon."

"Is it true you plan to retire after this season?"

"I haven't given retirement any thought. Right now, I just trying to help the Crowns reach the playoffs."

A female reporter from Portland's ABC affiliate beamed a bright smile at Jack, "So, how do you plan on proposing?"

Jack felt Kris' stare. "That's confidential until I do it."

"You guys set a date," a usually heavy-hitting reporter threw in.

"Not yet. Look, it'll be better to talk about this tomorrow."

"It'll be old news then, Jack," Kris said. "People want to know all about your plans to wed the woman who has been the cause of so much turmoil in your season."

Jack stood, wearing only a Crowns gray t-shirt and gold spandex shorts. "That's it. I'll be glad to talk about it tomorrow, when she's wearing the ring."

"Let's see the ring," Kris gave Jack a sly grin. "You bought it on West Burnside, right?'

Jack watched reporters jot down that little tidbit. "Doing your homework, huh?"

Kristen's smile dimmed. "I live right around the corner from Gene's."

"Let's see the ring, Jack," the female from ABC said. She fingered her cameraman to Jack. "It'll make great news. Women all over the state will be jealous."

Jack stared at Kris. Her eyes glossed, but she smiled. She was not hiding her hurt well, all though she thought the mask was working. Jack slowly reached up in his locker and brought down the box. Kris closed her eyes, she darted away crying. Jack forced his eyes front, and sighed.

"Bring it to your waist, and then open it," the ABC cameraman said.

"Wait!" yelled a newspaper photographer. "I gotta change film!"

In seconds, everyone was ready. The clubhouse silenced. Juris came out of his office. Jack opened the box, and it was empty. He panicked, until he heard his teammates laughing over in the corner, near the infielder's section.

"You fucking Puerto Rican!" Jack bellowed, forgetting the cameras were rolling.

Juan paused his laugh long enough to correct Jack, "Hey, I ain't no Puerto Rican, I'm Dominican, Baby!"

Jack rushed him, knocking over two reporters, and caught him after a short chase.

"I'm worried, Jack" Djuana said, frowning while cuddling into Jack on the sofa.

"About what," Jack answered, his fingers in her hair, eyes on the movie they rented.

"A job. What am I going to do?"

"Don't be worried," Jack's eyes never left the screen. "I'll call Karl in the morning, and he'll find you something."

Djuana didn't perk up. "I have to work."

"I said, don't worry about it."

Djuana snuggled into his chest, twirling her body to face his. Her body warmed as Jack planted light kisses on her forehead, nose, cheeks and then lips. As soon as his lips arrived to hers, she gave him a soul kiss that heated his furnace.

"Let's don't go out," Djuana panted between licks.

"We have to."

"It's late," Djuana worked her torso onto Jack's lap. " You have a day game tomorrow."

"We haveta go."

Djuana pulled his t-shirt down until the shirt's front stretched to reveal his chest. She flicked her moist tongue over his muscular breast plate. Jack held her hair, gently at first, then pulled the hair to get her away. Djuana's tongue extended its full length, arousing Jack all the more.

Her eyes flared with eroticism, "I don't want to go out. I want you in me."

Jack gulped, trying to shift his body so that his crotch wouldn't be so comfortable underneath hers. "It'll only take a minute."

"Jack."

"We'll be back before you know it."

"Jack," Djuana removed her shirt and reached behind her back for her bra.

Djuana was upset when they got in the Pathfinder. She sat with her arms folded and lips poked out.

"Why does Oscar want us to come over so late at night? It's almost 11:30 and you guys have a early game in the afternoon?"

"I don't know. You know how he is," Jack hid his joy.

Jack sped down the deserted Foothills Freeway. By the time he reached the Main Street exit, Djuana had fallen asleep. To Jack's delight, it had began to rain lightly before they reached Main and Tenth Avenue. Jack pulled over on Tenth, waited for a car to pass, then pulled the truck across the street, double parking on the wrong side. He got out, and saw Djuana stir.

"Where are we?" she said groggily as Jack reached her side of the truck. "You parked on the wrong side."

Jack opened her door. "I know. Come on out."

"It's raining, Jack. I only have on these shorts."

"It's just drizzling. Come on."

Jack backed away, and Djuana got out. She reached back in and grabbed Jack's baseball cap.

"I think you're losing your mind, Newhouse."

"Maybe."

He took her hand and led her across the doubled yellow lines in back of the Pathfinder and to the cross walk. Another car passed them, the passengers craning their heads to get a glimpse of the nuts walking in the rain.

"Jack. What are you doing?"

He stopped in the crosswalk, looking down, then out towards the buildings, approximating where he had found her four months ago. Djuana was flustered; feeling hassled and edgy.

She whined, "I want to go home."

Jack moved closer to her, putting her arms around his waist. "I thought I would never in my life see a more beautiful woman than the one I saw that night. But, each day you show me I was wrong."

Jack kissed both of her hands. "I love you, Djuana."

"Yes, I know, but-"

Jack continued, "When I met you here five months ago, my first impression was that you were the most beautiful woman I had ever seen. Now, I know that you are not only beautiful, but smart, caring and affectionate and a great lover when you are devoted."

Djuana's froze. She was puzzled, trying to swiftly pick up on what was happening. *Was he proposing?* She took in a quick survey of the area. *This is where he picked me up that night.*

Jack's right hand went into his pants pocket and pulled the ring out; it was in tissue, no box. He uncovered it, and took Djuana's hand. She quivered when he touched her, her hand jerking out of his. Her hands were hot, and became sweaty despite the damp weather. She rubbed them nervously. Her eyes moisten, but she wasn't crying.

"I want to marry you, baby," Jack calmly retook her hand. "I want you to be my wife."

Djuana couldn't stop the tears, or curb the blush, while Jack slipped the ring onto her finger with ease. Jack twirled it, noticing the ring fit loosely, yet was not coming off. It fit as Gene said it would.

Djuana's left hand burned, she had a feeling of streaking nerves from her heart to the hand. The ring was heavy on her finger.

"You like it, baby?"

"I love it," she said, the tears now flowing evenly and her nose leaking.

"Does it fit okay? I took one of you other rings and..."

She leaped into Jack's arms, his head knocking off her hat. "It fits wonderfully."

She squeezed him into a tight, snug embrace. Her wet nose, cheeks and lips rubbed against Jack's back. He held onto her.

"So, is that a yes?"

# 38

Djuana came out of one of the public ladies rooms in Adkins Stadium wondering if she really *needed* another hot dog. She looked over to the crowd at the concession stand, she was not going to wait on another line. It had taken nearly 10 minutes to relieve herself. Just as she turned to enter the concrete ramp leading to her seat, the voice with the hold of a vise on her soul called out to her.

"So you getting married, huh?"

Djuana cut her eyes in the direction of the voice. She didn't have to see Dexter Forns to know he was grinning. She turned away, to continue to walk, but he was on her very quickly.

Dexter grabbed her. "I saw that shit on the fucking news. Nice ring."

"Let me go, Dexter."

"If I don't? What, you gonna tell your man?"

"Dexter. Don't start anything."

He let her pull away.

"It's bad enough that you stole my money, but now you got that punk ass baseball player getting me jumped at a restaurant! What's up with that?"

Djuana sighed. She didn't want to argue, let alone talk to him, but if it was money he was after, she wanted to deal with it and be done with him.

"Dexter, what money are you whining about?"

"I gave you an envelope with $300 for an abortion. Did you have it? No. So, where's my fucking money?"

"You'll get your money. I promise you."

"Give it to me now."

"I ain't got it on me."

"You better have my money after the game, or I'm going to fuck you up."

"No you not. You are not going to put your hands on me ever again."

Djuana shook her head, fighting anger. "You spent $10 to get into a Crowns game to ask me for your money?"

"I go where I want to go."

Dexter's voice was unusually controlled for the anger that showed in his distorted face. Then, Djuana realized what was happening by watching and listening to her ex. But, she could not raise her defenses in time to fend off the hurt.

"You stole my fuckin' money. Spent it like a broke hoe. That's why you lost the baby. 'Cause you ain't worth shit. You don't deserve to be a mother. You stupid, low life bitch."

Djuana's heart sank, and the hurt seeped into her bones. Dexter laughed in her face. Her fist balled, and her eyes flamed.
"Go ahead and cry, you spoiled baby."

Djuana was afraid to leave the stadium after the game. She made her way down to the entrance of the clubhouse; most of the guards recognized her, the others flirted, and allowed her to pass. She stood in the doorway with other women, and some children waiting for the players. Usually, she waited in the Pathfinder for Jack.

She stood, leaning on the wall, outside of the clubhouse for Jack. How would she ask for the money? Should she say she spent it? Or, that she lost it? No, she wouldn't be able to lie to Jack. But, she had to pay off Dexter. The last thing Djuana wanted was more scandal in this, the worst and most trying season of Jack's career.

After a few players left out in street clothes, Djuana asked the guard at the door of the clubhouse if Jack was still in there. The young dark skinned guy smiled and nodded.

"He is, you wanta go in?"
"May I?"
"No! Ya, gotta wait here."
The guard chuckled to himself. Some of the others waiting also laughed.
"Idiot," Djuana fumed.
Jack and Oscar came out together, laughing. When his eyes caught hers, his smile broadened.
The guard nodded at Jack, and offered his hand. Jack slapped it.
"My man!" the guard pointed at Jack.
"Juanny, baby. Looking good, now!" O said as he went on out the door with one of the waiting women on his arm.
"He's an asshole," Djuana frowned.
Jack tensed. "Who, O?"
"No! That guard."
"What did he do?"
"Nothing. Nothing. He just thinks he's funny."
Jack smiled. "Yep. That's for shit-sure. Why you come in here?"
Djuana shook her head, looking for courage. "I have to tell you something."
She tensed, "Dexter is here, and he threatened me."
"What? Where is he?"
Djuana couldn't believe she was crying. "Jack, I owe him some money. He said he wants it now or he was going to hurt me."
Jack looked around. "Where did he say for you to meet him?"
"He didn't."

"Come on, let's go."

"Jack, I don't have it."

"Don't worry about it."

Outside were the usually collection of autograph seekers crowding the walkway from the stadium to the player's parking lot. Among them was Dexter. He moved forward when he saw them come out. He didn't say anything, just waited to be noticed. Djuana saw him. Jack had a guard let him in the lot.

"What the fuck you want?" Jack said.

The guard overheard him, and stood his ground close to the three of them.

"This is between me and your fiancee. Not you, superstar.'

"Let me tell you something," Jack moved in closer to Dexter. Dexter stood up, chin high and eyes piercing. "You come near Djuana again, and I'm going to fuck you up badly."

Dex laughed. "You a joke. A big overpaid joke."

He put his palm up to Jack, "Back off, Hank Aaron."

Jack turned to his woman, "How much you owe him."

Djuana weakly replied, "He said $300."

"Ten thousand," Dexter blurted.

Jack cut his eyes as he pulled out his wallet. He took out a wad of bills and counted out money.

Dexter watched him.

"I want ten thousand, or I go to the press and tell them that Djuana Newhouse claimed she was having my baby and took money for an abortion and didn't have it."

"Did you hear that, Kozell?" Jack said to the guard, not more than five paces away.

The guard nodded. Jack handed Dexter three crisp hundred dollar bills.

Dexter took them, licked his fingers, counted them and said, "This is short some duckets."

"Take it or leave it. That's all being offered."

"You'll be hearing from my lawyer."

"You are no good," Djuana said, wiping her eyes. "Why you doing this to me? I never did anything to you."

"Shut the fuck up."

In an instant Dexter was on the ground, and guards and police officers were running to Jack's aide. Jack had hit him so quickly, that Djuana did not see Jack move until he was recoiling.

Kozell and other uniformed men pounced on Dexter until they had him cuffed. They dragged him back into the stadium.

The Portland Crowns began their long climb out of last place in late August; coincidentally, it was around the time Jack rejoined the club. The team won 17 of 19 games before they realized they were back in the pennant race. They breezed by Seattle and San Francisco. The team entered September with eight less wins than first place Los Angeles.

Russ Jones made the Crowns and their fans forget about Cris. RJ was a better left fielder. His skills allowed Oscar to play shallow and not worry about every ball hit to his right. Also, Jones became the leadoff hitter the Crowns manager, Juris, always wanted Oscar to be. He got on base often and once on, he was a serious threat to steal a base or two. Russ set up the rest of the lineup by getting on base often. During the Crowns incredible stretch run, Russ reached base safely in 34 straight games.

Although the kid had a splendid mixture of talent and desire, he rarely spoke to his teammates, and when he did he addressed the veterans as Mister. Of course, the Crowns took advantage of his wide-eyed innocence. They took turns having him carry their luggage, buying dinner when the checks came and robbing him in poker. Still, RJ loved the attention, the acceptance. Luis Ratz, who was also a rookie, was basically ignored despite the fact that he was a Portland Crowns home grown product.

The major reason RJ was accepted and Luis was an outsider on this veteran, battle tested ball club was talent. RJ set up the rest of the lineup. Juris kept Pugsley second, and his bat skills were challenged by Russ' speed; and Pugs responded just about every time RJ got on base by moving him over with excellent bunts and crafty grounders to right. Oscar batted third, and loved it. He had two long hitting streaks, and his average zoomed over .300. Jack was the cleanup hitter by default. When Bingo left, there was no one to fill the void. Don replaced him at first base, but the Crowns had no power hitter. Jack stepped in, and although he didn't hit a homer, he knocked in runs any other way he could. Don batted behind him, and he had plenty of big, clutch hits.

The rest of the lineup did their usual job of opportunistic hitting. Juan, the Crowns ninth place hitter for the last three years, was also the league's most dangerous two-out batter.

The pitching was the huge surprise during the comeback. Without Lee to carry the unit, Danny and Floyd picked up the pieces. Both were forced to pitch more than they had ever in their careers because the young pitchers on the Crowns were of little help while they went through their growing pains. The pitcher the Crowns got in exchange for Cris from LA, Timm Peaston, was bombarded in his first three starts. This was no surprise, because he was one of the few pitchers on LA the Crowns would have regular success against.

Timm was thrown in the bullpen, buried by Juris. But, he came through in a few big situations to reclaim a spot in the rotation. He finished the season pitching as well as Danny and Floyd.

The bullpen was headed by one of the best firemen in baseball, Bobby Lyles. Lyles was one of the very few anti-social players on the Crowns. He was married, and he and his wife and three children rented a house in Portland during the season, but were virtually invisible. He was a family man when he was traded to the Crowns, and he chose not to hang out with any of the mostly single or promiscuous Portland players.

Lyles had the nastiest sinker in the game. He threw it often, mixing in a 90-plus miles per hour fastball and a late 70 m.p.h. changeup. Juris rarely used him for more than four batters.

A sober Mike Colbert was still the captain and soul of this team. He didn't hit that well after getting off the booze, but he was there to yell at anyone that didn't give the Crowns 100 percent of their heart.

Los Angeles had entered August in first place; the first time in three years that a team other than Portland was at the top of the West that late in the season. And, Portland wasn't the second place team. Portland was in last place, 17 games out on August 1. Each time the Trojans won a game, home or away, in late August and September, the team celebrated. They looked well on their way to finally getting past the Crowns and into the World Series. They especially thought so when they *stole* Cris Carpenter from the Crowns for a pitcher they thought would never live up to his potential.

The manager of the Los Angeles Trojans. Horace Johnson, feared the Crowns, a proud team, would be ready by the playoffs. In September, as the season was closing, and the Crowns won games in bunches, Johnson began berating his team after wins. No more celebrations, he proclaimed. He made it impossible for his players to forget that it was Portland who had knocked them out of the playoffs the past three years.

Johnson had the front page of the Los Angeles newspaper from the past October copied and placed on the stool of each player's locker. The headline of the newspaper, the day after the Crowns had come back from three runs down to eliminate the Trojans, read: "Trojans Choke Again."

For the most part, Johnson's players, a veteran bunch, ignored his motivational attempts. Some laughed behind his back. Some said at the time that they could feel it was their year to win it all. Cris even reasoned:

"How in the world can Portland catch us without Bingo, Lee, and, most importantly, me?"

When September began, Djuana was sure of what she wanted to do with the rest of her life. Marrying Jack was the easiest of her future plans. Loving him forever would not be difficult. But, she wanted dearly to go to college. Watching Tia struggle through exams, morning classes and studying had fired up her interest in furthering her education.

And, now was the perfect time. She saw that with Jack she was in the right environment; he was supportive, positive and financially secure. He was the first person she told, during dinner before a game at Adkins.

"You want to go to college? Baby, that's great."

She expected no less of an response. She put down her fork, and the excitement in her voice erased her appetite.

"I was thinking about it since I became pregnant. I need a better future."

"What you wanta study?"

Djuana wrinkled her nose, "I'm not sure, really."

Jack filled his mouth with the chicken gizzards and noodles causing Djuana to marvel at how he enjoyed such a simple meal.

He sipped some iced tea, then said, "It doesn't matter right now, I guess. You know where you want to go?"

"Tia goes to Portland State, she could probably help me get in there."

"Do you have enough time? It's already September?"

"No. I might be able to go now, but I really am not ready mentally. I think I should until January. Classes start in two weeks."

"Whatever makes you smile, I'm with."

Djuana watched Jack fork noodles into his mouth, chew them and add iced tea. He was the most positive-minded person she had ever known.

"These chicken gizzards and noodles are slammin'!" he suddenly declared.

Djuana laughed. "I can't believe you like that. I told my mother you wanted to try it and she said I better not cook it for you. She thinks it's a poor family meal."

"So? It tastes good, and that's all that matters to me."

When his mouth was clear, he said, "Maybe we can go over to Portland State and see what you'll need."

"I already picked up a class guide and financial aid information."

Jack shook his head, his mouth full again. "You won't need it."

"Jack, I can't ask you to pay for college for me."

"Okay. Then don't," Jack finished his tea and the ice chimed. "But just remember, if you need anything, don't be too proud to ask. Okay?"

"Yes." Djuana touched his right hand as he put the fork down to grab his glass. "It's not easy for me to live off of you. I want you to know that."

"You're not. And don't think of it like that. I love you, and it makes me feel great that I can help you do whatever it is you want to."

"I ain't no charity case, though."

"Relax. Djuana, you'll be my wife soon." His eyebrows pumped and he rubbed his fingers on a imaginary mustache. "I'll think of ways for you to pay me back."

Djuana smiled, "I might not say no."

Jack grabbed her out of the chair so quickly it startled Djuana. They rolled on the floor, her plate of food underneath them. She fought away from his grasp, and stood over him.

"Look at you!" she scolded him. "You got noodles all over your shirt. Now you have to change before we go to the game."

"You just want to get me naked!"

The game that damp Sunday afternoon ended up being the seventh win in a row for the Crowns. Jack, though, struck out three times and took his failure hard. And, in the clubhouse after the game, his teammates were merciless on him. He was the only starter to not get a hit.

He took their ribbing in stride; he had no choice. Even the reporters were laughing at him. Oscar and two other players invited him out for drinks; the team was off Monday, then would be flying out Tuesday. He wanted to hang out, but told his teammates he had Djuana with him.

"So, we bringing the dames tonight," Danny said.

"Yeah, man, bring 'em," Oscar added. "I'm bringing this chick from Miami. You know the one."

Jack grinned at the memory of the bronzed-skinned Hispanic cutie. "No can do. We got plans. Her moms is making dinner."

"Aw shit," Don intruded from his locker at the honored spot closest to the dugout steps. "You better let him go! You know his in-laws are timing him!"

"Damn," O laughed. "And you didn't get a hit today? They gonna make you sit with the children."

Jack tore opened the dry cleaner's plastic covering his suit, trying to ignore that he once again was the reason for the laughter in the clubhouse. His body was still semi-wet from the shower, but he didn't want to keep the Pioneers waiting. He did notice that among the jovial players and reporters, Kris Eisen was deadly serious. He ignored her as well.

"And look," Juan came over to point out, "He even rented a suit!"

"Leave him alone," Oscar finally said. "He in wuv."

Stacie loved the rain. She couldn't fathom people leaving Portland because of it. She stood in the steady drizzle, lapping her tongue out and taking in moisture. She enjoyed wearing light colored t-shirts and having the rain drops outline, then expose, her long nipples. She would nearly explode with excitement watching men stare at her breasts.

Stacie, wearing a sun dress that day, would have stood in the drizzle and waited for her date had she not seen Djuana get into Jack's Pathfinder. An anxiety attack rattled her bones and forced her to seek shelter. She went into the corridor leading to the player's clubhouse. And, Jack was one of the first players out of the locker rooms.

"Hey baby!" she beamed, revealing her perfect set of teeth, and waved.

Jack shook his head in disbelief. "You've got balls coming here."

"I don't have any, but I'd take yours any day."

Before Jack could reply, a female from behind them cleared her throat loudly. They looked back, and Don's wife Liela waved Jack over. He went.

"Don't, Jack. Okay? Because you gonna lose a nice lady in Djuana."

Jack gritted his teeth. "Now, why you think it's all about that?"

"I know how that hoe is, she be hypnotizing you guys."

"Right." Jack kissed Liela on the cheek and patted her shoulders. "Good looking out."

He resumed his walk to the parking lot. Stacie jumped ahead of him, blocking his path with her slender body in the doorway.

"I ain't here for you, although I wish I were."

"Move, Stace," Jack said, although not touching her.

Stacie moved with him. "How's your old lady?"

Jack tensed.

Stacie smiled, she had his attention. "You know," she took his silk tie into her hands, stroking it. "You should have given me a baby. I would have had it for you."

Jack stared into Stacie's dancing eyes. He bit his lip, trying to fight the urge to bash her skull in. The sound of his teammates snapped his anger.

"Move, bitch," he shoved her to the side, knocking her off balance.

"You bastard!" she shouted while trying to gather herself. "Don't call me no bitch! Your girl is a bitch!"

Oscar walked up to Stacie. "What are you doing, stupid? Shut the fuck up before I cram 12 fat inches down your throat."

"Fuck you too, O! Pencil dick muthafucka!"

Oscar grabbed a hand full of her small, round, firm ass underneath the dress, then continued out the door.

Luis came up from behind Stacie and hugged her.

"Hi, Daddy." She spun into his arms, her attitude changing instantly. She shoved her long tongue into his mouth.

"Yuck!" Liela said to her husband as he approached. "How nasty? Why don't you tell that rookie how many dicks she done sucked?"

"Nope. I minds my business, Momma."

Djuana had to park the Pathfinder two blocks from the building; in front of the private houses across 23rd Avenue on Tudor. The walk back wasn't bad at all. Jack engulfed her into his right arm, pacing her stride with his.

"You sure you don't mind eating at my mom's?"

"Nope. This is the first time she has invited me over. So, I knew I had better accept."

"You don't like her, do you?"

Jack looked down at Djuana while they walked hand-in-hand. "Did I ever say that?"

"You never said you did."

"Well, you know, I like that way she raised her only daughter."

"That's a cop out, but thanks for the compliment."

"It's your mother who acts like I stole something whenever I come over."

"Stop exaggerating!"

"Word. I'm serious."

"Just be nice tonight. She did invite you over."

"Okay!"

When they reached 657, Djuana slipped out of Jack's light hold to dig in her bag for the key to the building's front door.

"Now, I'm not going to let my mother bother you, but you have to be cool too."

"Ain't I always?"

"Hmmm. We'll see."

Djuana pushed the apartment's door as she usually did when someone was home, but the door was locked. Jack stood off to the side oblivious of this little change in the norm. Djuana mumbled as she reached back into her purse to get out her keys.

"I hope she's home, the door is usually never locked when she's home. You don't know how many times I had to complain to her to lock the door."

"Maybe she's changed."

Djuana glared at Jack as she unlocked the door. "Don't be smart."

Djuana swung the door open in to a house full of people.

"SURPRISE!!" everyone yelled in unison.

The surprise engagement party was a true stunner. 16 of the Portland Crowns, and many of Djuana friends, some of whom she hadn't seen in years, jammed into Emma's box-shaped living room, rectangular kitchen and long hallways. There were literally people everywhere in the modest five-room spread.

No one complained, though, except Djuana. She tried to take Tia to the side, and change venues.

"Forget it, girlfriend," Tia beamed, "The Crowns were going to rent a place, you know, but your Momma wasn't having it."

Jack hugged Oscar, who was there with the Spanish woman.

Jack said, "Man, I can't believe you guys held a secret."

"We had to threaten Juan, but besides that, we did okay," Don said, standing over Leila, who was sitting on the couch with four other people.

As soon as Jack noticed her, after Don spoke, he went over to Leila and kissed her cheek with more feeling than 40 minutes ago.

"Don't lose her, New." she whispered.

The players presented Jack with a miniature, solid gold, ball and chain. The chain had cuffs that hooked onto a pinky. They gave Djuana the key to the cuffs; she was not amused.

The music was handled by Calvin and his buddy, Ed. They were playing records and cassettes on Emma's antiquated rack system, but they were working a crowd that was there to party, so their mistakes were made fun of, then forgotten as the songs picked up.

Liquor and food were in abundance; although there were no leftovers the next day. The players brought rum, cognac, scotch and vodka. The women cooked fried chicken, fried fish, crabs boiled in beer and a variety of salads.

Emma basked in the joy of being the hostess, and mother of the bride-to-be. She accepted kisses and compliments from the players, and in return tried to stuff all of them with the delicious food. That night was the most Emma Pioneer had smiled in a long, long time.

If Emma was in Heaven, then Devon was in paradise. He had the players sign posters, balls and took Don in his room to see his wall poster of Don that was five years old. Eventually he had his friends come over to see the unbelievable.

Lyle Davis came into the party while it was in full swing. He gave Emma a light kiss, and hugged his son. Devon excitedly told him about all the ballplayers, and the autographs he had gathered. He didn't really pay attention to the boy, instead he searched the faces in the crowd. He was barely into the apartment, marveling at how crowded the place was.

Lyle wasn't surprised that when he saw Emma, nothing happened. No sparks, no desire. He found the enemy faces, and decided which way he could walk in his search for his daughter. He quickly cut his eyes at Cal, and Earline, hoping they would not say anything. He caught himself staring at Tia, who had grown into a sexy young woman since he last saw her.

"I knew you'd come."

He heard Djuana's voice before he saw her glowing smile. She hugged him, and he held on.

"Congrats, baby girl."

"Thanks, Daddy. You ready to meet him?"

"I guess so."

Djuana waved Jack over. He squirmed through the bodies that were now grinding to the rhythm of reggae.

Jack gave a friendly expression while Djuana introduced them. He stuck out his hand and gave Lyle's hand a hearty shake.

"Pleasure to meet you, Mr. Davis."

Lyle appreciated not being called Mr. Pioneer. "The pleasure is all mine, from what I hear."

His stare at Jack was not pleasant.

"I hope you have the right intentions for my daughter."

Jack's smile fell to a smirk. "Sure do," he quipped. "Butt naked and pregnant."

Djuana kicked Jack's ankle. He buckled over in pain.

"He's a funny man, isn't he, Dad?"

Lyle Davis did not smile.

Cal, drunk into slurs and staggering, demanded Jack and Djuana have the dance floor to themselves. He cleared a path, moving players and family members alike.

"Hey! Move your overpaid ass," he said to Danny. The rest of the players laughed and whooped louder than Djuana's friends and family.

Calvin dragged Djuana by her arm to the now empty center of the living room. The crowd formed a tight circle around them. Jack, who was holding a drink and wearing a party hat, knew better than wait for an escort. He scurried over before Cal got to him.

Djuana, blushing, whispered sorry to Jack.

"Don't be," Jack took her into his arms and kissed her neck.

"Wait for the music, fool!!" Cal yelled.

When he noticed Jack's drink he snatched it. "You don't need this, my man."

He gulped Jack's Remy Martin. Djuana hid her face in Jack's shoulder.

"Hit it, motherfuckah!!" Cal announced. Ed quickly press the play button and the beginning bars of Regina Belle's "This Is Love" quieted the room. Djuana gave in to Jack, and let him lead her in a slow sway.

Suddenly, the lights in the living room went off.

"Cal," Emma barked. "Cut those fuckin' lights back on or I'm going to crack your skull with this vodka bottle!!" Emma barked.

The lights came back on in an instant.

Djuana held Jack's hand tightly. He rubbed her knuckles, and squeezed her waist.

"They want us to pick a date," she whispered.

"Don't ask me."

"I was thinking that the season starts again in the spring, and goes through summer. How about this November? Before the holidays."

Jack pulled her closer, feeling her soft body melt into his. "It ain't soon enough, but I'll take it."

"We do need time to -"

"Babe, it's fine."

"November 5th?"

"November 5th it is."

Near the end of the song, other couples joined them. And, when the song and mood changed with a pumping rap song, O asked if he could dance with Djuana. Jack let him.

"My boy loves you," Oscar said as they danced apart to the music.

*He's a man*, Djuana thought. She smiled and nodded. She glided her hips closer to O, then the rest of her body.

"He's the best friend I have ever had," Oscar said, no longer smiling. "I love him and I am happy that you have made him as happy as he is."

Djuana sobered, her body slowed. "Thank you, Oscar. I appreciate that coming from you."

Jack was watching his best friend and woman dance, his body moving in unison with Dr. Dre's lyrics. He was caught daydreaming when Emma snatched him by his arm and returned him onto the crowded dance floor.

"Welcome to the family!" she shouted while waving her large body, her arms swaying and her feet flopping to the sides. She kept her short arms close to her body, and her devilish smile was made all the more weird by her bobbling head.

Jack, laughing at Emma and clapping to the music, sped his body up to keep pace with hers.

Lyle was not comfortable, but he stayed. He kept his eyes on Djuana, avoiding Cal or Emma. He wanted to get her alone, but it was impossible in the small apartment. Most of the night, he was the only person not dancing. It was amazing to him to see those millionaire ballplayers enjoy themselves in a little house party.

Finally, while Cal and his buddy were arguing about what to put on next, Lyle took his daughter by the arm and asked her to join him in the hallway. As they approached the stairwell, Djuana stopped to wipe sweat from her brow.

"I didn't realize it was so hot in there," she said.

"Yeah. It is," Lyle looked back at the door of the apartment.

"You okay, Dad?"

"Listen, I know it's not any of my say so, but I don't trust this ball player."

Djuana frowned, her eyes blaring. "Jack, his name is Jack. Why can't you say it? And what is it you don't like about him?"

"Forget it."

"No, what is it?"

"I just don't want to see you hurt, that's all."

"Daddy, I am going to marry Jack. He has been the only man to love me wholeheartedly."

Djuana brushed by her father, reentering the party.

# 39

On the last day of the season, the first Sunday of October, the Portland Crowns broke the hearts of a entire city.

The Crowns went into Buffalo, where the weather was chilly all weekend, never reaching 65 degrees Friday, Saturday or Sunday. When the Crowns got off the plane, there were thousands of Buffalo fans booed them. Their trail to the hotel, a 10 minute ride, was lined with men, women and children wishing them bad. The bus was pummeled with fruits and vegetables.

It wasn't until the team was in the hotel that the players realized that Danny was the reason for the greeting. Two nights before, a reporter following the Crowns run for the playoffs, had asked Danny what he thought of this weekend's series. He said, bluntly, "Buffalo is a last place team. They shot their load. We are going to beat them like bad children."

The Buffalo Soldiers had a club record 89 wins and were locked into second place in the East Division coming into the final series of the regular season. To make the playoffs for the first time in nine years, the Soldiers needed to defeat Portland in one of the three weekend games. Portland, the second place team in the west, had 87 wins; its lowest total in four years. One of the two teams would be the fourth team in the playoffs. For it to be Portland, the Crowns would have to win all three games.

By fate, Danny pitched the first game, on a cold Friday night. And, he was ready. The fans were brutal on him, but his curve ball was cruel. He threw it most of the night, dazzling the Buffalo batters. He fanned 11 of them, and gave up only three hits; all harmless singles.

Danny, a nine-year veteran, pitched a flawless game Friday night. He shut out Buffalo, 3-0. Don was the big batter. He hit two home runs and single to drive in all three runs.

Jack had three doubles Saturday, and Juan hit his first home run in two years as the Crowns won, 7-2.

Sunday was the coldest day. When the Crowns woke up, the temperature was 34 degrees and it was a very dreary looking day. When they left the hotel, it was 41 degrees. When the game started, there was a steady, bone-chilling breeze swirling snow flurries. It hurt Slight to have to ask Buffalo's owner Ron Capton could his players borrow parkas. Capton gloated, and rented Slight his team's extra down coats, and the players on the bench had to wear parkas that had the Buffalo team's colors and logo on them.

The Buffalo players, more accustomed to the weather, were confident they could win this pivotal, final game of the season. And, it seemed they would, leading the game 5-3 entering the eighth inning.

In the outfield, Jack and Oscar were near frozen. In left, though, RJ seemed oblivious. He was in his first pennant race, and was numbed by the experience.

"Man, I can't take this shit!" O yelled to Jack across the outfield while Juris went to the mound to bring in another pitcher. "Niggers ain't made for this weather."

Jack walked briskly to O. He slipped his right, ungloved, hand in his uniform pants. "Man, we can't go out like this."

"We ain't. Belee that. I'ma do what I gotta do. We ain't losin' to these fucks."

O looked into the infield where Juan and Pugs were talking just as he and Jack were. Jack followed his eyes.

"Hey, Juan!" O yelled, still agitated.

Pugs looked up first, then tapped Juan. Juan lifted his chin as if to say "what?"

"You ever seen snow before?!"

Juan put up his middle finger.

"New, that bitch got on three undershirts, two batting gloves on his left hand and three pairs of socks!"

Oscar laughed so hard he fell to his knees.

Juan cursed him in Spanish.

When the relief pitcher was near done with his warm-up tosses, Jack strolled back into position. O was still laughing when he left him, and when Jack looked across the well manicured lawn, he saw RJ apparently shaking his head at the fooling around. Jack understood the rookie's objection. But, he thought, this is how we do it.

When RJ led off the eighth inning with a weak ground out, the throng of over 50,000 spectators raised their noise level higher than it had been all afternoon. RJ dragged his bat back into the dugout. Pugs, the next batter, patted his rump, as did Oscar and Jack, but still he was near tears. Then, Pugs also grounded out. Oscar waltzed to the plate, glaring at the pitcher. The fans booed him barbarically. O just grinned and blew a kiss into the seats.

The catcher barked at O, "Why don't you just bat up?"

"Why don't you suck my bat?"

After the pitcher struck out O with three marvelous curves, the stadium rocked from a single, deafening roar.

Jack, facing the dugout standing in the on deck circle, moved just in time to avoid O's bat.

"Give me that fools glove," Jack said to anyone.

"You bastards don't deserve to fly home if you lose this game," Juris spouted as the Crowns took to the field. "I should have Slight bus your asses back to Oregon!"

Jack trotted out to Oscar, and handed him his baseball glove. "You made a lot of people happy."

"Shut the fuck up," O snarled.

Bobby Lyles came in to pitch the ninth for Portland, and he threw bullets by the Buffalo batters. He struck out the side using 10 pitches. Still, the fans gave their team a standing ovation as the ninth began.

Jack trotted in from right, and went directly to the bat rack. He selected his bat and moved out into the on deck circle. He drowned out his teammates words of encouragement, instead choosing to listen to the chants of the Buffalo fans. They wanted to see their team in the playoffs badly. Jack thought back to the first year the Crowns made the playoffs. Their fans were as desperate.

The pitcher for Buffalo was a talent rookie who had already won 21 games that season. He was the best of a young crop of arms that had propelled Buffalo back into contention. He was left handed, and threw a sharp slider to right handed batters. He had used his dazzling curve the inning before to fan Oscar. The kid had thrown a ton of pitches in holding down the Crowns, and Jack was banking he was told to get ahead of the hitters or he'd be removed from the game.

Jack dug in the batter's box intent on swinging at the first pitch, which he knew in his bones would be a fastball. And, sure enough, the kid unleashed a arrow of a toss belt high. Jack's eyes lit up. His hands raised, then he pulled the bat through the strike zone, drilling the baseball down the left field line. The ball whizzed by the third baseman before he could react.

Before Jack touched first, the base coach was yelling, "Two, New. Two!"

Jack got there without having to slide.

The stadium was silent as Don stepped to the plate. Buffalo's manager crept out of the home dugout and slowly walked to the mound. Just as he got on the dirt of the hill, he motioned to his bull pen for relief. But he got none from the pitcher he brought in. The guy, a veteran, walked Don, then hit Bryant Clark with a wild fastball on the thigh. Bryant, a notorious hot-head, took two steps toward the mound before Buffalo's catcher grabbed him. Both benches cleared, but a bit of shoving was all that happened.

With the bases loaded and the crowd cheering frantically for the relief pitcher to survive, Mike stroked the first pitch he saw into the wind. When Jack looked up from third, he knew it was gone. Mother Nature carried the ball high into the right field upper deck.

The Crowns went on to win, 7-5, ending Buffalo's season. The stadium was cold and silent while the Crowns were on the field celebrating after the last out. The party began on Buffalo's field, and ended in the wee hours of Monday morning. The team crowded into the visiting manager's office and watched Los Angeles survive a close game to end Portland's four year hold on first place in the West. Cris had three hits, and was talking to anyone with a microphone after the nationally televised game.

Djuana flicked off the television and let her head fall back onto the pillow. Loose leaf paper, crumbled and new, was all about the bed. Writing a letter to Jack was murder, but she felt compelled to answer at least one of his steamy love notes. She had tried to concentrate, but her mind would easily drift on the fact that he was a phone call away.
She called her man earlier than she had planned to.
"I saw the LA game," Djuana said as Jack answered the phone in his room.
"Yeah, we did too." Jack was on his back, laid across his bed fully clothed. A bottle of champagne in his left hand, resting on his stomach, while his right hand held the phone to his ear.
"So, you guys aren't going to finish first again."
"Nope, not this year. We have to go straight to Boston, you know? The first game is Tuesday. You want to come?"
"You know I do. But, Tia and I have shopping to do for the wedding."
"Don't worry about it. We will be back Thursday."
"I miss you."
"Djuana, I always miss you."
Djuana blushed. For some reason, she thought about the L.A. game.
"Why does that guy Cris Carpenter on the Trojans hate y'all so much?"
"To tell you the truth, I don't know."
"He said that you and Oscar sold him out to Honeywell."
"He has said a lot of stuff since he left. He wanted me and O to stand up for him, but not only wasn't he hitting, but his attitude stunk."
"He also said that it was wrong of the team to take you back and not Mike Colbert, and trade him."
Jack turned silent. Thoughts of Mike would haunt him for a while, but never did he think he could have done more to get him back on the team.
"I thought this guy was a friend of yours?" Djuana said.
"Yeah. I did too."
"Are you worried about the playoffs?"
"Nope."
"Why not? You said yourself that you guys have a weaker team than ever?"
"Because I have you to love. That's all I need."

Oscar came into their hotel suite moments after Jack hung up from Djuana.

"You still sippin' on that bottle? Give me some."

Jack handed over the bottle. Oscar downed the rest while he undressed.

"Don't tell me you're in for the night?" Jack, with his elbow over his eyes, asked.

"Come on, you know me. I ain't gonna fuck around too much during the playoffs."

Suddenly, there was a light knock at the door.

"As you were saying?" Jack craned his neck up to look at O.

"That ain't for me. You can gamble on that!"

Neither man moved for the door. The person behind the door shuffled, then knocked again with a faint tapping.

"Get that, man!" O said. "You see I'm half naked?"

Jack twirled out of bed and cracked opened the door. Kristen Eisen stood there teary-eyed.

"Hi, Jack," she said, her words choked.

"Hi Kris. What's up?" Jack felt uneasy. Her wet eyes, sliding eye liner and fidgety hands spelled trouble.

"I need to talk with you. It's important."

"What is it?" Jack's eyes blinked slowly, and a smirk grew on his chin.

"Can I come in?" she pointed into the room.

"No. Oscar's here."

"You can come to my room."

Jack stepped out of the room, and closed the door behind him.

"Bring her in here!" O yelled.

Kris began moving toward the elevator.

"No," Jack said. "Let's talk here. I'm not going to your room."

Kris looked around as if in a daze. When she looked into Jack's eyes he could see she her cheeks were raised in a blush.

"This is private, Jack."

"What is it? I thought you weren't speaking to me any more?"

"What gave you that impression?"

"The fact that you haven't said a word to me since I left Miami to be by Djuana's side."

"I have so spoken to you since then."

"Whatever. Just talk. Tell me what's up."

With her hands behind her back, she allowed herself to fall back to the wall opposite Jack's room. She stood there, her hands supporting her buttocks. She began slowly, obviously beating around the bush, yet Jack couldn't figure out what she was trying to say.

"Why you being so short with me?"

"Kris, you know why."

"I don't think what we did at my apartment was wrong," she put on hand to her heart. "I have feelings for you. Have for a long time."

Her hand dropped. "I just never thought you and I should be together because I'm a writer covering the team you play on. Then, I got tired of seeing you hurt. I hate it."

Jack shook his head defiantly. "I'm marrying Djuana. Period."

"You don't know how much I love you, do you?"

"Kris, Djuana is my heart. I love that woman. She loves me and nothing is going to make that change."

"She don't love you," Kris touched Jack's arm lightly. "She don't. She just loves the money. It's a way out for her. She ain't never had anything in her life."

"Look Kris, either we gonna stay friends and you support me, or you gonna stay outta my face with that bullshit.

"It's your choice."

Don came off the elevator and startled both of them. He excused himself and went into his room, the door nearest Kris. Kris leaned up, moving closer to Jack.

She stared in Jack's eyes the minutes Don took to disappear. She saw he was dead serious. She swallowed deeply, then closed her eyes and said: "Jack, I don't know how to say this."

Jack became edgy. "Say what?"

"Ah, I. I haven't had my period in two months," her eyes opened to find Jack unfazed.

"What are you saying?"

"Do I have to spell it out?"

"No, but you need to cut the shit."

"I ain't playing, Jack."

Jack stared down the hall. Three more teammates came off the elevator. They smiled at Jack and nodded to Kris.

"Knock it out the box, New!" Hector yelled as the three players cut between Jack and Kristen.

Ted Garrett giggled, "Giving exclusive interviews? Huh, J-New?"

Kris shook her head as they went into their rooms down the hall.

"Fuck them! You can't tell me you're pregnant by me," Jack said once they were alone again. "That's bullshit."

"You better think back!" Kris stood up to Jack's anger.

He had been, since their conversation began. The sex was enjoyable, and now he could recall her hips on his lap grinding as he came, her arms wrapped around his neck holding on.

"You wanted me to come in you," he said.

"Yes. It was good. But, I didn't think I'd get pregnant, to tell you the truth."

Jack shook his head defiantly and sucked his teeth, "Bullshit."

"What, you think I wanted to get pregnant?"

Jack just continued his piercing stare.

"No, Jack. Don't look at me like that."

"What do you want from me?"

"Of course I want you to be with me, help me raise this baby."

"I can't do that."

"I know, I know. But, I'm going to need you to be the father I know you can be to our baby. You're a great man, Jack Newhouse. A decent man. And, I want our baby to know that personally."

"Shit." Jack fought frustration, hurt and disappointment.

Kris moved to him, attempting to wrap her arms around his neck. Jack pushed her away. "No. Don't fight me."

She grabbed his head and moved it towards her eager lips. "I love you," she whispered.

The sudden sound of a door creaking startled Jack. He turned to see the door to his room close. He moved away from Kris, but she didn't let him go far. The noise had jarred Kris as well, but she hung onto Jack's pullover shirt, yanking it out of his pants.

"Jack, come to my room. I just want to talk."

"Kris, you can't have this baby."

"Why not?"

"You can't."

"I am. And, you'll be there with us. You know it and I know it."

She quickly sprang onto her tippy-toes and kissed Jack on his lips.

"You'll be with us. You'll marry me because you know I can take care of you and your babies. And, you know I'll give you beautiful babies."

"Why you doing this to me, Kris?"

"I don't need to do anything to you. Things happen for a reason. And, now you can be with me."

Jack went back in the room without cutting on a light and plopped on his bed. Oscar was awake, but said nothing.

Hal Juris entered the main clubhouse from the manager's office down the hall beneath Boston's ballpark. The room fell silent. The players were dressed, and ready for the game. He looked into every set of eyes wearing gray, burgundy and gold for what seem like eternity. When he finally addressed his men, the quiet in the room seemed to deepen.

"I shouldn't have to say shit," Juris began. His voice was barely about a whisper. "How many times we been here? This is our month. Our year.

"Las Vegas and Los Angeles are having nightmares about us. They know like I know. We are the best team on the planet and we got our shit together at the right time.

Jack heard every word. He was trying to. He didn't want to think about going back to Portland. He didn't want to think about Djuana's loving arms waiting there for him. He didn't want to think about how fast she would drop him when he told her.

Juris' speech hit the final lap. "Okay, ladies, let's saddle up. There ain't nothing but big asses to ride now. And, all them think we got little dicks 'cause we ain't fuck right the last five months.

"There ain't no more having fun. Ain't no more smiling and fraternizing with player's on the other team. No more grinning when you get a little fucking single. None of that shit.

"Boston ain't never beat us in anything. Now, they feel like top shit because they have a better record, and home field advantage.

"They ain't shit. Fuck them. We gotta ruin them. Destroy them. Make them wanna beat their wives.

"It's time to fuck hard or get fucked."

The first round series was easy for the Portland Crowns; with the nervous, younger Boston Seagulls defeating themselves, basically. The Crowns took advantage of every miscue the Seagulls made. In Boston, the scores were 9-3 and 7-4. The games were not as close as the scores.

The easy wins were a great fog for Jack to hide his hurt. He couldn't sleep or eat. The fear of losing Djuana was haunting his every move. He avoided Kris as best he could. And, since he was not a hero in any of the games, she, nor any other reporter for that matter, didn't need to ask him anything. He rented a car, and was never in his room. He would answer Djuana's pages with dead conversation.

Djuana put off his indifference on the telephone as being focused on playing baseball.

During the five-hour plane trip back to Portland Jack tried to sleep, but couldn't. He tried to read, no bet. He tried daydreaming up a way to tell Djuana without her soft, tender hand knocking his block off, no dice. He was in big trouble.

Oscar had wanted to let Jack simmer on his problems, but he couldn't. O, sitting in the aisle seat, with a seat in between him and Jack, unbuckled his seat belt and plopped down next to Jack.

"Listen New, talk to me, man."

"I'm straight."

O looked around, then whispered, "No you not. You know I know what's up."

Jack looked at O. "You were listening at the door?"

"Naw. Not really, but —"

"You ain't shit."

"Give me a break, will you? You my man, I ain't say shit until now. Have I?"

"Look, O, I really don't want to talk about this."

"She's lying, man."

"I don't know."

"Ask her to have a blood test, and go with her."

Jack exhaled. "Yeah, I was thinking about trying that."

"Yo, I'm telling you. That's the move."

Djuana had detailed plans for Jack's return. The first day back, the Crowns were off while Boston practiced at Adkins, she took him to Washington Park for a picnic. To her delight, it was a unseasonably warm day. She fried chicken and made his favorite salad, potato. She put extra relish in it for him. She also brought her portable cassette player, and had only brought slow music.

Jack didn't want to go out, but he chose to indulge Djuana. Besides, he didn't have the heart to do what he felt he had to do, and he damn sure didn't want Djuana to answer the phone if Kris called.

He followed her to a secluded spot she said she had found years before.

"I used to come here and just sit and think," Djuana said as they set up the blanket. "I would dream of the day I would bring a guy here."

"Why hadn't you brought anybody here before?"

"I guess my heart knew who I should bring to my spot."

While the Impressions crooned one of their least known jams, Jack watched Djuana from across the blanket. The way her shoulders and chest pumped with the doo-wop music soothed Jack. Even the way she ate her chips, one at a time, and always a wide chip, tranquilized his pain. She was a lot to lose. Jack thought he was smiling, but his dim eyes outweighed a light grin.

"Baby, you okay?" Djuana asked, her frown so sudden it brought Jack's back into full bloom.

"I'm fine, as long as I'm with you."

Djuana smiled. "And, where you think I'm going?" She stuck her hand out, Jack moved closer and took it in his.

"Nowhere. I hope."

She pulled Jack by his arm, and he let his body follow. She laid his head in her lap. Jack turned his body so his back would be on the ground. Djuana's fingers on his scalp was the best feeling in the world. Her free hand appear over his face, and her pointer finger outline Jack's lips. When his tongue appear she let him take her finger into his mouth.

They didn't notice a light drizzle begin. Drops of rain hit the leaves, then the grass about them; about the only sound audible. Jack covered Djuana's mouth with his, and manhandled her body. Turned on his side, supported by his left arm, he took in a handful of Djuana's body suit. His warm, soft lips left her mouth desiring more, and fell upon her shoulders. Jack licked and kissed her shoulders, all the while yanking down her sleeves to reveal as much skin as possible.

Jack unbuckled her belt, then flipped her snaps apart on her button-up denim shorts. Djuana grabbed his hands, letting his lips go down her shoulders and chest to her aroused nipples. She panted, moaned, then began pushing him away with little effort.

"No, Jack. Not here, baby. Wait 'til we get home."

The final win to knock Boston out of the playoffs came even easier that the first two. On a damp, cool Friday night, in front of 60,000-plus screaming, chanting Crowns fans wearing gold and burgundy, Portland routed Boston, 18-1, to take the series.

And, no one on the Crowns smiled during the ass-whipping. They were a veteran team going about their jobs expressionless as their manager had ordered. Realistically, they had no choice but to be focused; the Gamblers and Trojans were blowing out their opposition with little resistance as well.

After the game, Djuana met Jack inside Adkins. This had to be that game that snapped his funk, she thought. He was on base every time up, and he played well in the field. She wanted to greet him, then tell him he could hang out with his teammates as he had done before they met; but of course, he had to promise no women would be involved.

She hugged him at the door as he came out. Jack didn't hug her, though. He gave her a light kiss, and moved on to the truck.

"Wait, Jack. I know you gonna kiss me better than that."

Jack blinked. "Shit. I'm sorry, baby."

He pulled her into his arms and tongued her. He squeezed her into his arms hard, kissing her face and apologizing.

Djuana giggled, "Okay, okay!" But, then, she saw her man was serious. "Jack, what is it?"

He wanted to tell her, had every intention of telling her when the team returned to Portland.

"Djuana, I'm going through a tough time right now."

"I know baby, I know you got a lot of pressure on you. It'll be okay. You guys go to the next round now, right?"

"No. It's more than that."

Kris walked out of the stadium into the darkness, straddling her computer and purse. She saw Jack and Djuana hugging, and it burnt her chest. She made sure Jack couldn't see her, walking behind him. She stopped at the couple, they were now holding hands.

"You ready to talk?" she said, not looking at Jack.

Djuana thought nothing of it.

"Why you doing this, Kris?" Jack glared. The anger in his voice startled Djuana.

"Did you tell her that I'm pregnant?"

Djuana let go of Jack's hand. He turned to her, she looked at him and backed away. Djuana turned to walk away.

"No, Djuana," Jack started after her, but Kris dropped her computer bag and grabbed Jack.

"No, Jack, please! Let her go, I love you!"

Jack pushed Kris as hard as he could, and as she fell to the ground she held on to his button-down shirt, popping buttons and pulling it out of his jeans. Jack bent to punch her, but he couldn't. He unballed his fist and pinched her forearm. Kris reached for him, trying to grab hold, but dug her nails into his face.

Angry, Jack shoved her completely to the ground.

"No, Jack, please don't go," Kris cried.

Many people saw, but no one moved until Jack raced out of the parking lot. They gathered around Kris, she was fuming, causing her eyes to flame. She watched Jack run for his life after Djuana, realizing as guards and players helped her up, that he would never love her that way.

Jack ran to the bus stop, his first instinct. He hailed down a bus pulling off. It stopped, and he jumped on the crowded downtown special as soon as the doors opened. He walked in, and down the aisle. The driver had a horrified look, as did the passengers as he made his way. His voice was cracked, throat choked and he was near out of breath, so when he spoke, he sounded like a mute.

After a few seconds he could see Djuana was not on the bus. He slowly got off, oblivious to the talk that he began. He saw the cop rushing to him, but, he kept moving.

"You okay, Mr. Newhouse?" the officer asked.

"Yeah. I'm fine," then a thought came to his mind. "My fiancee and I had an argument, she's gone. I can't find her."

"We'll look for her, for you. You just take it easy."

Jack wondered why the cop stared at his face so peculiarly. Then, he remembered the stares on the bus. He touched his cheeks, and felt a sting on his left cheek, then wetness. He brought his hand down and saw the blood.

## 40

Jack sat quietly in the passenger's seat while Oscar ripped up the Foothills Freeway. The black Porsche did not go less than 90 miles per hour. He darted in and out of traffic singing along with the blaring music. The car cruised off the exit leading to Jack's place doing 75.

"Man, my shit is all fucked." Jack said, hiding his eyes with an open hand.

"No man, look," O said, turning in the driver's seat to face Jack. "You need to just gather yourself. You know what's happening. Kris is lyin'."

O continued, "Take my word for it, Chief. She probably thought like everybody else, that you wouldn't marry Djuana. Now, she makin' her move, trying to throw a wrench in shit so she can be Mrs. Newhouse."

"Where you get that from?"

"Man, I've watched that chick for years. She ain't nothing but poor white trash actin' like she got something. I peeped her game the first time I saw her. She wants to marry money."

Oscar swerved the car onto Jack's driveway. "You remember Joey? She tried to get him like that, told him she was pregnant before he got traded. But, you see, Joey was bonin' that shit everyday. He thought it was his, and I think he was going to marry her. But, when he got traded, all of a sudden her period came."

Jack unbuckled himself, and opened the door. His frown had spread to a scowl. "Wait a minute. You telling me that she did this shit to Joey?"

O got out of the car, keys in hand. "Yep."

"Where the fuck was I?"

They walked up the stairs to the house.

"Man, you don't pay attention to shit happening like I do."

"You mean, I don't gossip like you do."

When they got to the front door, Jack recalled he didn't have his keys. "We have to go around back."

"Damn! Does she have your wallet and checkbook too?"

"Suck my nuts, and come on."

O continued his lecture while they walked to the back of the house, "I ain't gonna ask you why she has all your shit."

"Then don't."

"Don't worry about Djuana, she loves you. She just don't want to be a fool again. When she finds out that it was just a scam, she'll be back.

"You see, Djuana don't understand that women are going to be after her man for a long time."

Jack glared an understanding stare at O as he slid the patio door open.

Oscar followed him in, changing the focus of his conversation instantly. "Why don't you lock this shit, sometime. This ain't New York, but this ain't paradise either."

"Whatever," Jack mumbled. He walked into his home hoping against all doubt that Djuana would be there. He didn't care if she hit him, cursed him, or even stabbed him, as long as she was there. Still there for him.

She wasn't.

Oscar went directly to the kitchen and took out two beers. "What you should do is kick Kris' ass. Fuck that bitch up."

Jack took one of the beers from O, and they sat in the living room. Oscar cut on the stereo.

"You hear me?" Oscar whined.

Jack gulped beer, popping the bottle out of his mouth and causing foam to rise up the long neck. "It ain't that easy."

"Maybe, what you should do is call her editors, get that bitch fired."

"Oh, yeah, who they going to believe, a pure white bread woman, or a nigger like me?"

"Then, bust her ass, like I said the first time."

Thane put his arms around Tia, and she warmed to his touch.

"So, do I finally get to see all of you, baby?"

His deep voice spawn goose bumps up and down Tia's slender arms.

"I think you've been good enough to get a peek," Tia cooed. She stood off his sofa and slowly began unbuttoning her oversized, flannel, button-up shirt. She undid each button with her eyes blazing through Thane.

He stood, finally, and pushed the shirt off her shoulders. The six-foot-six, solidly built Oregon State prison guard licked and kissed each one of Tia's bony shoulders. Then he swooped her off her feet with ease. He carried Tia's thin body into his bedroom. He let her fall on his bed, then undressed while she watched.

When Tia reached for her belt buckle, he barked at her to stop. The sudden order startled her.

"I'll do it," he commanded.

And, when he was down to his bikini briefs, he kneeled onto the bed and feverishly stripped Tia. She panted, and rubbed and caressed his defined muscles.

"Thane don't hurt me," Tia's faint voice pleaded. "Please be easy, it's been awhile."

Thane grunted, then grabbed Tia above her ankles; his coarse fingers locked to the bone and parted her legs. Then, the phone rang. By the third buzz, Thane was finished.

The answering machine picked up, and after the music and Thane's quick line, Tia heard the voice of her sister over Thane's heavy breathing next to her in the bed.

"It's my sister," she said.

"Don't answer it," Thane ordered, holding her arm.

"Let me just see what she wants?"

Tia dived over Thane, and picked up the phone to hear the click. She quickly dialed her home number.

"You know I want more," Thane uttered. His hand reached up to touched Tia's breasts.

Tia turned away as her sister answered.

"What's up?" Tia said.

Anesa, holding Tia's cordless, walked out of Tia's bedroom, leaving her mother to console Djuana. "I'm sorry to cut in, but Djuana is here, and she's crying like crazy. Me and Mommy are trying, but we can't get her to stop, or say anything."

"What happened?"

"All I can tell is something bad with Jack."

"Oh my God," Tia exhaled, covering herself with the sheet, and looking for her knee-highs.

"What should I do?"

"I'll be right there."

Tia hung up the phone, stood up and gathered her clothes off the floor. "I have to get home, my friend is there, she had some kind of argument with her fiancee."

"So?" Thane said, still laying in bed. "Why you have to go?"

"She's my best friend, she would do it for me."

Thane sat up, "This the one marrying the baseball player?"

"Yes, Djuana," Tia said, standing in her jeans and buckling them. "Can you drive me home?"

"Give me some more first."

"Thane. I have to go."

Thane's ride cruised up to Tia's family home in the Sellwood section of Portland. He rolled up onto the driveway of the Williams' place, one of the many large, restored Victorian homes in Sellwood.

"You coming in?" Tia she, reaching to open her door.

Thane put the car and park and rolled his eyes. "No thanks. You don't need me in there."

Tia stopped herself, and turned to Thane to give him a good-bye kiss. He grabbed her breast, and pinched her nipple.

Tia winced. "You have to be so rough?"

"You know you love it," he smiled. "When I'm going to get some more?"

Tia frowned, "I don't love it when you are rough with me."

Thane laughed. "Okay. Fine. Am I going to see you tomorrow?"

"Call me," Tia shortly replied.

Tia walked through the house to find it quiet and empty. She went upstairs, and again no one. She opened the door to her bedroom, expecting to find her best friend crying in her sister's lap. Instead, Djuana was asleep in her bed, her back to the door.

Now, Tia was mad.

It took Jack a good 40 minutes to find Tia's phone number while Oscar slept on the couch. He dialed it quickly, anticipating a conversation with the one person he knew could talk for him. But, as the phone rang, he wondered if Tia would this time.

"Hi, Jack," Tia said without emotion. "Djuana is here, but she doesn't want to talk to you."

Jack squeezed his glass of scotch. "How is she?"

"Jack, just give her some time."

Jack closed his eyes. "How is she?"

Tia paused. She looked over at Djuana's body under the covers in her bed. "She's fine. You hurt her, just give her some time."

"Yeah, I know I hurt her. For what it's worth, just tell her that I have never loved anyone like I love her. And I never will."

Tia was silent when Jack hung up.

He sat still for a long moment, holding the phone on his shoulder, near his ear. He then knew he would never hear from Djuana Pioneer again. His hand tightened around the cordless until he had all his strength centered on his hand. His hand shook, his teeth gritted, and his head pumped, but the phone didn't break, frustrating him all the more. He threw it against the wall above his stereo. It broke then.

Kris parked in front of her brownstone, oblivious to the Porsche parked across St. Clair. She opened her trunk and took the bags of groceries out. She started up the cement steps, her eyes and hands searching her handbag for the house keys, struggling to keep a handle on the two plastic bags. By the time she reached the top, she could smell the alcohol.

"You gotta be happy now," Jack said, standing down the steps.

Kris turned slowly, edging the bags to her side, away from Jack. He had been drinking, and with his temper, she knew he could kill her if he saw the box of Stayfree maxi pads on top of the bag in her left hand.

"No," she said, fighting fright and nerves. "Why should I be?"

Jack shrugged his shoulders, "I thought maybe because you got what you wanted."

"You really think I wanted to hurt you?"

"You did."

"Why don't you come in, Jack. We can talk inside, and I can put down these bags."

She turned to the door and struggled to put the key in.

"Naw, no. I might have twins then. I thought I'd come over here and beat the living shit out of you. Maybe even snap your neck. But now, I just feel like saying fuck it."

Kris' heart fell into her stomach. She dropped the bags inside, and stood in the doorway.

Jack turned to leave, walking off her stoop, but turned back.

"I just don't give a fuck anymore," he laughed. "You know something? You were right, all I had to do was be patient. I could die tonight and be happy because I found that one I was looking for."

He looked away and fought tears. "I just couldn't keep her, that's all."

Kris came down the steps. "Come on, Jack. Come with me, you've been drinking. I'm not going to let you drive."

"Right," Jack nodded feverishly as she neared him. "Now you care? Fuck you."

Kris took his left arm. "Come upstairs, Jack."

Her calm voice and light touch struck a nerve. Jack snatched her throat and pinned her to the Porsche. He held her in place, with his right hand's fingers wrapped tightly around her neck, and his left hand holding her right arm down on the car. She was squirming, and gasping for air, but he just glared down and her.

"Tell me why I shouldn't kill you?"

She began crying, pleading. Jack couldn't sustain his anger, listening to her. He let up his hold a bit, and fought off his tears.

"Why you do this to me?"

"I love you," Kris cried. "I love you."

Jack squeezed harder, she gagged. "Don't say that," he cried.

Djuana opened her eyes and was surprised to see she was nose-to-nose with Tia. She watched her friend for a second or two, listening to her light snoring, and admiring her clear, soft skin. Djuana turned onto her back and fixed her eyes onto the ceiling. Once again, she had to gather the pieces of her life and press on.

Unconsciously, her fingers twirled in her own curls while she pictured life without Jack. It would not be easy, she knew, but it had come to this. She had to leave him. She had to get Tia to borrow her father's car and help her move her things out of Jack's house. She had to pack her things and say good-bye.

Good-bye.

The word reminded her of when Jack had used it when he found out she was pregnant. He said, not meaning it as the end, but she told him not to use the term because it meant forever. She didn't want to lose him then, and she was realizing she didn't want to lose him at all, ever.

But, how many times could she be a fool? How many times can a man spring up with another relationship that she was clueless to? It can't keep happening. She can't keep allowing men the space to have another entire relationship while she was dedicated.

"Dammit," She bit her fist, the skin on her pointer finger just beneath her knuckle.

The darkness in the room was comforting, though. Tia, although dead asleep, would not be able to see the tears if she should turn in her slumber. Djuana reached onto the nightstand and retrieved the box of tissue. She tried to blow her nose quietly, and used another to wipe her eyes.

"You wanna talk?"

Tia's voice, although a faint whisper, startled Djuana.

"No. You can go back to sleep."

Tia sat up, behind Djuana. She was happy her friend wasn't ready to talk about Jack. It would be tit-for-tat; Tia had a problem with a man for the first time in a while, and wanted to get it off her chest with Djuana.

"No, I can't sleep. I had a nightmare."

Djuana smirked, "About my life?"

"No," Tia plopped her pillow behind her, up against the headboard, and sat back on it. "This guy I'm dating. He is not gentle in anything."

Tia looked down at Djuana, who still had her back to her.

*Gentle.*

Djuana let the word sink into her thoughts. Jack was always gentle, her mind reminisced. He would always caress her body, something she had craved for life. His kisses were always on time. How could she leave him?

Tia's eyes became focused in the dark, she was gazing across her room into the mirror mounted on a dresser. "I'm getting sick of guys who just want to bang, and that's it."

"Is that what your dream was about?"

"Yeah. I dreamt he had me pinned down and was cursing and slapping me."

Djuana's eyes widened, she was still facing away from Tia. "Did he do that to you?" she asked.

"No."

Djuana exhaled, rolled her eyes and shook her head.

"But," Tia continued, "He acts like he wants to."

Djuana turned onto her back. "Some women like that."

"I don't. I mean, I like it hard, in a nice rhythm, but Thane be drilling for oil."

"He is a big guy." Djuana pictured his muscular frame pounding Tia's slim body, her legs as wide as can be.

"You better believe it! Huge."

"So, you tried to tell him that it hurts?"

"Every time I do, he just picks up speed. Or, if it's afterward, he smiles, talking about I know I like it."

"Maybe it's time for a long talk, away from the bed."

"No. I'm just going to cut off his supply for a while."

Djuana smiled, and it felt good.

Tia slid down to face her friend. "So, now that we cleared up that matter, what happened with you and Jack?

"He called last night while you were sleep."

"I bet he did," Djuana frowned hard. "What he tell you?"

"To make sure I tell you he loves you more than anybody he had ever loved."

Djuana shook her head.

"What happened, Dee?"

"I'm surprised you ain't hear."

"Ansea told me he got that reporter pregnant. I can't believe that."

"Believe it. She just walked up to us, and blurted it out. She asked Jack if he had told me yet, like he had known for awhile."

Tia leaned her elbow on the pillow. "What Jack say?"

"Nothing. He was just frozen. He knew he was busted. He had been acting funny for a few days."

"Shit."

"Tell me about it," Djuana dropped an arm on her forehead.

"So, you going to leave him for this?"

"Why not? He was going to keep it from me. I ain't gonna marry him and he done got somebody else pregnant. How that look?

"And, he had to have been screwing her recently."

"Djuana. Did y'all talk about it?"

"I don't want to hear any bullshit. There's nothing he can say. What can he say? I'm sorry?"

"Djuana? Hear him out."

"No. Fuck him."

"You know you don't mean that."

"How you know?" Djuana turned, and got out of the bed. "He ain't never going to get fucking whoever he wants out of his system. Once a dog, always a dog. Just like my mother said."

Tia watched Djuana angrily plop into the winged chair. Tia slid onto the spot where Djuana had slept, and let her feet hit the floor.

"Jack is not like that, and you know it."

"Have you been listening?" Djuana said through the darkness. "He went and got somebody else pregnant!"

"How you know she's not lying?"

"Everybody thought I was."

"Ain't no everybody," Tia became animated. "Just one asshole. And, Jack stood by you all the way. Even though you had trouble telling him."

"Who side you on? Huh? Just tell me that?"

"You wrong. You should hear him out. That man has loved you through a lot of thick and thin. He deserves the same."

"I'm tired of being a fool," Djuana's voice lowered.

"Then don't be one. If you love him, act like it. Go stand by him. That man loves you, I can tell. He was hurting on the phone last night. He tells you how much he misses you every night when he's on the road."

Djuana, offended, became defensive. "Oh, men don't lie?"

"When he comes back, he shows you just how much he misses you, right?"

"It's so easy for you to say because you want a man like that. But, if it was you a man had done this to, you would have dropped him like a bad habit."

"I don't know that."

"Sure you don't," Djuana angrily nodded. Her voice lowered to a faint whisper, a mumble. "I'm sick of trusting men. Sick of it."

"Juanny, don't you know women can see what you have? They know Jack is a good man. He's got money, good looks and he carries himself well."

"So?"

"So, the grass is always greener."

"Why you making excuses for him?"

"Because I know he loves you."

Tia could see through the darkness Djuana had begun to cry. She got up from the bed, slowly, and dropped to her knees at Djuana's feet. Djuana fell back into the chair sobbing. Tia moved to the side of the chair, Djuana's right, and took Djuana's hand. She kissed it, and Djuana felt her tears.

"I know you love him. Just go to him and hear his side of the story. That's all I'm asking you to do."

Don stood up from the long bench in the hall of the Portland's detention center when he saw Jack approaching. He watched Jack rip open the manila envelope, put his wallet in his back pocket, and latch his watch on.

"You all right, Poppy?"

Jack said nothing, barreling through the revolving doors. He was oblivious to the reporters, cameras and lights. Jack and Don jogged down the jail's steps; the media moved with them.

"My car is over here," Don said, pointing in the opposite of Jack's tracks.

"Naw, I have to go get O's Porsche or he'll kill me."

"Let me drive you. Come on."

Jack glanced down at his watch, 2:37 a.m. He had spent two hours in jail. Jack walked with Don to his Land Cruiser, first Don took the baby seat out of the front passenger's spot. They rode to St. Clair.

"She dropped the charges," Don said, between yawns.

"So, you didn't need to come down and bail me out. I'm sorry I got you out of bed for nothing."

"Don't be."

When they got to the Porsche, Don watched Jack carefully.

"I'm going to follow you home," he said out of his driver's window as Jack got into the car.

"I don't need an escort, Don."

"Yeah, but I don't need to get home too quick."

Jack slammed the car door.

Oscar greeted them on the driveway. "Where the fuck you been? You go out and leave me here?"

Jack got out the same time as Don did. "Here's your keys, sorry."

O just stared at him. He looked to Don, "Is that all he's going to say? What you doing here? Y'all went out together and said fuck me?"

"You acting like a wife. Shut up." Don followed Jack into the house.

O, stunned, stood there a second, then darted up the stairs and into the house.

"So, is somebody going to tell me what happened? You guys go out or something?"

Don went into the kitchen, took down a glass, and filled it with ice and water. Jack disappeared into his bedroom. Oscar followed Don into the kitchen, where Don was sitting at the table staring at his glass. "The cops found your boy with his hands around Kristen Eisen's neck," he said as soon as he saw O.

"He kill her?"

Don finished his water and bellowed a satisfying sigh. "No, stupid."

"He should have. You know that bitch is lying, right?"

"Yeah, probably. But he shouldn't have fucked her."

"If she was throwing your old ass some leg, you would have sucked it dry."

"True," Don said, pointing a finger at Oscar. "But, I wouldn't have fucked her."

The phone rang, and before it could ring again, Jack dashed into the kitchen and snatched it off its cradle.

"Hello? Yeah. Nothing. Fine. Whatever. No, I don't give a fuck, actually."

O whispered to Don, "Who that?"

Don shrugged and poured more water.

Suddenly, Jack threw the phone across the living room.

"You breaking up all your phones, New," O said.

"Who was that?" Don asked.

"Honeywell," Jack said, glumly. "I have been fined and suspended."

Jack let himself fall back on the doorway leading from the kitchen to the hall. He rubbed his temples, and whispered, "I'll miss the first game in L.A."

Don and Oscar silently gazed in different directions, as if what Jack said was a empty statement.

# 41

The next morning, a misty, cool Sunday, Djuana cooked breakfast for the Williams family. After the talk with Tia in the middle of the night, Djuana couldn't go back to sleep. She stayed up, sitting on the back porch watching the sun fight its way through the clouds. She began cooking at eight-thirty, right after her favorite cartoon.

She had always thought it was incredible that Barney Rubble could make her laugh no matter what mood she was in.

Bernadette, Tia's mom, was the first to join Djuana in the kitchen. She was wearing a velvet jogging suit with a royal crest on the breast and tennis shoes donning the same crest. When she entered the kitchen, the stove was in full use, each burner held a pan or saucer, and Djuana was mixing a batter of pancakes.

"Now, you know you don't have to do all this," Bernadette said. She took a fork and turned the crisping bacon.

"I just felt like cooking. It gave me something to do until everybody got up."

Bernadette gazed at Djuana. When she turned into full view, Bernadette could see the bags under Djuana's eyes. "You didn't sleep well, did you?"

"Not exactly. But, I'm fine."

While Djuana poured the batter into the frying pan, she could feel Bernadette's eyes piercing through her. She continued working the stove, trying to ignore Tia's mother, hoping she wouldn't slip in a lecture.

She did. Bernadette was waiting for this chance. She had watched the television, read the newspapers, and believe she knew enough about Jack and Djuana to be of help to them. But, Tia, nor her father, would let her Bernadette get involved. So, with the rest of her family upstairs, Bernadette pinned Djuana down.

"Have you and Jack Newhouse broken up?"

Djuana bristled. She looked at Bernadette, whose eyes were fixed on Djuana's lips. "No. We need to talk about some things, but no, we haven't broken up yet."

"Why do you say yet?"

Djuana's left hand went to her hip, and she rested on it. Her right hand fiddled with the spatula and the pancakes. She stared at the four gold circles, mulling over the question.

"Don't let Satan break you two up. That man loves you, and the two of you have had to fight through so much that it would be a shame to see you to let some, some, sinner wedge between you.

"That's all that woman is, is a sinner. One of Satan's servants sent to keep garrison on you."

Djuana flipped the four pancakes, the last one broke, though, and stuck to the side of the pan.

"You have to remain strong, you have fought off Satan so many times, don't stop now. Everything the sinner has - time, strength, cunning - is spent to keep the devil on his throne. Don't give them the satisfaction."

Djuana, her eyes still only looking at Bernadette momentarily, finally spoke. Her voice was controlled; she forced respect and into each word.

"Mrs. Williams, I understand what you are saying, and I appreciate where you are coming from, but Jack has done something that I can't exactly take in stride. He cheated on me with someone I see every time I go to the stadium. Now she's pregnant by him.

"I just can't forget and forgive that easily."

"I have seen how people have reacted to you dating him since the beginning. Your mother didn't like it, and many of his teammates didn't either. People were saying you were a golddigger, were they right?

"People said he was a womanizer, a dog. Has he been?"

"No, but -"

"He hasn't. That man loves you, and what you don't understand is that Satan has enough devils to harass the whole earth. He can send a legion just to surround one person with enough doubt to not be a doctor, not be a lawyer, not be happy with a person they know they love."

Although Djuana had to scurry to get a plate to put the pancakes on, her heart was touched. What was being pointed out was clear.

"Yes, he had sex with this woman. He might have gotten her pregnant, although I seriously doubt it, but I saw the way this man was when you were in the hospital. He felt your pain like only a man in deep, true love would have.

"Sometimes men can be so weak. But, one has to take the situation for what it is. Get both sides, see what really happened. See where his mind was."

Djuana put the plate with the fresh pancakes in the oven. She poured more batter into the pan. She poured grits into the boiling water, then removed the sizzling, dark bacon.

"Why, Leonard will tell you," Bernadette continued, "Jack Newhouse is the only professional athlete playing in this city that I have seen interacting with our youth. Now, this does not make him an angel, but because he has given so much of himself, nobody has ever turned their backs on him no matter what he has done. The whole city rallied around him to get him back on the Crowns. Nobody is going to do that for Oscar Taylor. No way."

"Hmm, I can't think of a white player anybody here would do that for."

"Maybe you're right," Djuana finally said, leaning on the counter near the stove. "I should have listen to his side, or given him a chance to tell me what happen and what it was all about. I know he's a good man, and I know he loves me. But, all I could think about was, here I go again."

"Do you love him?"

Djuana nodded, "Very much."

"Do you trust him?"

Djuana paused, then worried if she should have answered that question immediately. She was ashamed to admit that all along she trusted Jack, but didn't want to seem like a fool to her family.

"It's difficult to have a relationship without trust," Bernadette interjected.

"I trust him. I do. I just let other people pull me away from him when he needed me."

Bernadette smiled a proud gleam, she walked around Djuana and took the banana phone off the hook. "Call him. Right now and tell him."

Djuana accepted the phone.

"Take it in the dining room, it'll reach. I'll finish breakfast."

Djuana sat at the foot of the rectangular, drop-leaf dining table. She mindlessly dialed the number, then sat back in the upright, wooden armchair. While the phone rang, she thought about what to say. Before she could decide her own voice came over the answering machine.

She said to the machine. "Jack, I really want to hear what's going on from you, I am at Tia's, and I will be there in an hour or two."

She paused, feeling her throat clog. She swallowed, then said, "I love you, bye."

After breakfast, and while Djuana was getting dressed, Tia ran into the bedroom and cut on the television.

"Your mother just called! Jack was arrested last night!"

Djuana closed her eyes, holding them shut as the reporter rambled on. She opened them to the sight of Jack and Don darting through a gang of media types.

Tia looked away from the telecast and at Djuana. "He tried to kill her."

"I don't think so, Tee. If he had, she wouldn't have dropped the charges so quickly."

"I don't know. Maybe the team told her to. They are in the playoffs, you know?"

Djuana blocked out Tia. She listened to the male anchor.

"...Jack Newhouse had an alcohol level of three point zero at the time of his arrest..."

"Damn," Djuana exhaled.

"...In a written statement released early this morning, the Crowns announced Newhouse will be fined and suspended for the first game in Los Angeles."

"Damn, damn, damn," Djuana moaned. "I can't believe all this."

"The Crowns are in trouble" Tia said. "They are going to need him against L.A."

The anchor switched to a reporter at the Portland airport standing near the boarding Crowns players. He interviewed a few of them, not Jack though.

"We all know Jack and we all know Kristen," said Danny Gross to the camera. "But, we don't know all of the story."

"I'm going to L.A.," Djuana blurted. "I'm going to get the Pathfinder and drive."

"No, that's a 19, 20 hour drive," Tia pointed out. "He'll be back Wednesday, right."

"I can't wait that long."

"Then fly."

"I don't have the..." *Money*. Djuana recalled the credit card he had left for use in case of an emergency. It was at his house.

Tia shook her head, "Just call him tonight, then you'll see him when he comes back."

"I have to go to his house, can you take me?"

Djuana had been in Jack's den once, and that was when he showed her where the credit card would be if she ever needed it. She recalled how she objected, not wanting anything from him but his love.

"That's fine and dandy," Jack smiled and said. "But, if I am out of town and you feel you need anything, you take this card and use it. I don't care what it's for."

She opened the top draw of Jack's roll-top desk, and saw a green business sized envelope with the *American Express* logo on the top left corner, opposite where a stamp would go. She felt the card inside. She opened it and was stunned to see her name on the gold card. Also, there was a small slip of paper folded in half. It read, simply: "I love you."

The Crowns charter to Los Angeles was delayed two hours before take-off. The line on the runway reminded Jack of the traffic during the bus ride over. Everything was moving slowly. Was it because it was Sunday, or because he missed Djuana?

Oscar was asleep, his head inches from Jack's, before the plane took off. Neither of them, O, Jack or Don had gone to sleep after Jack was released. Don had to go home to greet his daughters as they woke with breakfast, something he did before every road trip. O drove Jack to his mansion where he packed and changed clothes for the trip.

But, when the plane was in the air, Oscar looked over to Jack, who was still peering out the window, and struck up a conversation.

"While you were out trying to kill Kris, I called So."

Jack's head spun to face O. Oscar's eyes were fixed on the clouds. The voice of a stewardess passed them, and O twirled to it.

"I need a beer," he said as she passed.

Jack was uneasy. He watched his friend for a sign; did the conversation go well?

"What did she say?" Jack couldn't wait.

The stewardess handed O a beer, plastic cup and napkin. O popped it open and gulped as much as he could before filling the cup.

"Not a God damn thing," O finally said. "Her mother said she was out with some guy. You believe that shit?"

"Shit. I don't know."

O continued to drink from the can. "Do you blame her? If she had done half the shit I did to her, I'd have killed her."

"Yeah, I know."

"I love her, New. I really do. But, the bitch scares me."

"I know you love her."

"I mean, shit," he took another swig. "You know I married the pussy. She's fucking beautiful. The best looking woman I had ever seen. I just wanted to rent the pussy, wear that tight shit out."

Jack sat silently, watching Oscar tell the story he already knew. Oscar's head was back against the rest between drinks, occasionally, he would look at Jack, but mostly he avoided eye contact.

"I always thought she'd leave me, take half my money and divorce me. I never thought she would love me so much. The bitch loved me like crazy."

Oscar sat up, edging himself toward Jack, "I miss her, man."

"To hell with telling me, tell her. Call her when we get to L.A."

"Ahhh, please," O waved off Jack. "I can't, you know better than that. She ain't gonna believe me. She ain't never gonna trust me. Never."

Game time was 6 p.m. in Los Angeles. On the East coast, it was a prime time game, coming on the tube live at 9 p.m. The players were at the ballpark at three, around the same time as Djuana's flight landed in the city. The foul territory near home plate was infested with reporters during batting practice. And, it seemed, everyone had to speak with Jack Newhouse.

Jack, who was wearing his Crowns pants, cap, t-shirt, jacket and street sneakers, was calm, more subdued than anyone expected. But, the writers and television and radio reporters were animated. They pushed and shoved to get in better position as Jack stood there shaking his head. He was surrounded completely, standing maybe 10 feet from the batting cage. He took a quick visual survey of them to see if Kris was among them, and he was neither happy nor sad to not see her.

## LOVE'S HOME RUN

"Better not get too close," one of the L.A. players shouted from the first base side of the cage, "He fucks reporters, then he chokes them!"

Oscar, standing on the Crowns side of the webbed cage, shouted, "At least he gets laid!"

"Listen," Jack began, and cameras snapped. "I am only going to answer baseball related questions. That's it."

A frail looking man, Jack recalled seeing at least once before, threw out a question before his colleagues seemed ready, "Do you feel you have let down your teammates before the start of a series in which the Crowns will need to play above their heads to defeat the Trojans?"

"No. We have defeated them in the playoffs before. We can do it again."

"Are you going to play Tuesday?" another reporter fired out.

"I expect to."

"Is this your last season as a Portland Crown?"

"When the season is over, I will sit down and go over all my options."

"With Djuana Pioneer?" a male reporter shouted.

"Are you still getting married?" an attractive female pointed her black "Entertainment Tonight" microphone over another reporter and at Jack.

"Baseball related only," Jack said, giving her a easy smile.

"Just a yes or no?" Ms. ET drowned out other questions. "Did you hear Kristen Eisen recanted her story?"

Jack began moving away. "That's it. No more. I'm done."

Dozens of questions blew by his ears, but he could clearly hear that woman from the gossip station.

"She's been fired! She said she made it up! Give me a comment, Mr. Newhouse."

Jack removed his cap and darted into the clubhouse. He sat at his locker, in the quiet, hollow room. One teammate was getting rubbed down in the trainer's room, everybody else was on the field. He wanted to let loose a long sigh of relief, but, he wondered, what if that reporter was lying? He had to know.

Jack looked around, and saw Oscar had his cellular in his locker. He removed it, flicked the flip-top open and dialed Kristen's number from memory. He was wrong. He searched his locker for his phone book. It was back in his room at the hotel.

"Shit."

Djuana knew her day was going too well to be true. She got on a flight seconds after getting to the airport. She only had to call two hotels before finding the Crowns; and that hotel had a suite for her. But, when she got to the stadium, after a $22 cab ride, the game was sold out.

She tried to buy a ticket from scalpers outside the ballpark, but none of their prices were under $200 dollars. She ended up going to a sports bar a mile away from the stadium and sipping two glasses of wine through the three hour game. She was surprise that the crowd, mostly men, were more into the game than the women; especially herself. Although one man did send over the bartender with her second glass of wine when the Los Angeles Trojans scored three runs in the fourth inning.

It was tough for her to pay attention to the game since Jack was not playing. And, the Crowns were losing throughout. Every so often the crowd at the bar would erupt, Djuana would look up at one of the many large screen TVs and see more Trojans scoring. She watched men hug each other, high-five each other and declare Los Angeles the best team in baseball.

The Crowns lost game one of the series to the Trojans, 9-2. Djuana left the bar before the game was over. She had made up her mind to surprise Jack at the hotel, instead of at the ballpark; she reasoned that his demeanor would be better away from that place.

The Crowns got off the team bus in front of the Hilton in silence; most were pleased Juris had lost his voice arguing with umpires. Oscar was walking gingerly, leaning on Jack. Jack's replacement in right field, Hector Aponte, stepped on O's ankle in the outfield while they chased one of the many hard hit balls off of Danny.

At the elevators, Aponte tried to apologize once again, but O cursed him out.

"When I go for a ball, you freeze! Don't move," Oscar said, limping to get in the kid's face. "'Cause if I can't catch it, it won't be caught!"

The sound of Juris' cracking howl silenced the lobby. "Any of you leave this hotel tonight, and I will personally beat the living shit out of you and your roommate."

Jack answered the door to his and Oscar's room in a t-shirt and jeans. The woman at door was wearing a dark baby doll dress that reached the top of her bronzed thighs, with heels and lots of makeup. Before the outfit, her height was the first thing that caught Jack's attention. She was at least 6-foot-3, because Jack had to stand his full height to be at eye level.

"Hi, is O here?" the woman's voice squeaked, and her smile revealed her age.

Jack looked back at Oscar, who was sitting on the couch with his foot in a electric foot tub. "Your daughter is here."

"Let her in, man!" O barked. "My foot swoll 'cause you benched, and you got nerve to make jokes?"

"How old are you," Jack said after he close the door, frowning.

"Old enough to fuck without getting stuck," she replied near emotionless.

Oscar took the woman's hand, guiding her onto the couch next to him. "Who are you?" Oscar demanded, "My priest?"

"Whatever," Jack said.

"What's the matter with him?" she watched Jack go into his bedroom.

Oscar took his foot out of the warm water. "Don't worry about him."

"He's Jack Newhouse, right?"

Oscar nodded, now limping into the bathroom with the foot whirlpool.

"I feel sorry for him. What that reporter did to him was wrong."

"Yeah, I know. Sad, so sad. Now go in my room and get naked."

Jack listened to the phone ring, wondering if Oscar would answer it if he let it ring. No, but the thought gave his frown a rest. Jack clicked the sound down on the X-rated movie and rolled across his bed. He snatched the receiver off its cradle.

"Yeah?"

A cheery voice replied, "This is the hotel lobby, Jack Newhouse, please?"

"Yeah, you got me," Jack sat up. "What?"

"There is a message here for you. I forgot to give it to you when you came in."

"Who is it from?"

"Sir, it's sealed, and I am only supposed to give it to you."

"Throw it away."

"No. I mean, sir, you would want to see this," the concierge said.

Jack exhaled into the phone. He sat up in the bed. "All right. Open it and read it to me. If it's from a hoe, you can have her."

The desk guy laughed, "Okay, sir, but it isn't. I'm sure of that."

Jack felt like he could hear the fellow smiling along with the sound of paper ruffling.

"It says: 'My problem is I love you and I don't know how to handle it. If you love me, I'm in room twenty-one seventeen'.

"Sir, it's signed, Djuana Newhouse."

Djuana tried to stay awake, but the long day finally caught up with her. She was laid across the soft spread on the king-size bed, nude. She was snoring faintly in the dark room with the oldies station playing love music softly. She had bought a silk robe, panties and bra from the shop in the large lobby of the hotel, but she was too tired to bother putting any of it on.

Jack was about to give up after the third set of rapping knocks he laid on the door. But, when he pressed his ear to the door, he heard stirring. Djuana was panicking behind the thick, wooden door. She rubbed her fingers together, trying to collect herself. She grabbed the robe off the chair, darted into the bathroom and threw water on her face. She feverishly patted it off with a towel.

In the mirror, she brushed her hair; the curls just fell. She closed the robe around her nude body, hoping the long bath she had taken had not worn off. As she came to the door, the knocks came again. She flipped on the light switch near the door, and sprang onto her toes to look through the peephole. She tied the robe's wrap around her waist.

She opened the door wide, revealing her room. "Come in, Jack."

Jack watched her as he came in, thinking her attractiveness would never cease. She closed the door and came around Jack into the suite. He noticed in a quick glimpse that she was not wearing anything under the deep purple robe.

Djuana searched his face for a clue of his temperament. He seemed even, not smiling, but not angry.

"I'm sorry I walked away from you," she said, breaking the awkward silence.

"It's okay," Jack glumly said. "I might've done the same thing."

Although not evident, Jack was choking on his emotions, wanting to grab Djuana and squeeze her until all his frustrations were released.

"No," Djuana said, moving toward Jack in the center of the room. "I should have heard you out."

"No, look I was the wrong one."

Djuana's toes pushed her to his height. "Let me apologize." With her arms holding his neck, she kissed him gently.

Guilt had Jack handcuffed. He couldn't get himself to touch Djuana's inviting body. The smell of her body, it's natural flavor made Jack's mouth water. And, Djuana licked his wet lips.

"Djuana, I'm so sorry baby."

"Shhhh," she angled her head, and slowly moved her lips to his. Jack stood still, allowing Djuana all she wanted. When she felt his tears on her cheekbone she squeezed his neck and fired up her tongue.

"I'm sorry," Jack sobbed.

"Hold me, Jack," Djuana panted in his ear, kissing it.

His hands slipped between the robe and her body. They clasped around her waist, squeezing her soft skin between his fingers. He rubbed the back of her curving rib cage and her shoulder blades. His tongue followed her lead, his mind followed his hands. They were now in the front, caressing her breasts, fondling them, causing Djuana to pant even more. His touch was gentle, yet firm and direct. In one motion, he bent and picked her up by the soft cheeks of her buttocks. She clamped her arms around his neck and legs around his waist, kissing his face.

Jack placed her on the bed, and she spread her legs and arms, groaning and inviting him in. With his knees on the floor, he kissed and caressed her body. When he finally stood and undressed, she knelt on the firm bed and helped him.

"You still my lady?" Jack said while her lips attacked his face.

Djuana looked up, her eyes blazing with desire, and hummed, "I'm yours, just like you are mine."

They made love through the night. It would be their most erotic night together.

# 42

Djuana slept hard that evening, snoring louder than Jack had ever heard her do before. He attributed her deep slumber on the rush of the past two days; slightly, but proudly, to his lovemaking. Jack, on the other hand could not get himself to fall off. He kept her on his shoulder or chest. He would kiss her head every so often as a point of security for himself as well as her.

Jack listen to the radio, gazing out of the window into the bright stars. He visualized being married to Djuana for a long time. She was not a good communicator, but she loved him, and that night he promised himself to take control of their relationship. While rubbing her soft skin and listening to her snore, he vowed to be perceptive enough to know when she was bothered, when something he was doing was bothering her.

He pictured Djuana finishing college, himself at the graduation and proud, and doing whatever her heart desired. He hoped children would be a part of her dreams; although he knew she surely wanted to get pregnant again. He could see handling their children with ease. Her gentle ways and soft heart would make her both a pushover and devoted mother in Jack's eyes.

His face wrinkled in doubt as Kris entered into his mind. He hoped she wasn't pregnant. But, he considered, this season has been one rocking challenge after another. If she did have his baby, he was going to make sure there were no problems between Kris and Djuana. How exactly? He didn't know.

When he felt the flicker of Djuana's eye lashes on his chest, he hoarsely said, "I bet your mother loves the way I bring so much trouble in her daughter's life."

"What?" Djuana asked, lifting her head.

"Nothing," Jack sighed.

"No," Djuana stretched. "I heard you. Is that why you couldn't sleep?"

Djuana moved herself up to be face to face.

"You are not bringing me any troubles. My live wasn't no bed of roses before I met you.

"And, as for my mother, she loves you because I do and she knows you love me."

"Does she?"

Djuana kissed Jack's cheek. "Yes. Baby, please don't start doubting us. You have been the one who all this time was positive we'd make it. I'm there now. I love you with all I have. I believe we will be all right."

Djuana searched Jack's eye's. His expression didn't relax.

"Jack, if you start doubting us, and thinking we can't make it, we won't. I don't know if I am strong enough to carry us."

Jack closed his eyes. He couldn't picture a fairy tale ending for them.

Djuana and Jack enjoyed his day off between games. They went to one of Los Angeles' beautiful beaches, as far from the hotel as possible, and had a quiet afternoon. They ate sandwiches and sipped wine between dips in the Pacific. Swimming in the lukewarm water was refreshing for both of their souls. They avoided the television and the radio, even though Djuana was secretly interested in hearing Kristen Eisen confess.

Jack relaxed himself, trying to not think about that practice later that afternoon, and the media that will be there. He stood in the water, for the most part, watching Djuana gracefully navigate under the clear greenish blue water. Her legs, strong and soft, would pump her curved torso through the water as if she was raised in the sea.

Djuana saw Jack's legs under the water, and made a beeline for them. She stopped at his waist and pulled herself up using his arms. "Why aren't you swimming?"

"I enjoy watching you, baby."

Djuana blushed. She tugged at the midsection of his trunks. "Are you turned on, or is this a harpoon?"

"Well, you are a pretty whale."

Djuana threw her weight onto Jack's shoulders and chest. They fell backwards into the water with a huge splash.

Djuana was amazed that the beach was not crowded, all she had heard about sunny L.A. detailed the sandy dunes and rippling waves or gang violence. So, she assumed everybody would be out on the beaches or getting shot. Also, the people on the beach were oblivious to them.

"You think these people know who you are?" she asked while they laid under an umbrella in the sun.

"Nope," Jack said, half sleep on his stomach. "And if they did, I'm sure they wouldn't care."

"Don't be silly," Djuana smiled, leaning on her elbows, picking at her midlength nails. "Who doesn't like Jack Newhouse from the Portland Crowns?"

"You want names and numbers?"

Djuana's grin followed her eyes down to sand. "How come you didn't want to hear that woman apologize on T.V.?"

"For what? What would it change?"

"I heard your teammates in the lobby talking about it, they say she got fired."

Jack turned his head from Djuana, keeping his eyes closed.

"Were you dating her, Jack?"

The question stabbed through his heart. He bit his lip.

Djuana dropped her head onto the blanket. Although she could not see his face, the silence told her plenty.

"I'm sorry I asked that."

Jack turned, sitting up on his elbow facing Djuana. He rubbed her back, sliding his hand beneath the opening of the bathing suit. Her skin was soft, but hot.

"Don't be sorry. You wanted to know, so you should have asked. This is the deal."

Djuana looked up from the blanket, her eyes in the sun until she moved her into the shadow of Jack's head.

He said, calmly, "I thought Kris was a friend. I remember when she first starting working the Crowns. The guy before her had quit to go to a larger paper, and this was her big chance. She was covering us part-time, and doing golf.

"I don't know what happened, her first week she put a lot of guys in check, including me. She was all business. Then I started hearing rumors, even though she was acting the same to me."

"That's why you wanted to try her?"

"No!" he frowned at her. "It wasn't like that at all."

"Forget it. I don't want to know."

"Yes you do. Her and I only did it once. It just happened. Yeah, it was a mistake, but I had no clue she wanted me in any way."

"Was I at home waiting for you? That I think I do need to know."

Jack looked in Djuana's glare. He wanted to blast her with the fact that it was after she had stabbed him, but he held off. He simply shook his head. He tried to rub the black look off of her face.

"If I had you to come home to that night, I would've."

The next night, the Trojans and their fans were again laughing and taunting the Crowns. Portland was losing 5-0 and looking dead after seven innings. Juris was avoiding eye contact with his players. He spoke to his coaches about players that were either sitting or standing near.

"He is a star, right? Must be," Juris said as Jack selected his bat and walked up the dugout steps, grazing by Juris.

"He goes out on the beach during the playoffs, not worrying that this might be our last chance to beat the Gamblers. Not worried that my job is on the line as well as his.

"No, this ass must be a star."

Oscar, who chose to play on his swollen ankle, hit a two-run home run, he returned to the dugout, limping, with hard high-fives and slaps on the back.

"Let's go, fellas!" O shouted, the veins in his neck bulging, while he staggered down the dugout to an open spot. "We can bust this ass, easy!"

Jack was next up, and took a strike before ripping a hard liner into the right-center gap. He was surprised that while standing on second he could actually hear Djuana clapping and shouting his name over the sudden hush. Don worked a walk, then Mike followed with sharp single. Jack raced around third, watching the coach wave him on. He was set, in his mind and body, to run over the catcher, hurt him, if the ball beat him home. There was no throw home. Jack scored easily.

The score now 5-3, the Trojans manager changed pitchers.

Bryant Clark, a left handed swinger, was torrid for the last month of the season. He stepped to the plate against the relief pitcher, Don was on second and Mike was dancing off of third. Bryant jumped all over the first offering. The ball hit off the right field scoreboard a second after Bryant hit it. Now, the stadium was completely silent.

The Crowns led, 6-5.

The Crowns held that lead until the bottom of the ninth. Bobby Lyles, Portland's third pitcher that night, ran into big troubles. The Crowns closer could not put the ball over the plate. He walked two batters, then tried to groove a fastball by a good hitter. The Trojan batter ripped the pitch to Jack on two bounces. Jack snatched the ball, which was angling to his left, with his glove and twirled his body in position to throw. He was thinking third base, but when he looked there, the runner from second was just rounding past the base and heading home.

Pugs was yelling something at Jack from his cutoff spot, but Jack could not hear him because the crowd had exploded into wild cheers. Jack turned his body again, and fired the ball to home plate. Jack watched the ball, an arrow that Mike, standing in front of home plate, would catch on one bounce. It was the best throw Jack had made this season. The throw beat the runner by two steps, but when Mike tried to place the tag, his glove hit the sliding runner's knee, and the ball squirted from his glove.

The game was tied, 6-6.

Jack was stunned. His eyes were fixed on Mike, who was glaring out to him. The chants from the crowd grew as Juris came out of the dugout. Juris took Bobby out of the game without looking at the pitcher. The hurler Juris put in, a rookie who had used impressive tools to win a spot of the Crowns playoff roster, was not up to the task. He walked two batters, forcing a run home. The rookie then threw Cris Carpenter a first pitch fastball, a league-known mistake.

Oscar did not move as the ball CC hit sailed well over his head and into the center field bleachers. Jack slowly walked to the dugout, not worrying about getting hit by the flying rolls of toilet paper. It was a long walk, giving him time to consider that the Crowns reign as league champions could be over.

Jack spent his time in L.A. with Djuana in the room she rented. They came off the elevator into the lobby where his teammates had gathered. The bus arrived as he and his woman approached Oscar. O was standing by the lobby's seating area, wiping lipstick off his lips and cheeks.

Djuana chuckled, "He was happy to see me here, too. He had the room to himself and his freaks."

Jack elbowed her playfully. He gave O a tight hand shake, and light hug.

"Hey, Djuana, you looking damn good as usual," O's smile was warm.

"Thank you, Oscar."

"Sorry we couldn't win one here for you. But, we'll get them at home."

The players, scattered about the large lobby, were in a fair mood collectively, for the position they were in. Two more losses and their season would be over. Most of the normal folk, entering or leaving the hotel, just gawked at the stars. Some stood at the tinted windows watching players being interview by a television crew.

Slight and Honeywell came off the elevator with their usual entourage in tow. In their crew was the team's business manager, doctor, and travel manager. Slight, though, had them ride on the bus with the team. He always had a limousine lead the bus. Occasionally, when he was angry, he had Honeywell ride with him.

Jack watched the men come off the elevators. His eyes fixed on the travel manager, Herb Brooke, who snapped off from the group and went to the front desk. That forced Jack to think about how he was going to get Djuana on the team's charter flight. He knew Slight wasn't about to bend any rules for him. So, just then, he planned to get them another flight. And to take a cab there to avoid any conflict.

Slight clapped his hands and stopped at the center of the lobby, drawing Jack, and the rest of his teammates to his presence.

"Let's go fellows. Let's get out of this fucked up city and get home to wholesome Portland. A real city."

The players stared at their owner, who was smiling, and rubbing his hands together. Slight added, "When we get home, we are going to put something on their asses, aren't we?"

He patted Danny's back, who just happened to be the player closest to him. Danny patted Slight's back, mockingly.

"What is he so happy about?" O asked.

"Who knows?" Jack replied, shrugging his shoulders.

"I'm gonna haveta get us another flight," Jack blurted to Djuana.

"Why?" Oscar quickly injected.

Djuana knew why.

"Slight's not gonna let us ride with the team. You know that."

"Why not? Man, come on. I tired of this bullshit between you and Slight. He's going to make me hurt his old ass."

Djuana tugged Jack's polo shirt. Jack turned, and followed her head and eyes. The husky, balding Slight was now among them.

"Morning," he said brightly.

Jack nodded, and O mumbled.

"Good morning, Mr. Slight." Djuana said. She was smiling because she knew he had overheard Oscar.

Slight's smile widened at Djuana. "You are pretty like the day is long. And I love short nights."

Djuana blushed. "Thank you."

"You can thank me by riding in my limousine to the airport."

Djuana looked at Jack. He was off guard, looking puzzled.

"He don't mind," Slight said, still smiling. "He can't kick my ass. Shit, he can't even get a solid base hit."

"Oh, shit," Oscar said, turning his head away.

"No, that's okay Vinny," Jack said. "We were going to catch another flight."

"Hogwash!" Slight snarled. "Are you mad? You two'll ride with the team."

His temperament changed instantly, again all teeth, as his fleshy hand took Djuana by her arm. "And, you, Honey, will ride with me to the plane."

Djuana's body moved with the short, well dressed owner, but her head looked to Jack. She stopped. "No. Maybe I should ride with Jack."

Slight shrugged, "If you want to. But, I must tell you, they smell worse in that bus than they did on the field."

Jack shook his head, watching Djuana laugh. "Baby, if you want to ride in style, who am I to stop you."

"You sure?" She searched his expression for any hint of negativity. He seemed okay.

"Go ahead," Jack gave her a light push.

In the enormous limo, Slight sat across from Djuana, making her nervous. Every second, it seemed, she was fixing the straps on her royal blue sun dress, trying to keep her bra from being exposed. Or, her fingers were tugging the hem over her crossed knees. She wished she had worn leggings or pants, but Jack asked her to wear the dress because her legs had a golden tan from the beach.

"Some wine, or champagne?" Slight asked as the vehicle pulled out and lead the bus.

"No, thank you."

"How about some pop?"

"Sure," Djuana gave in. She wasn't thirsty, but felt like she should accept something.

"Jack is a wonderful man, isn't he?" Slight began while pouring ginger ale in a champagne glass.

"Yes, he is."

"He has a good heart. Never did I have to ask him to help out with the community, or volunteer his time with children in Oregon.

"He went out and did it himself."

Djuana nodded, sipping the cold soda.

"I watched him, on occasion, with the kids. He was great with them. Better than almost all the idiots I have on my team."

Djuana thought of the way kids swarmed them while out, even wanting to touch her because she was a part of their hero.

"I didn't want to cut Jack off the team. But, you see, he left me no choice. I knew he loved you, but he has an obligation to his teammates."

"And, I guess you saw the whole damn city come to his aid. Portland loves him. I'm glad I didn't trade him, they would have hanged me in Pioneer Square!"

Slight smiled. Djuana laughed.

"Jack thinks you hate him."

Slight closed his eyes, frowned and shook his head. "I was wrong. I admit that," he ducked across the limo and sat next to Djuana.

"Now," he pointed his thick finger at Djuana, "You don't tell a soul this, not even Jack."

He slid back in the thick leather seats. "I blamed him for us not winning last year, but none of them hit. I got caught up in all the media-hype on how he should have taken control. This year he has disappointed me. He looks bored with baseball. And, that I blamed you for."

Djuana squeezed her hand around the glass. "And, so, it's because of me that you have been so hard on him?"

Slight didn't hesitate, "I don't need ballplayers that don't put the team first during the season. Jack doesn't realize that many of the players look up to him. They love him because so many times he has stuck up for them on the field and off it.

"He thinks Oscar is the best player in baseball. No, Jack Newhouse is the best player in the game. He thought just because Mike was the captain of the team he ran it. No. Not at all. The players feared Mike, he's all intimidation."

Djuana felt an inner pride she had never felt before; for someone else.

"You know," Slight continued, "That was why Bingo was never comfortable here. He wanted the power Jack had over the players and the city. Jack is the man that controls the Crowns. We can't win without him."

Jack was silent on the plane. He held Djuana's hand, but without feeling. Djuana tried small talk, but he gave quick, blunt answers. She was the one sitting by the window, but it was him doing the sight seeing.

"Are you upset because I rode with Mr. Slight?"

Jack blew air, and let her hand go. "Naw. Not at all."

"Then, what is it? You sure are acting like it pissed you off."

"No. I'm just realizing we won't even get a chance to have Las Vegas bust our ass. We're done."

He finally looked her in the eye, "I don't think we will get past Los Angeles. And, then Slight is going to break up the team."

Djuana turned her body to face Jack. "I hate when you are negative."

"I'm just being real."

"But, you guys always beat Los Angeles in the playoffs."

"That was when we had Cris, Bingo and Lee."

"Mr. Slight said differently in the limo."

"Oh, yeah. Well, what did the boss man say?"

Djuana smiled, and snuggled into his chest.

"That you guys can beat the Trojans and the Gamblers without them."

"Right," Jack rolled his eyes, and his head fell back.

Djuana pulled Jack's hand to her lips, and brushed them softly on his knuckles. "And, guess how he said you guys will do it?"

"I give up."

"He said you are the one that can do it. You can carry the team. I believe he's right. I see how the players all respect you."

"I'm not that kind of leader."

"Yes you are, you just never tried. I bet if you called a team meeting, everybody would come, and they would listen to you."

"Slight said that, right?"

"No. I'm saying it. You can do it."

Jack finally gave her a smile. "I'm glad you think so."

"You taught me how to believe."

# 43

The Trojans won Game Three easily in Portland by the score of 11-3. The Crowns committed seven errors, Jack had two in the first inning. He dropped a fly ball that allowed two runs to score. Then he picked the ball up and threw it from right field into the third base dugout, allowing another run to score.

The dejected and embarrassed Crowns all but laid down for the remainder in the game. When they finally scored their three runs, the Trojans had nine of their own, and were cruising. Juris was speechless, just staring blankly away from his players. Jack and Oscar didn't speak during the game; not even on fly balls.

Adkins was silent after the third inning, when the Trojans scored four times, and by the ninth inning, the small stadium was near empty.

Devon watched the Trojans come out of the player's exit of the stadium. They were a jubilant bunch, all smiles, getting onto their huge bus with tinted windows. They were oblivious to the boos from the fans standing behind barriers. He imagined those same guys crying after the Gamblers destroyed them in the World Series.

"Hey Juanny, you think Jack can get us tickets to the World Series even though he ain't going to be playing in it?"

Djuana glared down at her brother. "How stupid is that question?"

"Seriously. I never seen the Gamblers play live."

"What makes you think the Crowns won't be playing them again?"

Devon craned his neck, and gave the sarcastic smirk he had seen his mother do so many times, "Now how stupid is *that* question?"

Djuana shook her head, "You're a real Crowns fan, aren't you?"

"They ain't gonna win four games in a row. Not these Crowns. They ain't got Bingo."

"And if they do win?"

"They not."

Jack came out of the shower and found the clubhouse near empty. Three players were left; Bobby and Luis were each dressing slowly, their lockers on the other side of the room from Jack's. Juris was still in his office fuming.

# LOVE'S HOME RUN

Don was sitting on one of the lounge chairs near the saunas, still in his uniform. He had a bottle of scotch in one hand, a Crown's souvenir mug in the other.

"You all right, baby?" Jack asked. He was now at his locker drying himself slowly.

"I don't know how much longer I can do this shit," Don replied.

It was an answer Jack was not expecting. "What you talking about? Losing?"

"All of it. Baseball is passing me by. There's fucking kids half my age throwing pitches I can't even see, let alone put the bat on."

"Later, fellows," Luis interrupted, waving and walking out the door.

"Tomorrow," Bobby said, dragging himself out behind Luis.

Jack and Don both waved and gave quiet good-byes. Jack slipped on his underpants, then sat on the stool to put his socks on.

"Listen," he said while Don poured more scotch into the mug. "You're doing just fine. Shit, you had a better season than I did."

"No I ain't. You bastards love me, so you won't tell me I stink."

"I don't love you that much," Jack smiled.

Don didn't, though.

"Come on, New. You know that had Bingo not been traded I would have still been pickin' splinters out of my ass."

"Maybe not," Jack stood and picked his pants out of his locker. "Who knows? You might have been playing."

"Naw. When they wanted to replace you, they went to the minors."

"Yeah, but they didn't release you, did they? They know they need you."

Jack buttoned up his shirt, and put the tails in his jeans. After he buckled up, he grabbed a mug out of Oscar's locker and rinsed it out at the sink in the sauna.

"Give me a taste of that," he said pointing the mug at Don.

Don sat up, and poured generously.

"Shit, Don! I can't drink all of that."

"You such a baby. Just sip it like I am."

Jack sat next to him, sipped and his face cringed up.

"Good, ain't it, Poppy?" Don's face opened into a wide smile, his tongue hanging out.

"Yeah, whatever. I can't be in here all night with you. Djuana is out there with her little brother."

"I know. I know. Liela is out there with the girls. I just can't leave. I feel like my days are numbered. If we lose tomorrow, I think I am going to retire.

"I discussed it with Lie, and she says what she always fucking says: 'Whatever you think is right'."

"Don't retire, man. Me and Oscar won't have nobody nagging us on the road next year."

324

"I'm serious, bro'. Very. I know she wants me to be home to be the live-in babysitter and homework helper. Shit, two of my babies were born during the summer. They hate that I miss their birthdays when we are on the road."

"Yeah, I can imagine that that sucks," Jack took in some alcohol. He licked his lips.

"I wonder about that when Djuana and I have some kids. As bad as I want children, I think I would be as upset as them that I'm traveling all the time."

"Yeah, you tell yourself that you all will get used to it, but I am still not over the crying when I start packing."

"They still crying?"

"Yeah, ever since they were watching the news and the sportscaster said Lee was sent packing it has gotten worse. They think I am going to get traded to East Bumblefuck and they have to stay here. Or worse, go with me!"

Jack grinned. Don poured more scotch into their mugs.

Don said, "Let's finish this bottle and get the fuck out of here."

Jack and Don left Adkins joking and laughing at one another. They split up in the lot, Don's station wagon parked on the other side, with its lights on. Jack walked over to the dark Pathfinder wondering if Djuana got tired of waiting and left. He walked up to the driver's side to find Djuana and Devon asleep. He tapped lightly on the window.

Djuana opened the door, "What took you so long?"

"I'm sorry. Don asked me to have a drink with him, and it got out of hand."

He gave her a light kiss, "I'll drive."

"No," she frowned and covered her face from his. "I better drive. Your breath reeks of liquor."

"Really?"

"Yes," she closed the door on him.

The smell of bacon and biscuits aroused Jack out of a deep slumber. Incomplete memories of a nightmare kept his mind occupied while his other senses caught up with his nose. All he could recall from the dream was the Trojans celebrating on the Adkins infield. He saw Cris laughing in his face, pointing his finger and declaring he told Jack it would happen.

Jack forced his mind off of baseball. He slid out of the bed, and dragged himself into the bathroom. He started the shower, but stood on the floor mat for nearly five minutes listening to the water before he got in. He stepped in, letting the hot water flow down his body, beating off his chest and arms. He let his thoughts drift, and a song he couldn't remember the name to chimed into his thoughts.

He hummed the chorus, dropping his head under the water.

Djuana knocked lightly at first, then rapped harder. She could hear the water, but no words from Jack. She finally tried the knob, turned it all the way, then pushed in the door. She saw him standing, his arms out in front of him against the wall, his head under the pulsating shower.

"You okay, Jack?"

She barely noticed him nod.

"I made breakfast. It's ready."

Jack stood up straight. He kicked in the knobs, then pulled open the curtain. Djuana instinctively picked up his towel and opened it. He stopped before her, though, his eyes fixed on the white, fluffy towel.

"Come, let me dry you," Djuana said.

Jack turned his back to her, and she rubbed up and down. "Lift your arms."

Jack sighed, following her orders. "I'm glad this season is over. I stunk up the whole town. Kids are probably burning my baseball cards across Oregon."

"Turn around. I oughta punch you in the nose, Jack Newhouse," Djuana became rougher with the towel, scraping his chest. "You sound like a loser. I ain't marrying a loser."

"I forgot to tell you. I'm a loser."

Djuana lightly, but directly, poked Jack in the groin.

"Shit!" he buckled over and sucked in air. "That hurt!"

"Well, then stop talking stupid!" She threw the towel at him. "Dry yourself."

Djuana was still irritated when Jack sat with her at the dining room table. Jack looked across at her until she looked at him from her plate. She scowled at him, and shook her head.

"Your food is in the oven," she said, cutting her eyes onto her fork full of eggs.

Jack kissed the top of her head, "Thanks, my love."

"Ain't no making up."

The ring of the phone caught Jack as he passed the new cordless hanging in its cradle. He plucked it up, holding it to his ear while opening the oven.

"Hello? Shit! God damn hot fucking..."

"The plate might be hot, dear!" Djuana giggled.

Bingo was on the other end, not amused. "Listen, I called to let you know how sorry I feel that I won't be bustin' your ass in the series, but hey, it seems you're too busy."

"Yo, Bing, lose my fucking number." Jack pressed the phone off and tossed it on the counter.

"Don't break that phone!!" Djuana yelled.

"How 'bout I break you!"

"Come try it, big boy!" Djuana laughed. "You'd get hurt up."

The phone rang again before Jack could sit down.

"Yeah?"

"New, baby. Losin' ain't easy, is it?"

Jack could hear the smile on Cris' face.

"Fuck off, C. I ain't in the mood."

"Don't blow your mind. That's what the fuck you get for stabbing me in the back. You faggot."

"Yo, C, check this out, obviously you didn't get the message when Floyd busted you with that fastball. But, if you fuck with me, I will bust you with a fist. Repeatedly."

Djuana got up from her food. She walked into the kitchen and stood behind Jack.

Cris laughed into the phone. "It's over tonight, baby. Over! You and Slight and that bastard O can kiss my championship-winning ass good-bye!"

He hung up before Jack could.

Djuana took the phone out of Jack's hand. She hung it back into the cradle. "Baby, I didn't know it was Pick On Jack Day."

Jack snatched up his plate, barely making it to the table before the heat sizzled his hands.

Djuana came to the table. "You need to take it easy."

"I'm fine. I'm just hungry. That's all."

The phone rang again.

"What is going on?" Djuana said as she answered it.

This time, it was for her.

"Hi Djuana, it's your mother."

"Hey, Mommy. We're in the middle of eating breakfast.

"I just called to let you know I had to curse out that no good father of yours."

Djuana sat, nibbling on bacon. "What are y'all arguing about?"

"He's losing the little bit of mind he has left! He called here upset because he saw Devon on television at the game last night. Talking about he should be in bed on a school night."

Djuana continued to eat, taking more food in her mouth. She would reply to her mother with mumbles.

"He also can't believe you are still with Jack. You know I let him have it. I told his sorry ass that not everybody gives up on relationships when things go tough."

Djuana smiled. "And what did he say to that?"

"He played it off. He thinks Jack is a dog because he is one. I just told him that Jack is human, and if you love him you should stand by him."

"You said that?"

"Yes, I did. Jack's a good man. Granted, he might be a puppy in some ways, but, shit, any man with pussy flopping up in his face every night would be one."

Djuana smiled at the words her mother continued to put together. She wondered if she would grow to speak to her children with the same zest some day.

Emma didn't break her stride, "I see how he is around you, and see that he loves you. I say give the man time to break off from his habits, and he'll be okay."

"I can't believe this is you talking."

"Why not?"

"I didn't think you liked Jack."

"I do. He's a nice enough man. Until he screws up. Then I have to crack his skull open."

Jack solemnly walked past the cheering fans and into Adkins. He was deep in thought, not hearing the children and teenagers yelling his name and waving things to autograph, thinking about last season ended. He couldn't recall what he was thinking the night the Gamblers defeated the Crowns for the championship. But, he was sure that he had to have been in a more positive frame of mind before the game started.

The guard posted at the door to the Crowns clubhouse, patted Jack on the back , as he had done each player that walked past that day.

"One game at a time, New," the guard said. "One at a time."

Jack entered the locker room, and was surprised to hear rap music blaring from Bryant's portable CD player. The room was loud and vibrant. And, for the first time in years, Oscar was there before him, in uniform.

"We ain't losing to these ass-wipes ever again," O said as Jack reached his locker.

Floyd came over just as Jack had begun to undress. He was not carrying his bible. "How you feel?"

Jack nodded. "I feel good."

"I feel like beating some sinners," Floyd said. "That's how I feel."

Jack's eyes followed Floyd across the room, he saw that Mike was banging his head on the cement wall inside his locker.

Floyd turned in the finest pitching outing by a Crowns hurler that season in Game Four. He shut out the Trojans for 10 innings. He struck out Cris three of the four times he batted, the other time he got him to ground out meekly. Each time he got Cris out, he would uncharacteristically pump his fist in the air.

Mike won the game with his bat, his mouth and his anger. Anytime the Trojans seemed on the verge of scoring, Mike would bark at his teammates. Then, in the tenth inning, with the game scoreless, he broke up the tense, pitching duel with a home run. When he hit the ball, a high arching shot into center field bleachers, the stadium erupted. The sound was more of a delight to the players than the hit. They mobbed Mike at home plate, slapping his helmet as hard as they could. The 1-0 victory sent the two teams back to Los Angeles for the fifth game.

After the game, most of the Trojans shrugged off the win. They had the collective thought that the proud ex-league champions *had* to win one game home before being dethroned.

Cris told reporters that the Trojans didn't mind losing.

"We just want to clinch the series at home in front of our fans," he said repeatedly.

Cris would not get another hit in the series.

The Crowns won game five, 6-3, behind Mike's suddenly hot bat. He set a league championship record with seven consecutive doubles during the course of two games.

The teams flew back to Portland, and the fans in Adkins were never silent in a thrilling 5-3 Crowns victory that tied the series at three wins a piece. They're loud cheering seemed to rattle the already nervous Trojans. Jack had his best game of the series with four hits, including the game winner in the bottom of the eighth. With the score 3-3, and runners on second and third, Jack hit a pitch he was fooled on between the second and first basemen to score both runners.

The game to decide who would play the Gamblers, who had destroyed a decent Maine baseball team in four lopsided games, was played in front a record crowd in Los Angeles. L.A.'s best pitcher was on the mound and Cris had guaranteed a victory for the Trojans.

But, Portland had regained its pride and spirit. Each starting player had at least one hit. Oscar's three hits were homers, and after each one he did a dance around the bases.

The Crowns won easily, 13-3.

The Crowns celebration was short. After the last out, a grounder to Pugsley at second, they hugged one another, slapped high-fives, and then dodged debris from the disappointed Trojans fans on their way into the dugout.

The clubhouse was draped with plastic to protect the players street clothes from champagne. But, any Portland player that had been around for the disappointing losses to Las Vegas, knew better than celebrate now. The veterans only wanted to party hardy after knocking off L.V.

The younger players, though, and those veterans new to Portland like Howie, who thought a trip to the World Series a big deal sprayed champagne on their teammates and raised a ruckus in the locker room. The cameras were on Oscar, the series Most Valuable Player for the third time in his career. Print journalist hovered over Jack, and he gave short answers. They tried to get him to comment on Cris, then Djuana, but he refused.

Don whistled him over to the showers when the reporters' questions died down.

"I got us some Trojans juice," Don said, presenting two bottles of champagne.

Jack smiled, "Where you get them?"

"The losers, bro'. Them scumbags won't be needing it."

The two men sat under an idle shower and drank the sparkling, dry grape juice. The sound of heels on the tiles was lost in the whooping of their teammates in the locker rooms. Don saw the woman walk toward them, her hips shifting with the swinging of her arms.

Jack heard the heels, turned his head, and saw the long legs first. On those long, creamy ivory legs were sheer white stockings, and a short sheath dress revealed all. Jack unconsciously licked his lips, and immediately felt guilty, then angry.

"Congrats," Kris' voice was pleasant and her smile inviting. "I didn't think you guys could do it again."

Don struggled to get up from the wet floor. He wiped off his uniform pants, then reached down to get his bottle.

"I'll be inside," he said to Jack. He walked past Kris, turning up the bottle and letting his head fall back.

Kris leaned against the cold, tiled wall, her hands shielding her beige skirt. "I tried calling you in Portland."

"Bullshit."

"True."

Kris took in a deep breath of the damp air. "I kept hanging up because that woman was answering."

Jack took a hearty swig. "Ah huh."

"Don't hate me, Jack. I don't want that."

"Whatever."

"I'm going to take a job here in Los Angeles covering the Lakers."

Jack drank some more.

"I guess what I'm trying to say is that I'm sorry. I'm sorry I caused you any pain."

"Apology accepted."

"If you ever needed me, Jack, I'd be there. I don't think I'd ever lose my feelings for you."

Jack slapped his palm on the tiles, and braced his body as he stood. "I gotta go."

Kris grabbed him, hugging into his ribs from the side, her head on his right shoulder. Jack looked away, feeling the effects of the alcohol.

"Kris, let me go."

"I love you, Jack. Please don't hate me."

"I don't. Just let me go."

"I can't," she slid her body into his chest, squeezing the gray jersey tighter. "When you walk away you're gone. I know that."

Jack sighed through his nose, "Kris, let me go."

"I will, after you hug me."

Jack looked to the ceiling for help. He wrapped his arms around her, and she cried softly.

Slight called Len Canisa from his limo on the way to the airport. He fought his giggling long enough to declare, "We're baaaack!"

"Welcome back to the show, Vinny," the owner of the best team in baseball said solemnly.

"Oh, I'm back! And I've got the best team ever waiting for your spoiled, overpaid humps."

"Vinny, please. I sent my boys to Hawaii for the three days it took you to finish L.A. We knocked out Maine in four easy games, if you hadn't heard. My boys didn't break a sweat.

"You think they are not ready?"

"Oh, I hope so. We've got something for you."

"What? What do you have? Don't tell me Danny and Floyd? Those two can't pitch to my team. You have no offense. New and O, and that's it. You had better give Mike a drink.

"Vinny, I'm begging you. Don't bet me."

"Los Angeles thought the same thing. You see where they are? Shit, we were the first team in history to come back from a three-game deficit in the playoffs."

"Vinny, goomba, we are not Los Angeles. We are not scared of your team."

# 44

Djuana was surprised to be invited to Las Vegas for the first two games of the World Series. She had thought Jack would consider her a distraction during the biggest games in baseball. But, she was proud when he told her he needed her there. She vowed to herself to be as quiet as a church mouse, and to not give him any sex... no mater how he begged.

She flew with the team into Las Vegas the day of the first game, a blisteringly hot Saturday. The Crowns stopped at the hotel for less than an hour, then it was off to the MoneyDome. She enjoyed the bus ride pass all the casinos. The city was lit up in the early afternoon, and Djuana was impressed. Jack let her sit in the window seat of the bus, expecting she would like the lights and action of Las Vegas Boulevard.

"If you want to check out the sights, you can," Jack said. "I'm sure some of the other wives will be going out after the game."

"You going?"

"No. The players will be under tight curfews."

"I'm not going without you."

Jack took her hand, "We'll come back after the series."

Djuana was amazed at how big an affair the World Series was. The players' wives and family were seated in the same small section, some 10 rows from the Crowns third base dugout. Directly across the field were the Gamblers' wives. Djuana was pleased to sit next to Liela and her three daughters. Liela took Djuana under her wing, telling her how the cameras were fixed on them, and how television would show her reaction to every thing, good or bad, Jack would do.

"Just be real, that's all I can tell you. Some of us aren't," Liela's eyes fixed on Bobby Lyle's glamorous wife. She was light skinned, slim, long hair and nails and was wearing diamonds on each hand and gold chains around her left wrist and neck.

"You'll see when the game starts," Liela continued, dragging Djuana's attention back. "How all of a sudden we have actresses on this row."

The MoneyDome was beautiful. Its roof was had dark, golden rafters from which 11 championship banners hung, along with the numbers of former great Las Vegas players. The seats, including the arm rests, were cushioned. The cement ground and stairs glittered with imitation gold dust. Most of the Gamblers' fans seemed well to do, dressed extravagantly and spreading big dollars around. They had to be, Djuana reasoned, the price of food at the dome was exceedingly high.

"Do you see how much they want for a hot dog?" Djuana asked Liela.

"What? Three fifty, right? Disgusting. I don't now why these people pay it."

"I guess they don't have a choice."

"We do. The Gamblers will have food brought to us three times during the game, and unlimited pop."

"That's the big difference between the owner of the Gamblers and Slightly rich, as I call him," Liela clued Djuana in. "Everything here is first class."

Emma had a huge party at her house for the opening of the World Series. She wasn't a sports fan, but she did watch the championship of just about every sport. Tia and Marla helped her with the cooking, Cal, of course helped with selection of the booze. Family and friends crowded around the two 27 inch televisions in the living room, with chips and popcorn all about. When the game began, the ladies were still frying chicken.

In the living room, they watched the pre-game show, falling silent when the interview with Jack began. NBC showed clips of Jack and Djuana in the hospital, and the reporter spoke of true love.

"On paper, Jack, this seems to be the worst season of your career," asked the charming and beautiful Amber Marie.

"I hope Jack don't screw her!" Cal chuckled.

He was hushed by the others.

Jack, sitting on a stool near the Crowns dugout in Las Vegas, calmly replied, "No. I don't see it that way. I didn't hit as well as I had in the past, but here we are in the Series again. I get hot now, and we win, nobody remembers what I did all year."

"What about the fact that you haven't hit a home run this year for the first time in your career?"

"Please!" Tia injected, from the doorway leading to the kitchen. "Why are they always talking about home runs?"

"Shhhh!!"

Jack said, "There are a lot of players in this Series that haven't hit a homer this year."

"None better than you," Amber retorted.

"Word up!" Cal shouted. He popped his friend a high-five. "Shit, what the man had been hitting 25 to 30 homers a year, now he has none?"

"Shut up, Cal!" Emma barked. "You ain't no genius!"
The room fell silent in time for Jack's reply.
"I hit the biggest home run of my life when I met Djuana Pioneer."

Before the game began, two bands played a few of their hits on the infield while showgirls danced. Afterwards, the entire Sounds of Blackness gospel ensemble performed "The Star Spangled Banner" to a roaring ovation.

Djuana enjoyed the player's introduction. First were the Crowns, and most of them were booed. All of the wives stood and cheered. Djuana took this opportunity show everyone how proud of her man she was. Liela and the girls cheered with her, and she also cheered loudly with them when Don was announced next.

After the Crowns, the MoneyDome went dark; all the lights shut off. Then a laser show began with the pumping bass line from the rap song, "Punks Jump Up to Get Beat Down" in the background. The announcer bellowed, "And now. Your Worrrrld Champion Gamblerrrrrrs!

"It's on!"

The roar of the crowd was deafening; as if the MoneyDome was hollow. Djuana had to cover her ears, she had never heard a crowd explode so suddenly. The Cruz girls giggled and followed her lead. The Gamblers, in white satin uniforms with gold and black trimming, came waltzing out of the dugout one by one as their name was shouted with zest.

"Welcome to the World Series," Liela shouted, and Djuana had to force her eyes on Liela's lips to hear her.

The Crowns went down in order in the first inning. Then, the Gamblers went to work. Danny walked the first batter, the next guy singled, and the number three hitter homered. The noise in the dome was louder than the introductions. The Crowns were down by three runs instantly.

Danny tried a curve to Bingo, and he rocked it. The ball went into the third deck of bleachers, some 500 feet away. Only the ninth ball ever hit there. The next batter waited until the cheering calmed before he stepped into the batter's box. This angered the already pissed off Danny. He had wanted to strike out Bingo badly.

When the batter was ready, Danny fired a fastball off his helmet, knocking the tall, slender hitter to the ground. Both dugouts emptied in an instant. Danny immediately dropped his glove and came off the mound. He waited for someone to come his way. And when someone did, he hit the guy.

Jack was fighting with the first player in white he ran across, when someone hit him from behind. He looked back to see Bingo hit him again. Before he could get up, Bingo shoved him and three other Gamblers pounced on him. They didn't get in too many hits before Jack's teammates came to his aid.

When the umpires finally got the field cleared, separating the men in white and gold from those in gold and gray, they ejected four Crowns, including Jack and Danny, and only two Gamblers, neither a starter. The batter Danny hit had to be taken out in an ambulance.

Djuana stood on her chair to see when Jack tumbled over and three players covered him. Liela noticed the blood on his jersey first, and she looked to Djuana, to find her crying.

"He's bleeding, oh my God," she stepped down, her hands shaking.

Liela held her arm and forced her to sit. "He's okay. He's fine. You see he's walking, right."

"Oh, my God. Did you see how those guys jumped him. The Gamblers ain't nothing but thugs!"

"Djuana, these teams don't get along, at all."

The Gamblers won the game easily, 9-0. Lee pitched his usual fine game during playoff time. He toyed with his ex-teammates, none able to touch his fastball or slider.

Djuana fumed throughout, as did most of the women she sat with and the Crowns players. She couldn't wait until the game ended to see for herself that Jack was okay. She patiently waited for Liela and the girls, though, the waited by the door of the bus while the other women waited on the bus.

She greeted the players as they walked by her, no smiles exchanged. When Jack appeared she was taken aback by his swollen lip. She grabbed him into a fierce hug. She felt her tears when her eyes closed in his embrace.

"I hate those bastards," she whispered in his ear between kisses.

Jack smiled. "Yeah, only their mothers love them."

"They jumped you like they were in an alley somewhere."

"I know, baby," Jack wiped her cheeks. "But, pay back is a bitch, and she's on her period."

Game Two on Sunday evening was no better for the Crowns. Jamie McLennon's sinker was working to perfection, and beat them for the fifth consecutive time in World Series play, 3-1. Jack had three of the team's five hits and he was playing determined. Floyd pitched well, and the defense behind him sparkled, but his one mistake, a belt-high fastball that Bingo crushed for a two-run home run, was too much for his teammates to overcome.

The plane ride home was silent, except for Floyd reading a passage on courage from his bible. Djuana laid in Jack's lap, but did not sleep on the late night flight. The Crowns flew out Sunday night, Slight wanted his team out of Las Vegas as soon as possible. The Gamblers didn't come to Portland until Tuesday; Game Three was on Wednesday night.

On the flight, her head nestled into Jack's lap and legs bent in the seat towards the window, Djuana daydreamed about Jack winning the games single-handedly and Slight loving him for it. Giving him a big bonus and signing him for life so they would never have to move out of Portland. They could get married, buy another house; Djuana did not want to make Jack's home theirs... too many memories.

    Jack looked down from the television to Djuana on his lap. They were sitting on the couch, watching yet another rented movie. Going out in public without being disturbed was becoming more and more taxing.
    He ran a finger over Djuana's wrinkled forehead, "You okay, baby."
    "Sure," she turned her head up to see Jack's face. "But, do you realize we are supposed to be marrying in less than a month?"
    "Shit."
    "You forgot? That's okay. It has been hard to think about with the World Series and all."
    Djuana closed her eyes and buried her head deeper in his lap. She tightened her grip on his thigh. "Maybe we should just cancel it for awhile."
    "No, I don't want to."
    Djuana's eyes opened. She exhaled a silent sigh of relief.
    "Naw," Jack said. "We've got time."
    Djuana watched Jack spin one of his patented smiles, but it didn't comfort this time. He kissed her frown.
    "Jack, how am I going to have enough time to get my dress, the bride's maid dresses and plan this right."
    "You want to push it back? Maybe the spring?"
    "I don't know."
    "Listen, you can do this, I know you don't want to do it alone, but I can't be of any help until after the Series."
    Worry kept Djuana's frown alive.
    "Maybe I should hire help."
    "If you want to, I surely don't mind."
    "I don't know," Djuana gave in.
    "Relax, baby. We're going to be all right."

    When Wednesday came around the city came alive with Crowns fever. The color burgundy was everywhere. T-shirts, pants, sneakers, blouses, skirts. Anything that could be worn. In grocery stores and in the malls, also at the Adkins, yellow hand cloths were being handed out for free.
    Djuana had remember October days like this, when any clothing item the color burgundy would sell from DeLux's. She had always thought the people to be a bit overboard with their love of the Crowns. But, now she understood after seeing Los Angeles and Las Vegas stand behind their ball clubs.

Throughout the morning, as Djuana drove around downtown, cars blew their horns at the Pathfinder and waved or pumped their fists, and pedestrians approached when she stopped. People shouted encouraging words at Djuana, even after finding no Jack Newhouse in the ride.

She picked up Tia from the Square before noon for a afternoon of shopping for the bridesmaids dresses. Tia did not take for granted that she would be the maid of honor, and took the responsibility seriously. From the moment Djuana had asked her, the night Jack proposed, Tia had been making sure Djuana kept an agenda and stuck to it.

"Damn, this year is crazier than any," Tia said as she got in the truck.

Djuana shook her head, "I guess it seems that way because we never were a part of it before."

"Yeah," Tia nodded, "And, you know, the city hates Bingo Wells and Lee Spencer for trading. Not so much Lee though. He didn't want to leave, I hear."

Djuana smirked as the Pathfinder joined traffic, "How you know all this?"

"I read the papers. I listen to the news. I'm there."

Tia dug through her school bag. "I got some ideas from that magazine you gave me."

"Really?"

"Yeah. And, Mable's Fabric is having a big sale."

Djuana swerved the Pathfinder across the lines, into the left-turn lane. She flicked on the indicator and wheeled the truck down Ninth Avenue. People in the crosswalk waved heartily. Djuana smiled and waved.

"You a star, girl." Tia gushed playfully.

"No even. All day people have been achin' to get a look at Jack."

"Hookers too, huh?"

"Of course! Some little young floozies tried to roll up, but stopped in their tracks when they saw me."

"Oh, you didn't smile and wave at them, eh?"

"Not."

Djuana slowed at a light, and found herself looking for people to wave to.

"You think Mrs. Spencer can have all these dresses ready?" Djuana wondered aloud.

"I think so. Her daughters will help her. Besides, she'll be getting paid up front for a change."

"Yeah," Djuana chuckled.

She turned the truck into a packed lot off Morrison, the first one they approached.

Tia pointed out the neon "full" sign above the attendant's stand. "This place is full, Dee."

The attendant leaped out of his seat when he saw them pull in. He raced over to the Pathfinder. Djuana eased down the window, lightly touching the button.

"Do you have any space?"

"Sure," the young man said, with a hint of a Spanish accent and a pleasant smile. "Just put it over here, Mrs. Newhouse."

Djuana turned to Tia and stuck her tongue out.

"Spoiled," Tia smiled.

They parked in a spot reserved for the owner of the lot.

Two blocks down Morrison, the ladies stopped in front of Stephanie's, an African American owned bridal shop. One by one, the bridesmaids arrived. Djuana selected Marla, Charlotte, Anesa and Liela Cruz to be in her bridal party. Liela was an easy choice, she and her husband loved Jack, and they were the first to make her feel a part of Jack's life in baseball.

Charese, who was promoted into Djuana's spot at Delux's, was not thrilled to be left out. She would be more upset when she wasn't invited to the wedding.

Djuana asked Pamela to be in the wedding, but she politely refused.

"I will not be a bridesmaid," she explained. "It's bad luck."

Instead, she offered a sharp discount to do the hair of all the women involved, and Djuana's free.

The women entered Stephanie's with no collective plan. Djuana knew what she wanted, and all the women had different ideas. Only Marla agreed with the color scheme; or at least she didn't complain. Four hours later, the women settled on the dress Tia selected, even though hers would be slightly different.

The dress was off the shoulder with a modest Princess neckline. It was fitted to the ankles, had a slit on the right, cut to the mid-thigh. It was made of raw silk, and Stephanie had six of them in forest green.

Surprisingly, not much altering had to be done. Tia was tall for her dress, which was nearly the same, just that it had a white shawl collar, and came with opera-length gloves.

Liela had the most difficult time being fitted. She had more hips and breasts than any of the women. She thought the final dress made her look hippy.

"It doesn't look right on me," she said into the mirror.

"Lord, you look great," Tia said. The other women nodded in envy.

"How many kids you have? Shit, I better go get pregnant so I can gain some ass."

The women laughed and touched.

"She's right," Djuana added. "You're beautiful, and you got a figure. No belly."

The ladies did agree, however, to purchase white shoes and dye them the color of the dresses.

Djuana treated her assembly to a late lunch at Hunan's, two blocks away. They laughed through a Chinese meal, telling jokes about men and marriage.

Before the game, Adkins Stadium hosted a humble string of festivities. The Queen of the Portland Rose Festival rode a convertible on the outskirts of the manicured playing field. The University of Oregon's marching band performed, and played behind Lisa Stansfield when she sang the national anthem.

Mayor Meier threw out the ceremonious first pitch from the mound. She was wearing a burgundy skirt suit with a yellowish-gold scarf. Security escorted her to a seat in the first row, behind the Crowns dugout. She chose to sit there instead of with Slight and Honeywell in Slight's skybox. Often, she would stand and waved her Crowns cap to incite the crowd to cheer on the Crowns.

Djuana watched her, recalling how far she had come since meeting the mayor. She knew that night, though, that she loved Jack Newhouse. And, here she was, deeper in love, and soon to be married to him.

From the end of the national anthem until the first pitch was thrown a strike, the fans at Adkins were on their feet cheering. They roared for every strike pitcher Timm Peaston threw, until the strikes starting come far and between a string of balls. Peaston walked three batters before Bingo strolled to the plate.

The booing from the crowd was loud, louder than the cheering had been. And, Djuana joined in, but, the stadium fell silent when Bingo pulled a fastball down the left field line for a grand slam. The ball seemed to be hit on a line, not rising more than 10 feet off the ground. It landed in the glove of a fan in the first row of the bleachers above the left field wall.

Timm settled after the blast, with those four runs all he gave up. From then on, whenever Bingo batted, Timm threw him nothing but slow curves, and Bingo popped up to Don at first and Bryant at third. Timm was far from a great pitcher, but he was experienced. He had pitched for six teams in seven years before joining the Crowns.

On offense, the Crowns could not put together more than two singles in a row against another solid pitcher on Las Vegas' staff. When the ninth inning came, the fans were still behind the Crowns, they gave Timm a standing ovation, waving their mini towels, as the team came up for their last at bat. They continued to cheer through the commercial break.

Down four runs, Juris sent Hector Aponte up to bat for Timm. Aponte, invisible on the Crowns team since he lost right field back to Jack, walked on four pitches to receive an ovation. On the next pitch, with Russ Jones batting, Aponte stole second.

The Las Vegas pitcher settled, striking out RJ on three wicked fastballs. Before Pugsley got out of the batter's circle near the dugout, Oscar grabbed his chubby arm, "Get on, man, I don't give a fuck how, but we ain't losin' this game."

Pugs just nodded. He hadn't had a hit since the Boston series, almost two weeks.

With the fans chanting "Here we go Portland, here we go," Pugs extended his arms and bat out on a fastball and slapped it past the first baseman. Aponte raced home from second, sliding in ahead of the throw from the right fielder. Pugs hustled to second on the throw home.

O snarled at Jack, waiting for Jack to come into the on-deck circle. "We ain't getting swept."

"I'm there," Jack said.

Oscar walked out to the batter's box, his head down, thinking it was time for him to carry his team to victory. When he looked up, the manager of Las Vegas was on the mound making a pitching change. O's first reaction was anger.

*They ain't getting me out.*

The pitcher brought in was the barrel-chested, Ray Tidrow. The 6-foot-5 ace of the Gamblers' bull pen had a terrorizing fastball. He threw it up to 110 mile per hour. It was straight, but tough to catch up with. Last year, in the World Series, Tidrow struck out 16 of the 19 Crowns batters he faced.

Oscar ran those numbers through his mind. He was fanned four times by Tidrow. The year before Tidrow struck him out three times. He had only one hit off of Tidrow in his career going into that at bat.

Jack went down to one knee in the circle. He watched Tidrow's fastball pop the catcher's mitt during his warm up. "Base hit, baby, that's all we need," he called out to O.

O stepped in the left handed batter's box and after one practice swing was set. Tidrow looked back to Pugs at second, who had a small lead off the base, then back to his catcher. He cocked and twirled, unleashing a blazer.

O turned on the pitch, connecting and driving the ball high and on a line. It landed in the hands of two fans in the right field bleachers.

The two-run homer put the Crowns within one run, 4-3.

Oscar did a side-stepping, hip-rotating dance down the line heading to home plate. Jack was the first to greet him, and O popped him with a hard five.

"He ain't shit, rock him, New!" O said.

The rest of the Crowns were out of the dugout, and O did another dance to them. He let them mob him, turning his body toward the mound and pointed his index finger at Tidrow.

"You going down, big boy," O yelled to the unshaven mountain of a man. "All the way down!!"

Tidrow stood on the mound, chewing tobacco and watching O the whole way.

Jack stepped in the right handed side of the box swinging his bat, gearing up for the heat. *Inside, inside*, his mind told him. *That's all that bastard can throw me. He ain't going to test me across the plate. He knows I can't hit the inside heat. But, I'm ready. I ready for your ass. If O can hit one off your ass, then I know I can.*

Tight, and high, heat was all any pitcher with a knowledge of Jack Newhouse threw him. He was a dangerous hitter, but Jack could not get his bat around quick enough to do any damage to good inside fastball.

The first pitch Tidrow threw Jack that evening was an inside fastball, high and inside. Before Jack could fully react, the ball hit his helmet near the ear hole as he cowered away. Jack was unconscious before he hit the ground. But, he sat up instantly, feeling around for his bat. He was oblivious to the almost immediate brawl that happened around him.

O had anticipated Tidrow may throw at Jack, and had hoped Jack had also. O's body was ready and as soon as he saw the ball was thrown at his best friend, he was on his feet. He was the first one out of the dugout when Jack hit the ground. He raced to the mound, where Tidrow fought him off. But, Don, coming from the on-deck circle, knocked Tidrow down with a hard tackle.

O and Don pounded the bigger Tidrow until his teammates came to his aid. Then, Don broke off, trying to hurt anyone in black and gold. O tried to hang onto Tidrow, absorbing blows from Gamblers. Mike was choking a Gambler into submission.

Djuana was on her feet instantly, hands covering her cheeks. She could not believe her eyes, grown men were fighting like dogs; many scuffling on their hands and knees.

"Shit," Tia said.

Devon was excited, joining in with some of the people around them in urging the players to kill one another.

"Fuck 'em up, O!" Devon yelled, standing on his seat spilling his popcorn. "Beat that ass!"

"Watch your mouth!" Djuana elbowed him. "I think you better sit down."

"You hear that boy?" Tia said in amazement.

"You see what they did to J-New? Naw, they gotta go to blows for that!"

Djuana was afraid the other baseball wives had heard her foul-mouthed brother, but their attention was on the field with their respective men. She found it difficult to watch Jack, his teammates were surrounding him as if he were their general in a combat. When the fighting was finally over, she followed his movements to first base. He seemed groggy, and stood on the base with his hands on his hips while another Crowns batted.

Djuana chose not to stop her brother from chanting "Bull shit, Bull shit," with the other 70 thousand fans in Adkins.

Don, Oscar and Danny were ejected from the game. Danny had come out of the Crowns dugout with a bat. He swung it once at a Gambler before two of his coaches disarmed him. Tidrow, his manager and one other Gambler were also thrown out for the remainder of the game.

Jack ran the bases and scoring the tying run, but he would never recall the finish of the game. The Crowns continued to rally, and defeated Las Vegas, 5-4.

During the drive home, Jack gave short answers to Devon's excited questions. When they dropped off the boy, Jack laid his seat all the way back and rested his hand on his head. While Djuana walked up to the building. Cal was downstairs waiting for them.

"Great game, Jack!" Cal yelled.

Jack waved.

"He all right," Cal asked his niece.

"Hello, Uncle Cal."

"I'm sorry, baby," Cal kissed her. "Is he all right?"

"He's tired."

Djuana got back in the truck, looking at her man.

"You okay, Jack?"

"I have a serious headache."

"You want me to stop and get you some aspirin?"

"No. I took two horse pills after the game. They should kick in once I get to bed."

Jack got out of the Pathfinder and climbed the stairs into the house. He went directly to the bedroom. He was naked and in bed before Djuana came up to the room.

Djuana undressed slowly, listening to Jack moan. "Maybe I should take you to the hospital. Wasn't that guy throwing the ball hard?"

"I'm okay."

Djuana sat on the bed, "No you are not. You're in pain."

"Pain is a part of life," Jack grimaced as he turned onto his back. "I have lived through worse."

"I don't like seeing you like this," Djuana said beginning to rub his temples with her hands on each side of his skull.

"Ah, now that's good," Jack said, his eyes closed, and his grimace relaxed into a comfortable grin.

"Let me get undressed, then I'll put you to sleep."

Djuana voice was as soothing her touch. She stood and dropped her jeans past her ankles. She slid her bra down her shoulders, turned it backwards at her ribs and unhooked it.

"I'm not ready to go to sleep," Jack grinned.

"Listen, now," Djuana chasten. "You are not feeling well, and there is another game tomorrow night. We can't do anything. Sorry."

"Come here."

"Jack! I need to take a shower, then we are both going to bed. I'll massage your temples, but that's it."

"Come here."

"Jack?" She took small, slow steps to the bed. She watched him pull back the covers, and let him take her arm and guide her in.

"Just let me take a shower, honey," she whispered.

Jack kissed her mouth, and whispered, "When I'm done, we'll both need a shower.

# 45

Djuana wheeled the Pathfinder down the rocky, dirt road called Timber Lane. Dust and pebbles kicked up behind the bucking truck. There were only two homes down the ancient path that led into the forest northwest of downtown, above Washington Park. The first home, a raggedy shack, had been guarded by an aged, shaggy dog that barked with a hollow woofing for as long as Djuana could remember.

Djuana almost panicked when the dog bolted out and chased the truck for a few feet. She watched the mutt give up, smiling at the thought of it choking on the dust and dirt the truck kicked back.

"Gotta move quicker, Fido!" Djuana giggled.

Mrs. Spencer's home was another mile beyond the shack. Her nest, a quaint retreat now, had been a ranch-style homestead when she and her deceased husband reared five children.

Djuana had gone to high school with the two youngest of the Spencer children, Deana and Dicey. She dated Dicey through junior year before Dexter made her his woman. Djuana enjoyed coming to the Spencer's place, plenty of space to roam, nooks to hide with Dicey or gossip with Deana and Tia.

The dirt road ended into a circle driveway, and the Spencer home. Djuana whipped the truck around the dying oak and the center patch of uncut grass. She parked near the steps of the porch, dust covering the Pathfinder once it stopped.

It wasn't long before Djuana was being measured.

"I'm glad you can do my dress for me," Djuana said, looking down at the top of the silver-haired woman.

"My joy," the white-haired woman said, battling to hold the tape steady across Djuana's hips. "Of course, you know I wish it had been my boy you married. That thing he wed, she ain't worth speaking of."

Mrs. Spencer sneered, marking down the findings.

"I'm proud of you. You have grown into quite a fine young woman."

"Thank you," Djuana looked around the unkempt living room. She felt pity grow in her. Old pictures of her kids were on the mantel, the same ones from Djuana's teenage visits.

She assumed they hadn't returned much to see their mother. The kids all live in or around Portland and they all had children. But, why no pictures for Grandma?

"You hear from Deana?" the frail woman asked before Djuana could.

"Not really. Not since she got married and moved to Beaverton," Djuana replied, holding her arms up.

"Oh, she's got a grand house out there," Mrs. Spencer smiled, the tape now around Djuana's bust. "They got five children, you hear?"

"No, the last I heard, Thelma saw them in a mall, and she told me Deana had four then."

"Yeah, well, she done had another. You can drop your arms."

Djuana watched the woman dodder to her chair, where she made notes in a worn, spiral note pad.

"Are you going to be okay doing this dress? It is kind of a rush order."

"Chile, please. You have paid me, brought me the material. Shoot, some of these modern women, that call themselves planning a year in advance, don't do me so well."

"I'll be fine."

"Okay, then."

Mrs. Spencer put her pad down, and removed her bifocals. "Sit down, baby. You want some sweet tea, or maybe a banana muffin. I just made a batch."

"No thanks," Djuana smiled. She sat on the couch, shifting a pile of magazines.

"Your mother's proud, isn't she?"

"Yes."

"Oh, that Emma used to be so worried that you'd be loose one day, then fret that you'd never get married the next."

"Yes," Djuana agreed, smiling genuinely then.

"But, you have matured well from what I don't hear. And, you picked a hell of a man."

"Truthfully, he picked me."

"Did he? Hmm. That's luck of the Lord."

"I think so too."

Floyd was a solid pitcher for the Crowns. He was a four-year veteran, and was always unflappable on the mound. He never showed anger nor pleasure when he was pitching. He was not at all an imposing figure with his mid-cut afro and thick sideburns. He had an average build, almost 6 feet tall with impeccable burnt almond brown skin.

He had the best assortment of "junk" pitches - curves, sliders, changeups and a nasty forkball - on the Crowns' pitching staff. Juris called it the best stuff he had seen in his 32 years of professional baseball. To Juris' anguish, though, Floyd would throw junk when common rule called for a fastball.

Floyd's even demeanor, and quotes from the scripture during games, also drove Juris batty. Floyd would become queasy whenever a player was hit by a pitch; he had never hit anyone, refusing to pitch inside fastballs.

No one could have ever said Juris liked Floyd Young, but Juris respected the pitcher's success at getting batters to swing at his stuff. His teammates hated the quotes from the bible, but liked him for the most part.

But, in Game Four of the World Series that year, Floyd cemented his place as one of the best teammates of any of those Crowns.

Floyd, pitching in a windy, steady drizzle, opened the game with a 98 miles per hour fastball off the helmet of the Gamblers lead-off hitter. All that season, Floyd's fastest pitch was clocked at 92 m.p.h.. The ball hit the helmet of the left handed batter so hard that it ricocheted six rows into the stands. The batter fell flat on home plate.

The brawl that ensued, was a more brutal team fight than the night before. It lasted 15 minutes. Gamblers stormed the mound from their third base dugout, but the Crowns had came to Floyd's side quickly. Mike dropped his mask and glove, and bodyslammed the first Gambler he saw. The Crowns formed a protective circle, the Crowns were eager to fight. Floyd backpedaled away from the attacking black uniforms.

Jack ran in from the outfield to join in, Oscar was already in it from his spot in center. All across the infield grass were mini-bouts. Jack wasn't sure who to help, nor who to fight. O was tangling with two Gamblers, Juan was on his back and Don was fighting along side Bryant.

Before Jack could get involved, he was grabbed from his blind side by two thick, huge hands. Bingo swung him away from the action by his jersey.

"I ougtha fuck you up," the barrel-chested slugger said, tightening his grip. "You little pussy."

Jack dropped his glove and tried to pry himself free. No chance.

"Do what ya gotta do," Jack said, holding Bingo's hands on his jersey. "But, if you let go, I'm gonna hurt you."

Bingo tighten his grip, pulling in more of Jack's uniform into his clamp-like fist. Their faces met.

"You know how many times I fucked Vivian? Shit, while you were out screwing hoes with O, I was opening Vivian up. She told me how you used to slide in and be wondering how it got so wide."

Jack cocked his arms back swiftly and swung them just as quickly, connecting with Bingo's ears. The league's most valuable player released Jack. Before Jack could attack, black uniforms swarmed him, then white uniforms were on top. Jack was crushed underneath a hill of bodies.

The umpires were quick with their decisions on who to eject. They threw Floyd, Juris, Mike, Jack and Oscar out of the game. L.V. lost three players, not Bingo, though.

Las Vegas erupted on the pitcher that replaced Floyd, Rod Murphy, scoring seven runs in the first inning. In the second, Pugs made two errors to allow them four more runs. Lee handcuffed his ex-teammates again, getting the win in the 17-4 rout.

The loss put the Crowns on the brink of ending another season with a loss. The sound of the Gamblers' players laughing and whooping it up in the visitor's locker room across the hall vibrated into the deafening silence that had become the Crowns clubhouse.

"We can't lose to these motherfuckers again," O said, in a weak mumble while nursing his swollen cheek with an ice pack.

Across the lifeless dressing room, the sound of Juris bashing the furniture in his office with a bat was ignored. So were the reporters, who soon had to scurry out, avoiding flying objects.

"Three straight years," Danny calmly said. "Three straight God damn years and no ring. I'm sick of this shit. I am out of here. I ain't playing here no more."

Jack was sitting in his locker, two unopened cans of beer at his feet, and one in his hand. He pictured his career in Portland ending within two nights in Las Vegas. O was on the floor next to him, bouncing a ball on the rug. He snatched Jack's can and guzzled it, beer pouring down the sides of his cheeks.

"I ain't going out like a punk."

"Me neither," Mike added. "They think they got us, like it ain't no thing to come in here and win it."

Jack got up and took another beer out of the huge beer can of a cooler in the middle of the room. He popped it, then leaned on the pillar near the cooler.

He took survey of his teammates. All frowns, with bitterness in their eyes. All of them except Floyd, of course. Floyd, was near completely dressed. He was adjusting his tie with his usual calm.

"Why you hit Rose?" Jack said, his voice barely carrying.

Floyd finished his tie, feeling all his teammates waiting for a reply. His locker was next to Mike's, and the catcher was soaking his hands in pickle juice as he did after every game.

Floyd put on his suit jacket, picked up his bible and turned to Jack.

He said, without emotion or a change in expression, "It had to be done."

Saturday the rain was steady, and Djuana listened to the drops hit the windshield of the silent Pathfinder in the PDX parking lot. There had been so many people there to see off the Crowns, cheering and urging them to force the series to return to Portland, that she chose to sit them out after the plane took off. Also, she was disappointed that she let the camera crews and reporters stop her from kissing her man the way she wanted.

Sitting in the truck, with it off, and the only sound being light, constant rain drops, relaxed Djuana's nerves. At home, and over on the southwest side of town, waited for her the first real steps toward a life as Mrs. Jack Newhouse. Tia was wide awake, and eager to do more shopping for the wedding.

"I'm ready, you kidding?" Tia said when Djuana called at 7:30 a.m. before she left the house.

"Relax, I still have to take Jack to the airport, then I will pick you up."

"I'll be outside!"

Djuana smiled to herself, seeing the image of her friend standing in the rain waiting. Djuana exhaled. It was real. She sat in the truck wondering about it all, telling herself the reason she wasn't rushing out of the airport was because of traffic; but, it died down quickly.

She felt devilish, hoping the Crowns would lose the next night, thus ending the World Series, and Jack's season. Then, he would be available full time to go over details for the wedding. And, he would be here to hold her when nerves rendered her thoughtless.

For the most important game of the season Juris put Floyd back on the mound, and moved Danny back a game, feeling the docile right-hander was up to the task. Then, in Game Six, of course Juris assumed there would be a Game Six, Danny would be pitching on an extra day of rest at home. None of the Crowns complained.

Las Vegas was more vibrant than when the Crowns left six days before. The city was gearing up to celebrate the towns fifth consecutive baseball championship - the ring for the thumb, as the players called it. No one in the state of Nevada doubted that by the end of the game that late Sunday afternoon, the partying would start.

The Crowns' bus bumped and churned through the city, and no one spoke. The players watched store owners boarder up windows, close shop early and give way to thousands of police officers. The casinos were lively, but outside the police were setting up barriers. There were thousands of police officers everywhere, different color uniforms; mounted cops, motorcycle cops. All in riot gear.

"Shit," Oscar quipped. "Is that our escort out this mother when we win today?"

A few players chuckled, but collectively they knew they were riding to slaughter. And, the only way they could avoid it was to play above their heads for nine innings against a much better ball club in a building where they had a 31-5 record during the playoffs.

While the Crowns dressed, Slight came into the clubhouse, something he almost never did. He walked into the center of the room, motioned to Juris, then took off his jacket.

"Gentlemen!" Juris bellowed. "Shut up and listen to what the man that signs your paychecks has to say."

The players continued to dress.

"I may have made some mistakes this year," Slight began, Honeywell at his side. "Got rid of some players that maybe I shouldn't have, tinkered with the team when maybe I should've. But, I love the city of Portland, and I love my team. Any player that is in this room is here because I felt you would do your best for the team and the city."

Slight looked around the room, and no eyes met his.

"The new players here have no idea how we that have been here the last three season feel. But, this goes for everybody. Forget winning for the team. Don't win for the city, or the fans. And don't go out there to win for your families.

"You have to go out there and play for yourselves. Pride and dignity has to come first. Do you want to be remembered as chokers, as the team that lost the most World Series games?"

Slight turned the floor over to Honeywell, who was short.

"Let's take this series back to Portland, and put them on the ropes."

O sucked his teeth.

"You got something to say, Mr. Taylor?" Slight said.

"No, you two put it elegantly enough already."

"I got something to say," Mike stood and the room fell silent, no movement.

"I am going out there and play the way I always do. I expect all of you to give 100 percent or I will kick your ass. No matter who you are.

"And remember I said it."

The fans in the MoneyDome booed every player in burgundy and gold, and Floyd the loudest. Floyd responded with his usual poise, and pitched a fabulous game. There was no score entering the ninth inning, and Floyd was tiring. He had gone deep into his repertoire in keeping the Gamblers off balance.

Meanwhile, the Gamblers Jamie McLennon's sinker was erasing Crowns batters with ease. The Crowns had only two hits through eight innings as opposed to the nine hits Floyd had yielded. The Crowns defense did a great job behind Floyd, turning three double plays, and Jack and Oscar each threw out runners at home plate.

The Crowns went down easy in their half of the ninth. The Gamblers, with the MoneyDome noise level growing with each batter, put together a modest rally. One run and the series would be over. With two outs, they had runners on the corners, first and third, with Bingo coming up.

Juris took off his cap and scratched his dry scalp. He then waved the worn, tobacco-stained hat until Bryant saw it. Bryant called time and trotted to the mound from his spot at third. Soon, all the infielders were at the mound killing time for Juris.

"Damn," Juris spit tobacco on the turf. He turned to the phone and press the button. The bull pen coach answered.
"Get Lyles ready, in a hurry."

Djuana covered her eyes. "I can't watch."
"They gotta walk Bingo," Cal said. "They can't pitch to him here."
"They're gonna lose," Devon said. "It's over. I told y'all."
Emma threw her soiled paper napkin at her son, who was laid out on the floor in the crowded living room.
"Little heathen," Emma said. "When the Crowns win you going to be beggin' to be on the bandwagon."

Juris walked slowly out to the mound. Floyd looked away from him. The hard-nosed Juris rubbed Floyd's lower back, "How you feel?"
"I'm fine, skipper." Floyd said, his head facing the Gamblers dugout.
"You think you and the Lord can get this asshole out?"
Floyd turned his head slowly, glaring at his manager.
"You don't have to throw him nothing good," Juris said. "Let him fish."
Mike added, "Throw what I call, and we get out of the fuck out of here."
Floyd saw glory. He saw himself throwing a fastball by Bingo three times in a row to end the game.
He tried it, and all he got to throw was one. Bingo exploded on the pitch, sending it sailing high and deep to right center.
Jack saw the ball well off the bat, and he trotted to the spot he knew it would land if it didn't carry out of the ballpark. He never saw Oscar, not thinking about his pal, knowing he wouldn't be able to hear him over the roaring of the crowd anyhow. What Jack did see was that the ball was going to clear the outfield wall, and not by much.
Jack stepped, bracing at his knees, and sprang up with his glove high over the wall. His eyes remained on the ball. He could feel in his heart, as he ascended, that he would be able to save Floyd's mistake.

Suddenly, as Jack's body bent as his rib cage hit the fence, a heavy object appeared by him, that at first scared him - he thought someone had throw some kind of large object from the bleachers. Jack closed his eyes and was overtaken by Oscar's body. Jack fell not far from where he had jumped, his right arm and right ribs sore from O's body crashing him into the hard padding on the top of the fence.

Jack looked to his left, he was facing the infield, and saw O land on his feet and balance himself. *This motherfucker just flew over me!*

Oscar stopped himself and dug his hand into his glove, pulling out the white ball. He held it up to show he had it. O's great, acrobatic catch ended the inning.

Jack held his ribs, and tried to stand. O came over to him, and helped him.

"You okay?" O asked.

"Shit, where did you come from?"

O smiled, "My mother."

Oscar led off the Crowns at bat with a walk. He felt Bingo's stare at first base, but ignored him.

"You robbed me," Bingo said as O took a lead off the base.

"Yeah, well tell your pitcher I'm about to pick his pocket too."

In a flash, Oscar stole second. The catcher didn't bother to throw down.

Jack and Don, behind him, struck out on pitches that were in the dirt.

Mike came to the plate next, and silenced the MoneyDome. He hit the first pitch he saw off the tall, yellow foul pole down the left field line to snap the scoreless tie. The ball bounced back onto the field, rolling toward second base.

Mike ran around the bases quickly, cheering himself.

Bobby Lyles relieved Floyd and got the Crowns the win, 2-0.

Game Six Tuesday night in Portland saw the Crowns use two big rallies, and a crowd that rarely sat, nor stopped cheering, to beat L.V., 6-3.

The damp weather was also a big help in slowing down the fast Gamblers. Their players ran with caution on the muddy basepaths, while the Crowns' runners, used to the conditions, ran with zest.

Danny pitched well, but it was O's four hits and Juan's home run that did the job.

Jack walked twice, but he was not happy that he was not contributing better.

And, Jack was the only Crowns player sulking at Alice's after the game. A few of the players accepted Alice's invitation for dinner. She set up two of her largest tables, the oval ones, and sat them in the back, behind the bar.

Don brought Liela, Jack and Djuana came, Danny and his wife - they loved Alice's cooking, and O brought a young lady.

The singer in Salese's band, Arri, came to the table and introduced himself to Djuana.

"I just want you to know that I would be indebted to you if you allow me to grace you with a song at your wedding."

Djuana looked to Jack, who shrugged his shoulders."

"I would be pleased to have you sing. Are you going to bring the band?"

"Sure, if you want." Arri said, he snatched a chair from another table, and joined them. He tried talking with Djuana while others spoke.

Most at the table, including Djuana, had taken Jack's silence as a sign he was still irritated about Bingo grabbing him. Jack got tired of the inquires, and offered his explanation about why he was glum:

"I'm not hitting the ball, and if I was maybe we would be winning this thing."

"Chill with that," O said. "You been getting on base, and playing your ass off in the outfield. Shit, we got them. They know we here for it."

"And, they gonna give it to us."

"I don't know," Jack fell back in his chair, taking Djuana's hand with him. She freed her hand, allowing it to fall into his lap while her attention was on the singer sitting on the other side of her. His lisp, and use of two-dollar words, were nagging at Djuana. He was a round man, no real definition to his six-foot frame.

She listened to him tell her of his credentials as a singer. Church choirs, some opera, and many blues bands.

"What's the theme for the wedding," he asked suddenly.

"I really don't have a theme."

"Oh, Djuana, you need a theme. African, traditional, European..."

"No," Djuana interrupted. "I don't think we need that."

"Which church are you going to have the ceremony in."

"My aunt goes to Mount Olive, on Creston."

Arri sighed, his chubby cheeks drooping, and large eyes darkening.

"I know that church," he said. "But, no offense, you guys need a much larger church. A grand church. I am a member of the United Methodist Church in Irvington."

Djuana nodded, holding in her rage. She dug her mid-length nails into Jack's cotton trousers. His attention came.

"Yes, I have heard of them, but I rather stick to Baptist, and my minister."

"Right. Nothing more, nothing less. I was just saying that two people with the aura popularis you two possess deserve an impressive house of worship to be married in."

"New, listen," Don chimed in, oblivious to the cat fight over churches. "The reason they walking you and not giving you nothing to hit is because I am stinking like day old Goya beans."

"Naw, that's not true," Jack replied.

Djuana turned her attention to Jack's friends, not exactly knowing what they were talking about, but it distracted her from telling off Arri.

"New, I'm telling you, they don't want to pitch to you, you the best power in the lineup. They're rather face me, they know I ain't shit."

"Don's right," Danny said with a straight face. "He ain't shit!"

Don smiled among the laughter. "I'ma fuck you up, Gross," he said across the table.

Liela nudged Don, "You guys curse so much."

"We are jocks, what you expect?" O said, picking up his glass of vodka. "Philosophical conversation?"

Arri rolled his eyes, "Oh, how true."

He offered his number to Djuana; she accepted it.

"I have some wonderful songs in mind. Give me a call and we'll choose one."

Djuana mildly grinned. "I have other singers I need to speak with first."

# 46

Big money was being bet on the Gamblers. They were the defending champions, they were at home, and they truly had the better team. The year before the Gamblers won the seventh game in Portland.

Some members of the media, tired of seeing Las Vegas win the title, gave the Crowns the edge. They noted that the Crowns were the first team to beat Las Vegas twice in a row that year. The Crowns had the momentum, and were due to finally win a championship.

All the gambling and predictions were irritating Jack; he believed. No, what was actually keeping him awake was the fear that he had to do something to get his ballclub a championship. Visions of Bingo laughing and the city of Portland in tears, haunted Jack throughout the night. He sat up in the hotel bed, his left hand on Djuana's soft back and his right hand grasping a glass of brandy; the bottle on the floor by the night table.

In complete darkness, he sipped every few seconds, and rubbed the curve of Djuana's backside. The brandy was an old remedy for the jitters his mother had began when he could not sleep before Little League games.

He wished Denise Newhouse could see him play for money. Like when he was child, all through Little League, Pony League, High School and on the sandlots in New York, his mother would have been the only one to bother to come to every game. His father was at Jack's debut in the majors; a sad Father's Day. Jack struck out six times, and the Crowns lost two games.

Afterwards, his dad said, "They pay you for this?"

The elder Newhouse came to a few more games that year, mostly losses. He had only seen his son live maybe 24 times in Jack's six years as a pro.

His sister, on the other hand, brought her two daughters to every game the Crowns played in New York and New Jersey.

The thought of his nieces, the way they hug him, and call his name, made him smile and caress Djuana's soft shoulder blade; and she turned to face him. Those two little girls worshiped Jack, and they were the only ones that made him feel like a super hero. They owned all the toy figures of Jack Major League Baseball produced, all his baseball cards, as well as Oscar's.

He looked over Djuana's body. Suddenly, there was something he wanted more than a World Series ring, or to beat Bingo and the Gamblers. He lowered himself down to face Djuana. He tenderly absorbed each one of her parted lips, and Djuana responded by flexing her arms and licking her lips. Her eyes opened quickly, then blinked a few times.

She groggily whined, "You should get some sleep, honey."

Jack lowered himself to meet Djuana's bosom, he nestled his face into her chest, parting her breast. His lips leading the way. His strong hands fondled her buttocks.

"I want a baby."

"Jack?" The statement didn't register.

"I want you to give me a baby."

The seriousness in the tone of his voice froze Djuana. She pulled back, lifting his face with her hands to see his eyes. No smile, no grin. He kissed her chest.

Djuana's lips hung, and her breathing slowed. She gasped, inhaling, then exhaling through her open mouth. She cut her eyes away from the moment. Her heart hurt, like a sharp, slicing.

Jack pulled her even closer. "I want a baby."

Djuana couldn't collect her thoughts, and fright held her speechless. She had to say something, but the right thing. Oh, yes, she wanted to give Jack a baby. But, what if she lost it? What if doctors found she could never hold a baby? They never said she could. What if God had destined her to rear only one child?

Djuana breathed in the questions, her eyes closed slowly, and she exhale no positive answers.

Jack moved Djuana, pushing her shoulders square on the bed. He slid his muscular thighs between her legs, and Djuana spread to receive him. His tongue licked a stream up from her pubic hair to her throat. He listened to her pant and sniff, helping him become more aroused by the second.

Djuana's wet palms squeezed the top of Jack's biceps, her nails dug into his muscles. Jack patiently licked the tears from her cheeks. He kissed her chin, and the corners of her mouth.

"I'm scared, Jack," she cried.

"Don't be."


No one in the Crowns locker room spoke before the game. There were no hellos, no jokes. The players got dressed, took batting practice, and refused interviews. To a man, they knew this could very well be their last chance for a ring. So many of them, including Jack and Oscar, were afraid of tomorrow.

The players understood that Slight was going to break up this team if they lost; especially if the Gamblers blew them out. Hate Slight or not, none of these Crowns wanted to leave Portland. None of them wanted to play elsewhere, with different teammates. Sure, they were spoiled in many ways - the press in Portland was very pro-Crowns. And, the fans loved them because it was truly Portland against the world. A large town, rather than a small city, with only two professional teams.

Oscar would complain, but the two previous times his contract was up with Portland, he chose to resign with Slight rather than go to Las Vegas, New York or Los Angeles; teams that had offered double what Slight could afford to pay. The Crowns sat in the dugout and studied the Gamblers while they practiced. Bingo looked over into the dugout often, pointing and laughing. When it was his turn to bat in the cage, he would call over to his dejected looking ex-pals and point to where seconds later the ball would land hundreds of feet away.

"I hate that motherfucker," Pugs whispered. None of the Crowns responded verbally, but Pugs knew he had plenty of empathy on that bench.

Oscar wanted to say something, something powerful. Something that would be remember for years as the rallying cry for a desperate team in a desperate situation. But, he could think of anything that hadn't been said. And, he damn sure didn't want to sound corny at a time like this. He patted Jack's leg, not making eye contact when Jack looked over to him from his spot on the bench next to him.

"Baby, we can do it."

Jack was leaning forward, elbows on his thighs. He slowly turned his head back to the direction of the Gamblers. He returned his concentration on the hatred he had for Black and Gold. "Hits, I gotta get hits," he faintly said to himself.

Juris shifted his wad of tobacco from cheek to cheek, spitting every so often. He avoided watching the Gamblers put on a show for his players. The silence in his dugout was wearing on him, although he hoped his team was gearing up for war, quietly. He waited until the Gamblers headed for their dugout, and the grounds crew at the MoneyDome prepared the field for play to snap the funk.

Juris moved to the center of the dugout, "This is it fellas. Don't leave shit in this dugout. When you step out there, go with the anger of a team that has never won a championship of any kind."

He spat out of the dugout and onto the turf. "Go out there with the memory that no one picked us to come this far. That no one respected us. And that we are the greatest team ever assembled.

"Go to work."

Lee was chosen to pitch the deciding, and final game of the season. An honor, the owner and manager of the Gamblers told him. He was selected over the other highly paid pitchers, most believed, to further the hurt in Portland. Lee had won all his playoff games for Las Vegas, and he wanted, as much as his new owner, to beat Slight for trading him.

Juris had Floyd come back on four days rest, his usual, to pitch for Portland. But, he was not sharp. He allowed two baserunners in the first inning, and would have gotten out of trouble had it not been for a error by Pugsley on a sharp ground ball.

In the second inning, the same problem arose. Floyd walked two batters, then Pugs dropped and kick a ground ball. The next batter hit a slow roller to Pugs, he picked it up without a problem, but then he threw it wide of Don at first.

Before the third inning began, the Crowns were losing, 9-0. The crowd was enlivened, giving Pugs a standing ovation when he batted. With each out, Bingo would laugh heartier at his ex-mates. After the third inning, the score the same and the Gamblers taking the field, Bingo called out to Jack as he pasted on his way to the dugout. Jack instinctively looked in his direction.

"You guys are losers!"

Jack bristled.

Don answered the man he replaced, "You an ass!"

"Fuck you, Don. You'll be retiring this year without a ring."

Jack lead off the fourth inning thinking Lee would give him something to hit. Lee had a big lead, and Jack had watched him throw down the middle of the plate the previous inning, challenging everybody.

Jack waited for his fastball, the one Lee had thrown him in practice so many times. And, there it was. Jack jumped on it, his sweetest swing of the year. Running down to first, he missed seeing the ball land. He looked for the left fielder, and saw him stop running.

Jack clapped his hands and rounded the bases quickly. He got in the dugout, and found his teammates on the top steps waiting for him.

"Come on, guys! It ain't over yet!"

Jack's words were followed by other encouraging chirps. But, the Crowns had seen this scenario too many times. Lee was tough to beat, especially when he had a big lead. Unless he beat himself. And, the players knew they had played their best ball to get to another World Series where a better ball club was waiting.

Jack took some Gatorade, and selected a seat next to Oscar.

"You finally hit one, huh?"

Jack grinned, "I'ma hit another."

Pitching was the biggest difference in this squad and the team the year before. The Crowns pitching staff was weakened by trades and free agent defections. Two of their best bull pen pitchers left before the season started for more money elsewhere. When Lee was let go, it left a void that Slight seriously thought rookies could fill.

When Juris selected Rod Murphy from the bullpen to relieve Floyd, the players conceded the lost. Murphy had been the worst pitcher in the majors last year. But, he was a Crown for life; Slight loved him, but none of the players did. During his warm up pitches, Mike defiantly threw each return into center field.

Jack watched O throw the ball back in.

"That bastard is doing that on purpose!" O yelled.

"Yeah. He ain't crazy about Rod."

"Neither am I, but shit, this is the World Series!"

After Jack's homer, Lee did not allow another base runner until the sixth inning. Mike started the inning with a single. Bryant singled after him. Lee came back to strike out the next two batters before he walked R.J. on a boarder line pitch.

Lee wanted that third strikeout in the inning. He knew it would have destroyed the hopes of his ex-teammates. He walked off the mound toward home plate. He asked his catcher where the pitch was and the umpire, standing at the catcher's side answered him.

"Don't question my calls," the husky ump said, putting on his mask.

"I didn't ask you," Lee snapped.

The umpire snatched off his mask. "One more word, smart ass, and you won't be a hero tonight!"

The catcher took of his mask and tried to talk with the umpire. Lee walked all the way up to them.

"What's your problem?" Lee asked, his arms spread, ball in one hand, his glove on the other.

The ump pointed to the field, "Go back to the mound, pitcher."

L.V.'s manager came jogging out of the dugout, and he intervened.

The Crowns dugout became silent. They watched Lee intently, praying this would become one of Lee's patented tantrums.

"Lee's losing it," O said, sitting next to Danny on the bench.

"Yeah, he got high last night. Always does before a game."

"You sure?" Jack asked, looking back to the bench. He was seated on the dugout steps.

"I know him like I know my wife," Danny bent, and spat out a wad of tobacco. "They are both fools for some blow."

Mike jogged down the line from third base and called Pugs over while the argument grew. Just as Mike clamped his thick, muscular arm around Pugs' chubby neck, the crowd erupted in boos. Mike looked back, directing Pugs with his turn. L.V.'s manager got ejected.

Mike spun Pugs away from the action. "You know how Lee is, that cokehead. Bunt him. He'll be so pissed he'll probably throw the ball through the roof!"

"What if he goes home? It's two outs."

"Pugs, bunt the fucking ball. If he throws it home, I will kill that pussy-ass catcher."

The Gamblers argued for another minute or so, before the umpires demanded the game continue. Pugs waited for Lee to stand ready on the mound, but the umpire told him to get in the batter's box. Lee coiled a tossed a hard fastball. Pugs squared his body, and put his bat on the ball.

Lee seemed unfazed, he hopped off the mound and gobbled up the ball. But, when he threw it to first, the ball sailed past Bingo and down the line. Mike and Bryant scored. R.J. raced from first to third.

O stepped to the plate next, glaring at Lee. Lee fired him the same fastball, and O dragged the ball down the first base line. Bingo, playing deep, had no chance. Lee ran over to the ball, but when he picked it up halfway between first and home, R.J. had scored, Pugs was on second and Oscar was past first.

The score was then 9-4.

The pitching coach, now acting as manager, came to the mound hoping to calm his team.

Lee greeted him, "Don't say shit to me. I got this."

"Walk Newhouse, and get Don Cruz," the coach said, agitated.

"I can get Jack."

"Do as I say. Walk him.

Lee looked back to the Gamblers' bull pen to see two pitchers warming up. He bit back his anger, and glared past Jack into the catcher. When Jack was set, the catcher sprang up and stood outside the plate with his arm extended to signal a intentional walk. Lee lobbed the ball out to him.

Jack looked at Lee in amazement, "Pitch to me, baby!"

Lee snarled a curse, then rolled his eyes from Jack.

"Do this!" O shouted among the boos.

Jack could not make out what O said. Feeling it must be important, he kept eye contact with him while tapping his cleats with the bat.

O, standing on the bag, tapped his right thigh, then pointed his chin to right field, "Do this!"

Jack smiled. He looked out to right, the right fielder was walking toward center as if to talk to the center fielder.

Lee slowed his pitching motion and lobbed the next pitch outside to the standing catcher and Jack lunged his arms across the plate and tapped the ball in the air toward first. Bingo moved late, but the ball was out of his reach anyway. He stuck his glove up, and the ball landed on the turf and skidded away from him.

The right fielder raced to the ball, which continued to bounce away from him. Pugs was running as hard as he could, his meaty legs churning and his arms flailing as he rounded third. O, who was off with the pitch, caught up with Pugs at third and ran a step behind him all the way home.

Jack slid into second before the right fielder's throw. He stood up, asked for and got time out. He wiped the dirt off his uniform, proud that he silenced the crowd.

The Gamblers changed pitchers, and Don was ready at the plate. He was angry, and tired of being disrespected. Lee was going to walk Jack to pitch to him. The whole league was watching, and he was determined not to give them the satisfaction of seeing this aged superstar fail.

He could hear the sound of his girls cheer, they would yell "Daddy!" together, and he would tell them after games who he heard the most. He would make sure neither won more than the other.

He gave them plenty to clap for when he hit a high and long home run to bring the Crowns within two runs of the Gamblers.

The score remained 9-7 for one inning.

Bingo hit a blast that landed over 600 feet from home plate, a two-run homer that changed the mood of the Gamblers' fans. They began chanting good-bye to the Crowns. But the relief pitcher the Gamblers put in was wild.

He walked two, then gave up a hard single to R.J. that loaded the bases for the Crowns.

Pugsley strolled up to home plate trying not to think; telling himself to just hit the ball hard, somewhere. He knew he was a key batter; the Gamblers had to get him out before they faced O, Jack and Don in succession.

*Just hit the ball hard, just hit the ball hard. That's all I have to do.*

"You the best, Pugs," Mike called from the dugout.

The thought that helped Pugs relax was the fact that he had made five errors in the World Series, and still the Crowns were close to winning it.

Tidrow threw a blazer to Pugs, and the round, short second baseman connected with a beautiful, compact swing. Before the ball landed in the left field bleachers, barely clearing the fence, Pugs was jumping up and down. He slowly jogged around the bases, savoring every moment. He dove into the waiting arms of each and every teammate. They slapped his helmet as hard as they could, making the celebration last.

Pugs' grand slam tied the game, 11-11.

"It's on, now," Oscar said as they walked back to their dugout. "Look at them, they don't know how it feels to be challenged. They gonna fold."

The Las Vegas Gamblers had breezed through the American League. They had won a record 117 games, had winning streaks of 31, 24 and 18 games. They had four hitters with more than 30 home runs, three pitchers with 20 or more wins. And, more importantly, the Gamblers had never lost a game they were winning after the seventh inning all year.

The Gamblers did not give up. No, they kept coming, hitting the ball hard. But the Crowns were playing with fire, and the zest of a team that could smell victory. Every ball the Gamblers hit, a Crowns' fielder caught. Some were spectacular, some routine, either way the plays were made. And, the Gamblers frustration took its toll.

In the ninth inning, with Bobby Lyles pitching for Portland, Bingo jumped on a fat pitch, driving it into right-center. Before he dropped his bat, he saw a streak Oscar leave his feet and catch the ball. O slid on his chest for a few feet, jumped up and fired the ball in. Bingo threw his bat to the ground, cracking it.

The game went into extra innings, and the longer it went the more the Crowns confidence grew. The opposite happen with the Gamblers. Bingo, as he was prone to do, was barking at his teammates. But, those guys were the best in baseball, they didn't take kindly to him berating them. The Las Vegas players were arguing in the dugout in the 10th and 11th inning.

Jack had his first chance to win the game in the top of the 11th with Tidrow pitching. There were two runners on and two outs, and Tidrow threw Jack a serious curveball with two strikes. Jack struck out meekly The fans cheered wildly.

Going back on the field, Jack felt tired for the first time that night. The walk to right seemed to take too long. He refused the warm up tosses to rest instead. When Oscar saw him sitting on the turf, he jogged over quickly.

"You all right?"

"Yeah."

"You tired?"

"A little."

"You fucked last night?"

Jack smiled. "What? Shit, that wore off. You know, I had a hard on last inning."

"That chick in the halter above the Gamblers dugout?"

"Yeah, you saw her?"

"Think I didn't?"

Pugs called the men back to duty.

With one out in the top of the 13th, Pugs hit a booming shot off the top of the wall in left. The ball hit off the wall and bounced back to the infield rapidly. Pugs rounded first, but thought better of trying for second.

After the game Las Vegas' coaching staff, which had to manage the team when their skipper was ejected, admitted that they were shocked the game went on so long. They used that as an excuse for using Tidrow so long. The prized reliever was into his fourth inning, he usually pitched to three or four batters. They finally thought to get another pitcher ready when Pugs, of all Crowns, drove a Tidrow fastball.

LV's pitching coach went to the mound and asked Tidrow if he could get Oscar out.

Tidrow nodded slowly and evenly.

He had to, there was no one else ready to pitch.

Oscar trotted to the plate confidently when the pitching coach left the field. He dug in, looking for nothing but a belt high fastball. He wasn't going to swing at anything else, so he thought.

Tidrow blew away O with three high pitches that were clocked at 101, 103 and 104 miles per hour respectively. O threw his bat at his dugout, missing the bat boy by inches.

"Pick me up, New," Oscar said, tears in his eyes.

Tidrow waited for Jack, and when he saw Jack look into his eyes, he pumped his body into a ball and unleashed a pitch Jack did not see. Jack missed the next one also, and was in the hole with two quick strikes.

Jack stepped out of the batter's box, mumbling to himself.

"Can't hit what you can't see," the catcher said.

Jack stepped back in, glaring at Tidrow, biting down on his bottom lip. Tidrow unleashed another fastball and Jack froze. His heart ached. He thought he was out, but the umpire was silent and he heard a chorus of boos. He looked back at the same time as the catcher rose.

"Outside," the umpire snarled.

Jack swallowed his heart back into place. He released a deep breath. The next pitch should have surprised him, as it did two innings previously, but he wasn't thinking, just watching Tidrow. Watching his arm, watching his hand, watching for the ball.

He followed the rotation of the breaking pitch, holding his body for the last second. Jack's hips moved first, then his arms and wrist poked the bat outside. The ball carried high and lazy into right center.

"Shit," Jack moaned immediately.

He dropped the bat, and trotted slowly down the line. He watched the center fielder go back on the ball, his movements fluid and easy. *Miss it, you bastard*! Jack dropped his head and continued to first.

*I suck.*

When Jack reached first, he looked up, a deep grimace on his face, and he saw the center fielder still backing, but slower now, and his neck was bent far back, looking to the roof. The building fell silent as the ball disappeared.

Jack was puzzled. His body kept going, rounding the base and moving toward second; Pugs was running around the bases and was near third. Jack looked to the second base umpire who was out toward center. He turned to the infield and raised his right arm to signal home run.

Jack leaped and screamed. He exploded into a spirited run, dancing and pumping his fists as he touched second base. He looked up into section 109 and he thought he could hear Djuana. She was clapping, in the midst of the only people cheering. When he reached third, all of his teammates were out of their third base dugout. The third base coach slapped Jack hard on his back and followed his down the line.

Mike was crying and shoving his way to home plate. He had to be the first to touch Jack. Gray uniforms surrounded the base, Juan fell to his knees and wiped it clean with his cap. Once Jack touched it, they mobbed him.

Mike grabbed him by his waist, squeezing Jack as hard as he could.

"We got these moefoes!" Mike cried, his tobacco spilling out of his mouth and down his chin and jersey. "They dead! Those bastards are dead!"

Juris, burning inside to hug somebody, pushed and shoved his players back into the dugout. He pumped his fists together, holding his joy.

"Not yet, girls!" Juris shouted, "We ain't there yet!"

The Gamblers were now losing, 13-11. Tidrow was taken out of the game, and his replacement struck out Don easily to end the inning. But, Don walked to his spot at first with a wide grin.

"Yeah, boy," Don turned to his dugout and pumped his fist as the Crowns raced to their positions with renewed life. "One-two-three. And, it's all about us!"

The Gamblers walked off the field in a stunned, sober state. Cameras showed Tidrow knocking over the Gatorade jugs and tossing his glove in the stands. Bingo sat on the bench, eyes wide, speechless.

Once the inning began, all any of the Crowns thought about was the fact that Bingo batted third in the inning. None of them wanted him to be the one to beat them. Rookie Steve Bartkowski was on the mound, his first appearance of the World Series.

Bartkowski, a bundle of nerves, started off poorly. He fell behind the first batter of the inning, two balls and no strikes. Mike bolted up from his crouch, and raced to the mound.

The young pitcher, sweating profusely, reached out his glove for the ball. Mike punched it into the dark brown mitt.

"Walk him and I fuck you up."

The rookie nodded. Two weak fastball strikes followed, then the batter grounded to Pugs. Pugs ate the ball up and fired it to Don at first, who squeezed it in.

"Yeah, Pugs!" Jack yelled. "We can do this, we can do this!"

Two more outs to go, almost every Crown thought in unison.

"Come on, kid," Don chatted from his position. "We behind you. Just let 'em hit it."

The number three hitter in the Las Vegas line up was a singles hitter, no power. Jack cheated in on him, a right handed batter, hoping he would hit it his way. The batter pulled it to R.J. instead, and Jack watched the ball into R.J.'s glove. Jack pumped his fist and looked over to O.

Oscar bowed his head and prayed for one more out.

Bingo stepped to the plate, and Mike kicked dirt onto his cleats.

"Ain't this fucking ironic," Mike chuckled. "You about to make the last out and us losers are about to do what you won't."

"Shut up, you wife beating faggot."

Mike bristled, then laughed uneasily. He fell into his crouch. "Yeah, ain't that funny. Some women like it when I spank them. Your wife didn't complain.

"How is her ass, by the way?" Mike said looking up from within his mask. "Oscar said it was getting wider."

Bingo let the head of his bat tap home plate, and his eyes fell on Mike.

The umpire, bowed his head, biting his laugh, "Come on, let's go."

Jack watched Bingo. This was the ball he wanted to catch.

Bingo turned his anger toward the pitcher, exploding on the rookie's first pitch. The ball was on a line to right. Jack moved in instinctively, thinking he would have to dive to catch the sinking liner. But, suddenly the ball vanished. Don had leaped high off his feet, arching towards the outfield and snagged the ball out of the air.

Jack kept coming. He headed for Don, who had gained his footing, and was now jumping up and down. Pugs got there first and knocked Don down. The Crowns piled up on the veteran, hugging and groping one another.

Bingo stood, near first base watching his ex-teammates. He wanted to look away, walk away, but he was frozen.

During the celebration in the clubhouse, Slight hugged each one of his players individually into a warm embrace. He saved Jack for last. When he took the taller man into his arms he thanked him.

"You are the best player this franchise has ever had," Slight said. "We were nothing until you got here."

Jack, a smiled stamped on his face, shook his head. "No, you and Honeywell deserve the credit. You brought us together and taught us to depend on one another."

Slight looked into Jack eyes, ignoring his words. He wanted to say the word, but it wouldn't come up from his guts. But, he was deeply sorry for the way he treated Jack Newhouse that year. Right then, he planned to make him the highest paid Crown ever. To sign Jack for the rest of his playing days. And, he dared anyone, Oscar Taylor, Mike Colbert or Danny Gross, to question it.

Djuana came into the clubhouse with the other wives and children. She searched the wide grins for that handsome smile she loved. She was taken into a hug by Oscar, and let him kiss her on the cheek.

"Your man did it!"

Djuana blushing, quietly replied, "I know."

She looked over at a makeshift platform, with a white backdrop in the middle of the locker room and saw Jack being interviewed by NBC. Jack's jersey was out of his pants, and it looked soaked. He had on a white cap that read: World Champions.

Another man, well-dressed, joined them. He was carrying a long, wide gold trophy. It had a batter as its top piece, and a four bar base.

"I must say I am very proud to be giving you this Most Valuable Player award," the suited man said.

Jack accepted the trophy and turned to the cameras. His teammates hooped it up behind him. Djuana clapped and cheered. The reporter moved closer to Jack.

"This has been some season, hey Jack?" the smiling, tanned man said, point the microphone in Jack's face.

"Oh yeah," Jack said his eyes fixed on Djuana. "Most definitely."

Jack turned to the reporter, "It was trying, and for a time I thought I was not going to be playing again, but, I'll tell you Bob, I wouldn't trade this year for the world."

Mike sprayed the reporter and Jack with champagne from behind, then stepped up on the stage and sprayed the cameras. Oscar jumped up on the stage, and handed Jack a bottle.

"We gettin' fucked up!" O yelled into the camera, before kissing Jack on his ear.

The reporter begged the station to switch out of the locker room.

Jack handed the bottle and trophy to O. "Hold this for me."

He stepped down from his dancing teammates to hold his woman.

"And you thought we couldn't do it," he whispered.

Djuana's mouth gaped open, her smile continuing. "I never said that! I outta pop you, Mr. Newhouse."

Jack hoisted her off her feet, "Come on, pop me. Right on the mouth."

And, she did. With a long, wet kiss.

Back in Portland, the city went wild. It was the first championship in over 30 years for a city with only two professional teams.

Cal, his running partner, Ed, and Devon shook up beer cans and popped them open. They sprayed each other in the crowded living room in their version of a championship party.

Marla, Cal's wife, was the first to tell them to knock it off.

"Who is going to clean this mess, there's no ground's crew here!"

Emma popped the cork on a bottle of champagne she had bought for the occasion. Tia was the first on line, with her glass. Emma spread it thinly throughout the house full of family and friends.

She raised her glass, stopped suddenly when she saw Cal sipping. She hit her brother on the shoulder with the bottle.

"Your ass can't wait?!"

Cal, smiling widely, licked his lips. "Well, stop stuttering and make the toast."

Emma waited for all eyes to meet hers. Devon took a quick sip of his bubbly.

"To my new son, I hate that son-in-law nonsense," Emma said, blushing. "To my second son. The champion."

# 47

"How's my tie?" Jack asked for the third time. He had struggled to get the red and blue silk tie straight after taking fifteen minutes to tie it. Djuana shook her head and frowned, her man was nervous. "You look like a fool," she smiled, trying to ease him.

"Thanks. Just checking."

They walked down the steps leading to the entrance of Mount Zion Baptist Church. The large doors opened into a foyer. On the right were more double doors that lead into the church. Opposite was a staircase leading up.

"We have to go upstairs," Djuana said. "He said he will be in his office."

"Okay," Jack said, but he went to the doors. He opened them and went into the church.

The auditorium was huge. Wall-to-wall red carpeting, and red upholstery on the divided benches. The benches, arching on each side to form a semicircle around the pulpit. Jack looked around, feeling the well cushioned benches.

"I'm sorry, I forgot you have never seen the church," Djuana said, walking in behind him.

"I like it. Not too big, or too small. Is there a back door?"

"Why?"

"In case I have to dip."

Djuana hit him with her small handbag, "You're real funny."

"Excuse me," a voice came from above. "You two aren't fighting all ready?"

"No, Pastor Reid," Djuana grabbed Jack's hand.

"Good, then come on up," the minister said from the balcony.

Pastor Orenthal Reid was a slim man, with a large head, pushed in chin and serious eyes. He was the youngest reverend among the Portland Baptist community of churches at 36 years old. He was laid back and very modern, but when it came to marriage he was hard nosed.

"Listen," he began after being formally introduced to Jack and having them sit across from him at his desk. "I usually put the couples I marry through a nine month learning session, that I call the birthing of a wedlock.

"The only reason I chose to marry you two was because of Sister Earline. She is a most devoted member of my congregation. Has been long before I got here."

Jack squirmed in the wooden chair. He had glanced around the office while the pastor spoke. It was modestly furnished, and the walls held the

# LOVE'S HOME RUN

pastor's college degree from New York University, pictures of Pastor Reid with Mayor Meier, the governor and various children at their graduations or award ceremonies.

"Reverend Reid, I understand this," Jack began, twisting the bulb of his tie at the collar. "But, I truly believe that Djuana and I have had quite a period of getting to know one another." "Maybe so, but I take my job of marrying couples seriously. While the rate of divorce goes heavenward, I, praise the Lord, have never had a couple split after I have brought them together."

"I love Djuana with all my heart. I was ready to give up my livelihood for her. I don't want to be without her."

Djuana slid her hand into Jack's, on his lap.

Pastor Reid smiled, a warm grin.

"Mr. Newhouse, I wasn't trying to say you don't love this woman. I am merely trying to let you, and Djuana, know that marriage is a lot different than living together.

"Problems among married couples seem to be taken with much more sincerity than when they are just going together."

Jack nodded, "I understand."

The pastor turned to Djuana, "Are you ready to have this man as your husband. To stand by him faithfully, and love him through the thick and thin?"

"Yes."

Djuana turned to meet the eyes she knew were on her. She tightened her grip on Jack's hand. Her breathing quickened. She looked back at the pastor.

"I thought I was in love once. I thought I could marry that person. But, I have never loved a man the way I love Jack Newhouse. And, I would be proud to be his wife.

"I know that when I marry him, I will be happy because he loves me, and he makes me happy without trying hard, or buying me gifts."

Pastor Reid scratched his scalp through his low cut patch of hair. His eyebrows raised his forehead into a wrinkle.

"Okay, then. You guys seem ready. Let's talk details."

Jack and Djuana's wedding was three weeks and a day from the end of the World Series. During that time, Djuana encouraged Jack to go on the talk shows in Los Angeles and New York that were calling Berger while she finalized plans. Berger even had an proposal from "Good Day, Portland" to follow Djuana on her quest to be ready in time.

Djuana rejected the offer, and the $10,000.

She did, however, ride in the team's parade down Burnside. She sat, not waving that much, in the MVP float with Jack. It was the float of honor, the last of the six carrying the players. Mayor Meier gave Jack a key to the city, and Djuana a kiss. Jack's speech on the steps of City Hall was short, but well accepted by the thousands of fans spread out across downtown.

Jack liked talk shows, but the main reason he went was to stay out of Djuana's way. Being with his bride to be now that he was off from baseball was all he wanted to do. He admired how settled Djuana became. She worked without panic, controlling details as if she had been a wedding planner for years.

None of the women could hear the knock at Emma's door until the laughing and chattering died down. The ladies were sharing stories about wedding disasters, and linking them to Djuana's hasty decisions.

"Listen, nothing is going to go wrong," Djuana stood. "I have a daily agenda, and I check off each thing after it's taken care of."

"Oh, like nobody else did that?" Marla injected.

Djuana moved toward the steady raps. She opened the door, and choked back the shock.

Dexter, leaning on the doorway, fought back the tears.

"What do you want, Dex?"

"I need to talk to you," he whimpered.

"Close my door, Juanny!" Emma barked.

"Please, Djuana. Just give me a second."

Djuana searched his eyes, she felt the hurt and no anger.

"You got a minute," she looked back the ladies. "I'll be in the hallway."

"Djuana!" Tia squeaked.

"How stupid is that girl," her mother complained.

Dexter walked to the far staircase. Djuana, in thick socks, Crowns sweat pants and t-shirt, followed. Dex stopped at the banister, and leaned his back on it.

Djuana kept her eyes on his.

"I've missed you," were his first words.

Djuana was not sure what to say. She crossed her arms at her chest.

"Shit," Dexter touched the Crowns emblem on Djuana's sweat pants.

"I can not turn a corner, drive a block or cut on the television without hearing or seeing about the Newhouse wedding."

"Is this all you have to say?"

"No. No. Not at all," he swallowed deeply. He looked into her inpatient eyes.

"No matter what, I want you to know that I love you."

"Dexter, that's bullshit. I have to go."

Dexter ran in front of her, "No, it's not bullshit. I love you, but I made a mistake. I need you, come back to me, please Djuana. I need you in my life again."

That was when Dexter cried. "I need you, baby. I hate that I lost your love."

"Don't do this, Dexter."

He grabbed her arm, unfolding it, "I have to. I can't give you up. I can still smell you on me. I need you. I need to be inside of you."

"Let go of me, Dexter."

Emma swung open her front door, "Jack is on the phone," she snarled.

"I gotta go, Dexter. Have a nice life."

"Why you doing this to me?"

"You're married. Go tell your wife you love her. Your children need for you to do that sometimes, instead of breaking their mother's heart."

Djuana walked down the hall, her mother moved from the door, wedging a the broom's handle in it.

"You don't know shit! I didn't get married for love, just like you're not. The only difference is you're going to be rich."

"Hey, babe," Jack said when Djuana picked up.

"Hi."

"What's the matter? Why'd your mother call me and say you needed to speak to me?"

Djuana glared at her mother. Emma took the cue and slipped into the kitchen.

Djuana exhaled, "Dexter was here."

"What? What happened?"

"Nothing. I really rather not talk about it."

"Okay. But, I need the truck. Can I come get it?"

"Jack? You know I have to go to my last fitting."

"I got a ride for you."

"No! You can't take me!"

"Relax."

Jack wheeled the brand new car beside the Pathfinder. He got out, jumped into the truck and moved it out of the parking spot. Then he parked the car in the space. He opened its truck and took out the body cover, and covered the car.

"Hey, Mom, can I speak to the ball and chain?" Jack said as he sped his Pathfinder away from Tudor.

Emma wasn't amused. "Ball and chain? Jack, we need to have a long talk."

Jack laughed to himself.

Djuana came on the phone all attitude, "Well, will you come on? We need to go before it gets dark."

"Baby. Honey. Sweetums. I done came and went. I left your ride in the spot."

"Jack. Stop playing, please. All you and your men have to do is go to the tux place and walk out."

"Just go on. I'll talk to you when you get home."

"I love you."

Djuana, Tia and Emma came down stairs, the Pioneer women complaining from the elevator to the street. Djuana, knowing where the Pathfinder was parked, saw the beige cover and huge red bow on top of the car first.

She ran over to it and yanked the cover off of her two-door, red convertible BMW 325i.

"It's beautiful!" Tia gushed.

Djuana pulled up the right wind shield wiper, and plucked the envelope away. She tore it open. The key was in it, along with a note.

"This is my wedding gift!" she announced.

"Oh, he gets you a small put-put, so he can keep his truck?" Emma said, hand on hip.

"A BMW put-put," Djuana said.

"Let's get in and roll down the top," Tia begged.

"Bet!"

"I'm sitting in the front," Emma said.

Djuana had begged Jack not to have his bachelor's party the night before the wedding; and he didn't.

Oscar, his best man, held it the weekend before, and thankfully so. The players got drunk and were tossed from the Tunnel. Mike started it, of course. After one of the numerous toast to Jack, Mike fired his glass across the club, against the farthest wall to him. Others followed his lead.

The night before the wedding, though, they didn't behave much better. The men in the wedding, Oscar, Danny, Mike, Don and Juan, stayed at Jack's house, drinking a bottle of 37 year old scotch Slight had given Jack, and watching pornographic movies.

"New, can I have your phone book?" Mike said during a riveting sex scene.

"No."

"Why not? You don't need it."

"Neither do you. You should be cleaning yourself up so you can get back with your wife."

"What, are you a fuckin' doctor of marriage now? For your info, and anybody not stroking themselves, I will quit drinking, for good, January one."

"Shut up that lying before you get us all struck down by lightning!" Danny said, sitting in the recliner with the bottle in his hand.

"You don't need Danny in the wedding, do you?" Mike asked.

"Speaking of stroking," O said, laid out on the couch, one hand in his unbuckled black slacks. "We need to call some women over. You know, kick out the old habit tonight."

"Forget it," Jack said. "If I didn't want none of that at the party, what makes you think I'd do it now, in my house?"

"Yo," O sat up. "I know this kinky light skinned babe, she'll do all of us."

"Call her!" Mike jumped.

"Damn!" Don grimaced, "Do you ever eat white meat?"

"Wait a second, Rico," Mike retorted. "I ain't never seen you with nothing but Black chicks when you hang."

"Shhh, stupido, you know Liela got a hidden mic in here somewhere!" They all laughed.

"Listen," Jack said to Oscar. "We can't do that."

"What's this we shit?" O said. "You got a mouse in your pocket? Me and Mike can do her, y'all can watch."

At Emma's, the scene was much more subdued. The ladies had wine, cheese and grapes. The sat in the living room, lights out, burning several candles.

"You nervous?" Liela asked, sitting forward on the couch.

Djuana sipped the wine. She was sitting on the rug, back against the chair Marla was sitting in.

"Very. I just hope everything goes like it's supposed to."

"That's the least of your worries," Marla said, patting her back.

"Yeah, you have to perform tomorrow night," Tia laughed. "Knock them boots. Let him know what he's got into."

"Oh. He knows that already, for sure," Djuana blushed.

"I hope you're a lady sometimes," Emma said, pouring her fourth glass.

Djuana shook her head. "Nope. I give it to him raw!"

Emma was embarrassed, but laughed with the others.

"You think he's going to like the dress?" Marla asked.

"Oh, yeah. I think so."

"Yeah, he will," Tia agreed.

"But, you know," Djuana started, looking down in her glass. "What if we don't last? What if he gets tired of me? What if we start fighting. Arguing over little things that escalate?"

Liela chimed in, "I don't think that will happen with you two," she said, wanting to shed a positive light on the situation before Emma ripped in.

"Jack loves you very deeply. He is the type of man that will talk things out, and he usually doesn't stay mad for long."

"That was before," Emma broke in. "Let's see how he does married."

"He'll be fine," Tia added. She turned to Djuana and winked.

Liela then said, "Jack won't break his vows. All that fooling around was his way of killing time until he found the right one to settle with."

Djuana raised to her knees, walked on them to the couch. Liela met her and they embraced.

The taste in Mike's mouth woke him. It was raunchy, and dry. The sun burned his eyes, but he had to get something to drink to kill the unsavory flavoring going on in his mouth.

Oscar heard dishes in the kitchen, looked around the sleeping men to pick out who was missing. Mike appeared with a beer.

"What time is it?"

Mike looked at his watch, then leaned back into the kitchen. He calmly said, "It's only eleven fifty-seven."

"Shit!" O jumped off the couch, nearly stepped on Juan. "Fuck! We suppose to be at the church at one!"

Emma stepped back from her daughter. She had to smile.

Djuana sucked in her bottom lip, "How do I look, Mommy?"

"Too good to leave me."

Djuana cried for the first time that day.

"Where the fuck is that limo?" Oscar barked at anyone willing to answer. The men, though, were too busy dressing.

"Who got on my socks?" Juan asked, darting across the living room.

"Shit, I can't find my watch!" Don barked. "I need that watch, bro'?"

"You two sound like bitches!" O said, running to the bedroom.

Jack was sitting on the end of the bed, elbows on his thighs. He was fully dressed in his tux; the same as Oscar's. It was a black, single breasted tux with a double lapel. Their vests were black. The groomsmen had midnight blue vests to match the bridesmaids.

"I gotta call the limo guys, where the fuck are they?"

"Relax," Jack said. "We are already late."

"Relax? Man, we ain't supposed to be late, they are."

"Sit down, O."

Oscar sat, not before catching a glimpse of himself in the mirror.

"I need to tell you how much you mean to me," Jack began. "You my man, and I love you. You have always been there for me. You, Don, Mike. Shit, all y'all."

Oscar took his hand, and they shook the Crowns handshake. "Let me tell you something, before I met you, I never trusted another guy. Fuck that."

"But, you've been true. You earned the respect."

"Thanks, man."

"But, also," Jack's eyebrows raised. "I want to be the first to tell you that when I come back from the honeymoon, I am going to sign a five-year deal with the Crowns."

O smiled, "I knew that."

"How you know?"

"Slight told me," O stood. "He asked me if I would mind the money he was going to offer you. He said I could renegotiate, saying that I wouldn't get as much as you either way.

"You know what I said?"

Jack stared up at O.

"I told Slight he could not have picked a better player to give the money to."

The still photographer, and the video man hounded Djuana while she got dressed, while she got down stairs and while she was greeted by thousands of people when she exited 657 Tudor.

November 5 was a gorgeous, clear day. It was 57 degrees, no rain.

"Mom," she said as the limo pulled out. "Dad's not going to come, is he?"

"Don't count on it."

Djuana looked away, inhaling deeply in an attempt to slow the tears.

"He knew I wanted him to be here."

"Djuana. Mother had him, mother fuck him."

Liela grimaced, and looked away.

The phone rang loudly in Pastor Reid's secondary office, behind the pulpit. He answered with two yesses. He calmly put on his kente cloth neck band. He picked up his Bible, and looked at Oscar, then Jack.

"The music is about to start, brothers."

Jack swallowed deeply. He rubbed his soaking hands together roughly.

O patted him on his shoulder, then grabbed him into a deep embrace. He kissed Jack's cheek.

"It's over, and it's starting, baby."

Jack watched his teammates escort Djuana's beautiful bridesmaids down the aisle. The church had shrunk, was his first impression. There was not a seat available, and people were still coming. He looked against the wall, where people he had to assume were Djuana's family or friends were lined two deep.

Djuana was in the hall, listening to the wedding march. When it ended, and a second later picked up again, Djuana looked up from her veil to her uncle.

"You ready, doll?" He said, a bright grin revealing his teeth.
"Thank you, Cal."
"No, thank you. This is the biggest privilege of my whole life. And, I mean that."

Jack heard oohs and ahs, then cheering. He looked up the aisle, and his heart leapt into his throat. He exhaled a loud gush of air.

O patted his back, smiling, "You okay, baby? I got the car out back running if you want to split?"

The walk seemed to take for ever. When she came down to the three wide, circular steps, Calvin stopped her.

Pastor Reid asked who gives the bride to be married, and Cal stepped in to the spot light.

"I do, your honor. The proud uncle of the most beautiful woman God bestow this earth."

He stepped away. Djuana stepped up, Jack was to meet her, and escort her up the steps. But, he was frozen. Her gown was more than he expected.

Djuana's white gown was off the shoulder with a sweetheart neckline. Her cleavage excited Jack. The bodice was highlighted by hand beaded lace trim with Austrian crystals. The dress was made of Italian silk.

Her hair was pinned in a French roll.

O whispered, "Get over there!"

"She's beautiful," Jack mumbled.

"I thought you knew that?"

Jack stepped to her, and lifted the veil. The stream of tears magnified her warm smile. He wanted to kiss her passionately, but held off.

While the pastor read from the Bible, they held hands and gazed into one another's eyes. Djuana would not notice Jack's hands being sweaty, although he could feel the trembling in her fingers.

Jack mouthed the words, "I'm a lucky man."

He reached and wiped the new tears.

Djuana glanced at the pastor, he was looking above and beyond them. She sucked air, fighting nerves, and was immediately eased by Jack's smile. The smile she was proud to be a part of for the rest of her life.

"Yes," she faintly whispered. "You finally realize that, huh?"

For additional copies of

# LOVE'S HOME RUN
## AN AFRICAN-AMERICAN ROMANCE
## BY THOMAS GREEN

please contact the publisher

**TURTLE COVE BOOKS**
3695F Cascade Road, Suite 166
Atlanta, Georgia  30331

**(404) 344-6862**
**(404) 346-0072 FAX**